PROGRESS IN ORAL CANCER RESEARCH

PROGRESS IN ORAL CANCER RESEARCH

FREDERIK L. NIELSEN
EDITOR

Nova Biomedical Books
New York

For permission to use material from this book please contact us:
Telephone 631-231-7269; Fax 631-231-8175
Web Site: http://www.novapublishers.com

NOTICE TO THE READER

LIBRARY OF CONGRESS CATALOGING-IN-PUBLICATION DATA

Progress in oral cancer research / Frederik L. Nielsen, editor.
p. ; cm.
Includes bibliographical references and index.
ISBN-13: 978-1-60021-865-1 (hardcover)
ISBN-10: 1-60021-865-2 (hardcover)
1. Mouth--Cancer. I. Nielsen, Frederik L.
[DNLM: 1. Mouth Neoplasms. 2. Carcinoma, Squamous Cell. 3. Mouth Neoplasms--therapy. WU 280 P9645 2007]
RC280.M6P38 2007
616.99'431--dc22

2007026673

Published by Nova Science Publishers, Inc. ✣ New York

CONTENTS

PREFACE

Oral cancer is any cancerous tissue growth located in the mouth. It may arise as a primary lesion originating in any of the oral tissues, by metastasis from a distant site of origin, or by extension from a neighboring anatomic structure, such as the nasal cavity or the maxillary sinus. Oral cancers may originate in any of the tissues of the mouth, and may be of varied histologic types: teratoma, adenocarcinoma derived from a major or minor salivary gland, lymphoma from tonsillar or other lymphoid tissue, or melanoma from the pigment producing cells of the oral mucosa. Far and away the most common oral cancer is squamous cell carcinoma, originating in the tissues that line the mouth and lips. Oral or mouth cancer most commonly involves the tissue of the lips or the tongue. It may also occur on the floor of the mouth, cheek lining, gingiva (gums), or palate (roof of the mouth). Most oral cancers look very similar under the microscope and are called squamous cell carcinoma. These are malignant and tend to spread rapidly. This book presents important new research in the field.

Chapter I - Oral cancer is one of the most widely prevalent cancer types in developing countries, and tobacco use and/or alcohol consumption are known to be risk factors Significant improvement in the survival rates of oral cancer patients has not been reported in years. A major reason for the lack of progress is the high incidence of regional and/or distant metastases, recurrence of the primary cancer, and development of a second primary cancer after treatment of the primary cancer. Although recent research has provided deeper insights into oral cancer, the molecular mechanisms underlying oral carcinogenesis remain largely unknown. More molecular-based studies are needed to provide a better understanding of susceptibility to oral cancer. It is therefore essential to identify the key targets for the diagnosis and therapy of oral cancer. In this chapter, the authors focus on the new candidate molecular targets for oral cancer, which will allow clinicians to identify the patients most likely to benefit from adjuvant treatment and potentially spare many patients from unnecessary therapy.

Chapter II - Oral cancer is an increasingly prevalent disease in the United States. Although it accounts for only about 3% of all malignancies in this country, it encompasses approximately 30 percent of all head and neck neoplasms. It is estimated that 34,360 Americans will be diagnosed with oral cancer in 2007 and of these, 7,550 individuals will eventually succumb to their disease. Despite recent advances in surgery, radiation, chemotherapy, and the shift toward multi-modality treatment, the overall 5-year survival rates have not improved from the 1970s (50-55%).

Oral cancers often begin as premalignant lesions, such as leukoplakia, erythroplakia, and, less commonly, lichen planus. Because clinical evidence of such lesions may be visible with a thorough physical exam, dentists, oral surgeons and otolaryngologists all play an integral role in early detection and prevention of cancers of the oral cavity. Ongoing technological advances have facilitated radiological detection of primary tumors and surveillance for the early detection of recurrences. While computed tomography (CT) and magnetic resonant imaging (MRI) have become the mainstay imaging tools for surgeons, the widespread availability of positron emission tomorgraphy (PET) has allowed for whole body surveillance where applicable, and has brought new hope for cancer detection. On the surgical front, the utility of sentinel lymph node biopsy (SLNB) for staging malignant melanoma and breast cancer has served as an impetus for its early experimental use as a potential procedure of choice for staging oral cavity cancers. However, the effectiveness of SLNB for oral cancer staging has yet to be proven. While radiation therapy continues to evolve in its precision in the treatment of oral cavity cancers, chemotherapy adjuncts have remained largely unchanged in the agents administered, but the duration and timing of chemotherapy regimes continues to be investigated and evolving. One of the main drawbacks from the use of radiation therapy, and to a lesser extent, chemotherapy are the unique treatment-related sequelae of the oral cavity.

In this chapter, the authors review current practices and investigate some future directions for the diagnosis and treatment of oral cancers.

Chapter 3 - Oral cavity tumors account for the sixth cause of cancer in the world and rank second in the head and neck, after skin cancer only [1]. In Brazil, the estimate incidence for the year 2006 was 10,060 new cases among men and 3,410 among women [2]. In the United States there are over 21,500 oral carcinomas diagnosed each year, causing 6,000 deaths. About 90% of all oral cavity cancers are squamous cell carcinoma, and its etiology is the well established exposure to carcinogens present in tobacco and the synergistic action of ethanol. Smokers have a 7 fold risk of developing oral cancers; heavy drinkers have a 6 fold risk; and those who abuse both alcohol and tobacco have a 30 fold risk. Other factors involved are chewing tobacco or betel nut, poor oral hygiene and dentition, and poorly fit dental prostheses.

Chronic exposure to tobacco carcinogens results in the field cancerization effect, as proposed by Slaughter in 1953 [4], and there is a higher risk of developing other upper aero digestive mucosal cancers, as pharyngeal, laryngeal and esophageal tumors. The chronically exposed mucosal cells tend to develop genetic abnormalities, activating proto-oncogenes and down regulating tumor-suppressor genes. Cell cycle becomes abnormal and mucosal cell population becomes instable with rapid cell cycling and decreased cell surveillance, with impaired capacity of cell repair and apoptosis, evolving to premalignant and malignant cell clones.

Although not directly related to smoking, there are other mouth neoplasms such as minor salivary gland cancers (mostly adenoid cystic tumors) and soft tissue sarcomas, which are very rare: less than 1% of all head and neck malignancies. Their primary treatment is also surgery, often combined with adjuvant Radiotherapy.

Chapter IV - Morbidity and mortality from oral cancer are high and this has not improved in decades in spite of extensive research. A significant portion of research is concentrated on chemoprevention. However, advances in this field have not translated into a visible change in mortality and morbidity. In addition, existing chemoprevention strategies have two important obstacles: toxicity and reversal of the effects after cessation of treatment. Chronic infection and inflammation have been linked to carcinogenesis in a few organs. For oral cancer, substantial evidence has accumulated for the role of *human papillomavirus* (HPV). However, the development of an effective preventive vaccine strategy for oral cancer is still years away and the target population is largely unexplored. Therefore, safe and practical additional approaches are necessary to change the status quo of oral cancer. Periodontitis is a chronic oral infection caused by inflammatory reactions in response to gram negative anaerobic bacteria in the endogenous dental plaque. It leads to irreversible destruction of tissues around teeth clinically detectable as periodontal pockets and alveolar bone loss. Periodontal pockets have been suggested as reservoirs of HPV. Chronic proliferation and ulceration of the pocket epithelium may help HPV's initial infection and persistence. The Authors preliminary results from existing data at Roswell Park Cancer Institute suggest a robust independent association between the history of periodontitis and incident oral cancer. The authors next step is to test the synergy between periodontitis and HPV for the risk of oral cancer. If this is true, it will translate to practical and safe prevention and treatment strategies. This chapter will review the evidence supporting the association between chronic periodontitis and oral cancer as well as HPV-periodontitis synergy.

Chapter V - The aim of this article was to review and describe techniques for reconstruction of the lower lip defects after resection of malignant tumors with emphasis on the cosmetic and functional outcome. The lower lip reconstruction must be considered individually because the methods employed are not always applicable to every defect conditions. Lip defects may be classified as partial (involving only skin or mucosa) or full thickness, which involve both skin and muscle (with or without mucosal involvement). The size of the defect is often the most important consideration because it is usually a strong indicator for the optimal method of reconstruction. Therefore, a defect of approximately 30% of the lower lip can be reconstructed with primary closure because of the great elasticity of the lips. If a horizontal defect is greater than 30% of the lip, the use of adjacent tissue is mandatory to reconstruct the deficiency. If there is total lower lip defect following tumor resection, other adjacent or distant flaps may be needed for lip reconstruction. The reconstructive procedures can be classified as follows:

1. Cutaneous defects
2. Defects of 30% or less of the lower lip
3. Defects of 30% to 50% of the lower lip
4. Defects of 50% to 75% of the lower lip
5. Transverse narrow defects in the lower lip
6. Total lower lip reconstruction

Chapter VI - Epidemiology is often seen as a rather remote entity, far removed from the real world of patient care. While it is frequently identified with narrow epidemiological aims such as the publication of large tomes of incidence and mortality rates, epidemiology has a critical role to play in the fight against cancer. It is difficult, if not impossible, to properly organise and implement a response to a specific disease without detailed information on its aetiology, epidemiology, natural history, therapeutic options and patient outcome. This is particularly true in the fight against oral cancer. Analysis of relevant patient details may lead to the identification of aetiological factors, regional variation in incidence and mortality rates, and assist in the development of preventive strategies and improved services.

However, epidemiological analysis can only be as good as the quality of the data collected. The validity of the incidence data depends on full case ascertainment with microscopic confirmation, accurate ICD classification including sub-code or 4th digit, as well as exact dates of diagnosis and death. Meaningful comparative survival analysis requires treatment related details, and accurate staging data. This is dependent on three issues: (i) the accuracy, completeness and availability of the original medical notes, (ii) intensity of the diagnostic work-up and (iii), the regional cancer registration protocols. While international research has continuously highlighted the importance of appropriate staging of tumours to facilitate stratification of definitive treatment and evaluation of results, the availability of tumour-related variables such as staging and sub-site location is generally disappointing.

A high resolution study of Oral and Pharyngeal Cancer in Southern Ireland revealed sub-optimal recording of vital details. This phenomenon is by no means unique to Ireland, or even, to head and neck cancer. Indeed, international reports indicate that survival comparisons are frequently limited by the quality of the staging information available and the accuracy with which it is recorded. Clearly, the current level of missing data undermines the power of epidemiological research and the evaluation of patient care. We must all accept responsibility for ensuring that accurate and complete data on disease stage, management and outcomes are recorded as information collection and audit are crucial to improving services.

Chapter VII - Toxicology and risk assessments rely upon various testing systems to estimate risks of adverse effects from chemical exposures. In this regard, genotoxicity tests have become a fundamental tool for regulatory decisions, since the data have typically been important in regulatory schemes and decisions involving the identification of potentially DNA-damaging agents and in supporting concerns for carcinogenicity. Recently, a number of dental materials have entered the market. Such compounds have the potential to be in contact with oral tissues over extended periods of time. However, studies on the genotoxicity of dental agents are limited and contradictory. The purpose of this paper is to provide an overview on the genotoxic potential of compounds currently used in dentistry, such as fluoride, chlorhexidine, endodontic compounds, dental bleaching agents, and glass ionomer cements based on recent research. Some of these compounds appear capable of exerting noxious activity on the genetic material. The action mechanisms are discussed. Therefore, this is an area that warrants investigation since the risk assessment of these substances with respect to genotoxicity certainly will improve oral health as far as will prevent oral carcinogenesis.

Chapter VIII - Oral cancer (OC) is a tumor with a fairly large male to female sex ratio in most populations. Moreover, OC develops in older age in females as compared with males. The conspicuously larger incidence of this tumor among women than men may suggest some endocrine involvement in its development. Until now there are no available literary data, which explain definitively this gender specific incidence rate of OC.

A case-control study was performed to analyse separately the data of the male and female OC patients to clarify the role of the suspected endogenous risk factors, namely estrogen deficiency and elevated fasting glucose (>5.5mmol/L).

Significantly older mean age of OC females as compared with OC males, significantly lower ratio of young (<45 yrs) OC women as compared with OC men may allow an assumption that women are defended against OC in their reproductive period. Almost exclusively postmenopausal state of OC women and a long interval (17 yrs) between their menopause and tumor diagnosis suggest also an important role of estrogen deficiency in OC epidemiology. The mean age at tumor diagnosis of OC women with premature ovarian failure was significantly lower as compared with that of all OC women. Hysterectomy, with or without oophorectomy was significantly more frequent among OC women as compared with those of control female cases, which supports also the estrogen deficiency hypothesis. The results of the present study underline that elevated fasting glucose is also a strong risk factor for OC among estrogen deficient postmenopausal women, but not in men.

The presented results raise a new concept: not estrogen but its deficiency may provoke OC initiation, especially in postmenopausal insulin resistant women. The estrogen deficiency theory may explain the lower ratio and older age of female cases among OC patients. On the other hand, the continuously increasing prevalence of insulin resistant states (metabolic syndrome, type-2 diabetes) all over the world and the close correlation of glucose intolerance and OC risk among women may explain the increasing ratio of non-smoker non-drinker female cases among OC cases.

Chapter IX - During the past 30 years, great emphasis has been placed on the determination of prognostic and predictive factors in cases of oral squamous cell tumors. Numerous systems have been devised, and numerous investigations have been performed, not only on the clinical parameters relating to the patient and the tumor, but also on histological, immunohistochemical and biological markers.

In the authors present study, 60 patients with tumors of the floor of the mouth or of the tongue ($T_2N_{0\text{-}1\text{-}2}M_0$) were randomized into three treatment groups. The first two groups participated in low dose inductive chemotherapy, surgery and then radiotherapy, while the third, control group underwent only surgery and radiotherapy. In all three groups, studies were made of the stage, grade, gender, the localization, the extents of expression of the pretreatment laminin and syndecan-1 and the disease-free survival rate, and the correlations between these.

The response to neoadjuvant chemotherapy was assessed by means of a method that the authors themselves developed, involving measurement of the degree of histological regression observed in response to chemotherapy.

Immunhistochemical methods were applied to investigate the changes in degree of expression of laminin and syndecan-1 in response to the medication, and their correlations with the survival.

As concerns the overall tumor-free survival rate a significant difference was not found between the two chemotherapeutic groups. However, there was a significant difference between the survival indices of those who participated in cytostatic treatment (70%) and the control group. (40%).

In the clinical and immunhistochemical examinations the initial laminin and syndecan-1 levels obtained from biopsy samples could be used as *prognostic factors*.

The authors model measuring the extent of histological regression clearly demonstrated that the survival indices of the patients who responded to the neoadjuvant cytostatic treatment with adequate tissue regression were better than those of the patients who responded to the treatment to only a decreased extent or not at all.

The changes in the expressions of laminin and syndecan-1 in response to cystostatic treatment proved to be important *predictive factors*. The increase or stagnation of these clearly forecast a good prognosis, whereas their decrease was a definite indication of poor prognosis.

Chapter X - Oral epithelial carcinogenesis is multifocal carcinogenesis and multistep carcinogenesis. This concept decides the biologic rationale for chemoprevention in oral cancer. The authors demonstrated the strategies for clinical treatments of oral premalignancies. The authors reviewed the current status of chemoprevention and addressed a new approach of integrating traditional Chinese medicine (TCM) and western medicine in the chemoprevention of oral carcinogenesis.

In: Progress in Oral Cancer Research
Editor: Frederik L. Nielsen, pp.1-9
ISBN 978-1-60021-865-1

Short Communication

EPIDEMIOLOGICAL CORRELATION BETWEEN DIABETES MELLITUS AND ORAL TUMORS

M. Ujpál and Zs. Suba
Departement of Oral and Maxillofacial Surgery Semmelweis University, Budapest, Hungary.

ABSTRACT

Diabetes mellitus is a risk factor for the development of periodontal diseases and various inflammatory lesions in the oral mucosa. The literature data revealed a relationship between diabetes and cancers in different sites. A possible correlation between diabetes and oral premalignancies and tumors was examined in this study.

Stomato-oncological screening was carried out on 200 diabetic patients in the medical departments; the control group included 280 adult dentistry outpatients. The lesions found were classified into three groups: inflammatory lesions, bening tumors, and precancerous lesions. A retrospective diabetes screening of 610 inpatients with histologically confirmed oral malignancies was also performed. The control group comprised 574 complaint- and tumor-free adults. Fasting blood glucose levels were determined in both groups, and the tumor location was registered in the cancer patients.

Benign tumors were found in 14.5% and precancerous lesions in 8% of diabetic patients. In the control group these values were significantly lower, a 6.4 and 3.2%, respectively ($P<0.01$). Earlier Hungarian screening studies indicated similar frequency of these lesions in the general population. The proportion of oral cavitiy lesions was higher among diabetic patients compared with that of the control patients. In the oral cancer patient group, diabetes was present in 14.6% and an elevated blood glucose level in 9.7%. These values are significantly higher than those for the tumor-free control group ($P<0.01$). The gingival and labial tumor location was significantly more frequent among diabetic cancer patients than in the nondiabetic group ($P<0.01$). The combination of diabetes and smoking means a higher risk for oral precancerous lesions and malignancies.

Diabetes may be a risk factor for oral premalignancies and tumors.

Introduction

Correlations between diabetes and inflammatory oral lesions were first published in the 19th century [1]. Gingivitis and destructive periodontitis with a rapid loss of the teeth were described as cardinal, pathognomic oral symptoms of diabetes [2,3].

The discovery of insulin treatment justified a close correlation between the disorder of the carbohydrate metabolism and oral inflmmatory complications [4].

The inflammation-mediated carcinogenesis is well-known empirical fact, but the exact pathway of this transition has not been perfectly clarified until now [5,6].

The literature data reveal a relationship between diabetes and cancers in different sites [7,8,9].

Hyperglycemia promote tumor genesis by several pathway and increased the cancer risk in men and women [10,11]. The insulin resistance in the type 2 diabetes mellitus (DM2) means also an enhanced risk for breast, pancreas, liver, colon, kidney, prostate and oral cavity cancers [12,13,14,15,16,17].

A possible correlations between diabetes and oral premalignancies and tumors was examined in this study.

Our first investigation involved the stomato-oncological screening of 200 diabetic patients.

This was followed by a retrospective study of incidence of diabetes and tumor location in 610 in patients with oral cancer.

Patients and Methods

Stomato-Oncological Screening of Diabetes Patients

Between 1 March 2002 and 31 January 2003, stomato-oncological screening examinations were carried out on 200 diabetes patients at the medical departments.

Both inpatients and outpatients were involved: 82 patients had type 1 diabetes (DM1), and 118 had type 2 diabetes. A total of 131 were women, and 69 were men. The average age was 45.8 years (range 19-80). The mean age of the patients was 36.3 years in the type 1 diabetes group, and 55.3 years in the type 2 diabetes group. The control group comprised 280 adult, otherwise healthy dentistry outpatients (109 men, 171 women). Their mean age was 47.2 years (range 17-82).

Screening took place on a voluntary basis. Two physicians performed the examinations, and the data were recorded on a specially prepared questionnaire. Besides the relevant personal data, the recorded information of laboratory values related to previous treatment of the diabetes, possible complications, as well as alcohol consumption and smoking habits were also recorded.

This was followed by a clinical examination, including a thorough examination of the oral cavity and bimanual palpation of the cervical region. Details were recorded, mucosal lesions, precanceroses, and tissue accumulations considered clinically to be benign or malignant. The examiners were not aware of the patients' diabetic state.

Diabetes Screening of Oral Cancer Patients

We studied 610 inpatients (435 men, 175 women) at the Department of Oral and Maxillofacial Surgery, Semmelweis University, with histologically confirmed malignant tumors in the oral cavity, between 1 January 1998 and 30 June 2002.

Histologically, 606 of them proved to be squamous cell carcinomas and 4 were adenocarcinomas. Their mean age was 59 years (range 36-85). The control group consisted of 574 tumor- and complaint-free adults (351 men, 223 women) who volunteered to participate in stomato-oncological screening. Their mean age was 51 years (range 32-78).

Fasting blood glucose levels were determined repeatedly within 4 days. The level was regarded as elevated only if it was repeatedly elevated; if the repeated measurements included at least one negative result, the case was not considered pathological. All determinations were made using automatic analyzers (Hitachi 717/912; Roche Diagnostics Boehringer Mannheim, Germany). Based on the findings, the patients were classified into three groups: 1) patients with a normal fasting blood glucose level (<6.1 mmol/1), 2) patients with an elevated fasting blood glucose level (6.1-6.9 mmol/1, impaired fasting glucose), and 3) patients with diabetes (>6.9 mmol/1).

The frequencies of malignant tumors at various locations in the oral cavitiy in the different groups were studied. The x^2 test was used for the statistical analysis, and probability level of 5% was taken as the limit of statistical significance.

RESULTS

Stomato-Oncological Screening of Diabetes Patients

The results are presented in Table 1. The lesions found were classified in three groups: 1) inflammatory lesions, such as cheilitis and glossitis, 2) benign tissue accumulations, and 3) precancerous lesions, such as leukoplakia and erythroplakia. Malignant lesions were not found among these 200 diabetes patients nor in the control group.

Some form of lesions of the oral cavity was found in 51.5% of the diabetes patients. In both types of diabetes, inflammations were the most frequent, followed by benign tumors, and then by precancerous states. In the control group, the frequency of all lesions was significantly lower ($P<0.01$).

The proportions of inflammatory lesions (31.3 vs. 25.6%), benign lesions (16.9 vs. 10.9%), and precancerous lesions (11 vs. 3.6%) were higher among patients with type 2 diabetes than among those with type 1 diabetes (Table 1).

Fifteen percent of the examined diabetes patients were active smokers: 23% had given up smoking; the corresponding data were 12 vs. 16.9% and 21 vs. 24.5%, respectively, among those with type 1 and type 2 diabetes. The 11% incidence of leukoplakia in the DM2 group was noteworthy. The proportions of active smokers and of those who had given up smoking in this group were 38 and 32%, respectively, i.e., a total of 70% who still were or had been smokers. The smoking diabetes patients were found to include 16.6% with precancerous lesions and 13.3% with benign lesions.

Table 1. Distribution of lesions by type and sex in the control group and in the type 1 and type 2 diabetic patients

	Control group			
Lesion	Men	Women	Total	%
N			280	
Cheilitis, glossitis	11	15	26	9.2
Benign tumor	8	10	18	6.4
Leukoplakia/erythroplakia	4	5	9	3.2
Total	23	30	53	**18.8**
	Type 1 diabetic group			
Lesion	Men	Women	Total	%
N			82	
Cheilitis, glossitis	6	15	21	25.6
Benign tumor	2	7	9	10.9
Leukoplakia/erythroplakia	2	1	3	3.6
Total	10	23	33	**40.2**
	Type 2 diabetic group			
Lesion	Men	Women	Total	%
N			118	
Cheilitis, glossitis	12	25	37	31.3
Benign tumor	6	14	20	16.3
Leukoplakia/erythroplakia	4	9	13	11
Total	48	48	70	**59.2**

Diabetes Screening of Oral Cancer Patients

Blood glucose levels were elevated (6.1-6.9 mmol/1) in 59 (9.7%) of the 610 patients with oral malignancies, and diabetes was present in 89 patients (14.6%). Seventy-two of the diabetes patients were known cases, whereas 17 (2.8%) were newly diagnosed. Of the 72 known diabetes cases, 20 were being treated with insulin, 52 with various oral drugs, and 2 were on diets. Eighty-seven (97%) of the 89 diabetes patients had type 2 diabetes.

The mean age in the diabetic group was 60 years (range 42-81). The control group was found to contain 32 (5.6%) individuals with DM2, 6 (1%) of whom were freshly diagnosed cases.

Of oral patients with malignant tumors in the oral cavity, 14.6% had diabetes, whereas 9.7% displayed an elevated fasting blood glucose level, i.e., overall, 24.3% of the patients had abnormal glucose metabolism. There were significantly more diabetes and elevated fasting blood glucose cases in the tumor group than in the control group: 5.6 and 5.5%, respectively ($P<0.01$). The distributions of the malignant tumors in the oral cavitiy according to location for all of the patients and for the diabetes group are shown in Table 2. The most frequent malignant tumors among nondiabetic patients were sublingual carcinomas (146 patients, 28%), followed by lingual tumors (100 patients, 19%). By contrast, the most frequent oral cancers among the diabetic patients were gingival tumors (26 patients, 29%), followed by lip cancers (21 patients, 24%). There were significantly more gingival and lip cancers in the diabetic group than in the nondiabetic group ($P<0.01$).

In this study, 68% of all patients with malignant tumors, and 30% of the tumorous diabetes patients were active smokers. The proportion of smokers in the control group was 27%.

Table 2. Occurrence of oral cavity cancers among diabetic and nondiabetic patients

	Location of oral cavity cancers						
	Labial	Lingual	Sublingual	Gingival	Buccal	Other	Total
Nondiabetic patients	73 (14%)	100 (19%)	**146 (28%)**	83 (16%)	21 (4%)	98 (19%)	521 (100%)
Diabetic patients	21 (24%)	16 (18%)	13 (15%)	**26 (29%)**	3 (3%)	10 (11%)	89 (100%)
Total	94	116	159	109	24	108	610
Date are *n* (%)							

DISCUSSION

The chronic inflammatory processes in the gastrointestinal tract have an important role in carcinogenesis [6,18]. Considering the well-known oral manifestations of diabetes (1-4) both the inflammatory processes (gingivitis, periodontitis) and the atrophic lesions (chronic cheilitis and glossitis) are possible precursors of malignant epithelial transformation.

The first step was a stomato-oncological screening study to clarify the incidence of benign tumors and precancerous lesions in diabetic patients.Our examinations revealed an higher incidence of benign tumors than reported by other authors. Bánóczy et al. [19] found a frequency of 3,7% for the most common benign oral lesions. This was substantially lower than the 14,5% among our diabetes patients (10,9% for those DM1, and 16,9% for DM2 patients).

Albrecht et al. [20] found leukoplakia in 6,2% of their diabetes patients, whereas in the present study, an incidence of 6% for leukoplakia in diabetic patients was observed. Of the 16 precancerous lesions that were screened out, 4 proved to be erythroplakia, i.e. 2% of the 200 diabetes patients. This is markedly higher than the literature value of 0,1% [21].

The incidence of both precancerous lesions (leukoplakia and erythroplakia) was 8% in our diabeteic patients: 3,6% in DM1 and 11% in DM2. This value is essentially higher than the data of other Hungarian authors, who screened the general population for premalignant lesions [19].

An assotiation between diabetes mellitus and premalignant oral lesions among women has been observed in India by Dikshit et al. [22].

The higher incidence of benign and premalignant lesions in DM2 suggest, that hyperglacemia is not primarily responsible for the development of oral tumors and precancerous lesions. The insulin resistance in the DM2, among other factors, may have an important role in the intraoral tissue proliferations.

The present study confirmed the well-known fact that smoking is a deciding risk factor for precancerous oral lesions [20,22,23]. Seventy percent of our diabetes patients with leukoplakia were or had been smokers. The incidence of 16,6% for premalignant lesions (leukoplakia and erythtroplakia) in this group of patients was extraordinarily high as compared with data of Albrecht et al. [20]. They reported an incidence of 11,5% for leukoplakia among smoking diabetes patients. It may be stated that smoking diabetes patients are a high-risk endangered group from the aspect of oral premalignancies.

The other aspect of this study was the diabetes screening of 610 inpatients with histologically confirmed oral malignancies. A majority of them had oral squamous cell carcinoma. There were significantly more patients with an abnormal glucose metabolism (24,3%) in the tumor group than in the control (11,1%) ($p < 0.01$). Among our 89 tumorous, manifest diabetes patients, 87 (97%) had type 2 diabetes. Smoking and alcohol consumption are additional well-known risk factors for oral malignancies [23], so smokers and alcoholics among diabetic patients construe an extremly high-risk group.

The incidence of oral premalignancies and malignant tumors is higher in persons of disadvantageous social status; these persons also are more likely to have undiagnosed or insufficiently treated DM [24]. Also the inadequate dental state and poor oral hygiene are independent risk factors for oral cancer [25], wich are deteriorated by DM.

As concerns the location of oral malignancies, in the nondiabetic group, the lingual and sublingual tumors were dominant. In the diabetes group, the most frequent locations of cancer were the gingiva and the lower lip, wich are also preferentially affected by inflammatory lesions in diabetic patients [26].

The precancerous and tumorous oral lesions are more frequent in DM2 than DM1. Possible etiological factors may be partly the insulin resistance, the decreased sensitivity of peripheral tissues to insulin, or partly the fact that DM2 cases are generally diagnosed and treated after a longer delay, as the complaint-free latency period can take several years [27].

A disturbed oxidation equilibrium has been confirmed in DM [28]. The elevated glucose concentration, the excessive formation of free radicals and the protein glycation depress the activities of the antioxidant scavengers and enzymes. These noxious processes can cause serious damages in the biological structures even at molecular level. In response to the chronic hyperglycemia, increased amounts of glycated end products may be formed, which promote the formation of further free radicals, induce the production of cytokines and growth factors, and damage the structures and functions of various extracellular matrix materials [28]. The expression of the receptor for advanced glycation end products (RAGE) is enhanced by the increase in advanced glycation end products (AGE). RAGE expression is a newly recognized factor regulating cancer cell invasion and metastasis. Its expression appears to be closely associated with the invasiveness of oral carcinoma [29].

Hyperglycemia provokes agglutination of the formal elements of the blood, resulting in microembolization and thrombotic obliterations cause tissular hypoxia [30]. The metabolizm of tumor cells is characterized by nonoxidativ steps of anabolic pathway, these cells are capable of multiplying even under conditions of hypoxia [31].

Insulin resistance is a proven risk factor for colorectal and breast cancers and a possible predictive role in the development and the progression of oral cavity cancers as well [7,32,33]. A number of reports have confirmed a connection among insulin resistance and carcinomas of the prostate, liver, pancreas and kidney [7,12,13,14,17,34].

Tumor necrosis factor (TNF)-alpha is considered a potential mediator substance of insulin resistance, because it blocks signal transmission by the insulin receptor [35]. Studies have demonstrated that the prevalence of insulin resistance is significantly elevated in patients with gastrointestinal cancer, and the level of insulin resistance correlated with the serum level of TNF-alpha [36].

The exact pathomechanism of the diabetic tissue disorder or that of the malignant transformation is not clarified, but the microvascular changes, the secondary hypoxia, the breakdown of the oxidation equilibrium, the insulin resistance can play a complex role in the development of oral precancerous and tumorous lesions.

Confirmation of these findings and relationships requires further research.

References

[1] Glickman J: *Clinical Periodontology*. Philadelphia, PA, Saunders, 1972; 386-389

[2] Oliver RC, Tervonen T: Periodontitis and tooth loss: comparing diabetes with the general population. *J AM Dent Assoc* 1993; 124:71-76

[3] Tervoven T; Oliver RC: Long-term control of diabetes mellitus and periodontitis. *J Clin Periodont* 1993; 20:431-435

[4] Kleinman DV, Swango PA, Niessen JC: Epidemiologic studies of oral mucosal conditions: methodologic tissues. *Community Dent Oral Epidemiol* 1991; 19:129-140

[5] Hussain SP, Hofseth LJ, Harris CC: Nitric oxide in cancer and chemoprevention. *Free Radic Biol Med* 2003; 34:955-968

[6] Tsuji S, Kawai N, Tsjusi M, Kawano S, Hori M: Review article: inflammation-related promotion of gastrointestinal carcinogenesis: a perigenetic pathway. *Aliment Pharmacol Ther* 2003; 1:82-89

[7] Bloomgarden ZT: Definition of the insulin resistance syndrome: The 1st World Congress on the Insulin Resistance *Syndroma. Diab Care* 2004; 27: 824-830

[8] Inoue M, Iwasaki M, Otani T, Sasazuki S, Noda M, Tsugane S. Diabetes mellitus and the risk of cancer: results from a large-scale population-based cohort study in Japan. *Arch Intern med* 2006; 166:1871-1877

[9] Bowker SL, Majudamar SR, Veugelers P, Johnson JA. Increased cancer-related mortality for patients with type 2 diabetes who use sulfonylureas or insulin. *Diabetes Care* 2006; 29:254-258

[10] Jee SH, Ohrr H, Sull JW, YunJE, Ji M, Samet JM. Fasting serum glucose level and cancer risk in Korean men and women. *JAMA* 2005; 293:194-202

[11] Rapp K, Schroeder J,Klenk J, Ulmer H, Concin H, Diem G, Oberaigner W, Weiland SK. Fasting blood glucose and cancer risk in a cohort of more than 140,000 adults in Austria. *Diabetologia* 2006; 49:945-952

[12] Adami HO, Chow WH, Nyren O: Excess risk of primary liver cancer in patients with diabetes mellitus. *J Natl Cancer Inst* 1996; 88:1472-1477
[13] Lindblad P, Chow WH, Chan J: The role of diabetes mellitus in the etiology of renal cell cancer. *Diabetologica* 1999; 42:107-112
[14] Hammarsten J, Hogstedt B: Hyperinsulinaemia: A prospective risk factor for lethal clinical prostate cancer. *Eur J Cancer* 2005; 41:2887-2895
[15] Nagel JM, Goke B. Colorectal carcinoma in patients with type 2 diabetes mellitus. *Z Gastroenterol* 2006; 44:1153-65
[16] Kuriki K, Hirose K, Tajima K. Diabetes and cancer risk for all and specific sites among Japanese men and women. *Eur J Cancer Prev* 2007; 16:83-89
[17] Ujpál M, Matos O, Bíbok Gy: Diabetes and Oral tumors in Hungary: Epidemiological correlations. *Diab Care* 2004; 27: 770-774
[18] Munkholm P: The incidence and prevalence of colorectal cancer in inflammatory bowel disease. *Aliment Pharmacol ther* 2003; 2:1-5
[19] Bánóczy J, Bako A, Dombi C, Ember I, Kosa Z, Sandor J, Szabo G: Stomato-oncological screening examinations: possibilities for early diagnosis. *Magy Onkol* 2001; 45:143-148
[20] Albrecht M, Bánóczy J, Dinya E, Tamás G: Occurrence of oral leukoplakia and lichen planus in diabetes mellitus. *J Oral Pathol Med* 1992; 21:364-366
[21] Ben Slama L: Léseions précancereuses de la muqueuse buccale. *Rev Stomatol Chir Maxillofac* 2001; 102:77-108
[22] Dikshit RP, Ramadas K, Hashibe M, Thomas G, Somanathan T, Sankaranarayanan R. Association between diabetes mellitus and pre-malignant oral diseases: a cross sectional study in Kerala, India. *Int J Cancer* 2006; 118:453-457
[23] Johnson NW. Etiology and risk factors for oral cancer, with special reference to-bacco and alcohol use. *Hungarian Oncol* 2001; 45:115-122
[24] Hashibe M, Jacob BJ, Thomas G. Socioeconomic status, lifestyle factors and oral premalignant lesions. *Oral Oncol* 2003; 39:664-671
[25] Rosenquist K, Wennerberg J, Schildt EB. Oral status, oral infections, and some lifestyle factors as risk factors for oral and oropharyngeal squamous cell carcinoma: A population-based case control study in southern Sweden. *Acta Otolaryngol* 2005;125:1327-1336
[26] Ponte E, Tabaj D, Maglione M, Melato M. Diabetes mellitus and oral disease. *Acta Diabetol* 2001;38:57-62
[27] Gibson J, Lamey PJ, Lewis MAO, Frier BM. Oral manifestations of previously undiagnosed non-insulin dependent diabetes mellitus. *J Oral Pathol Med* 1990; 19:284-287
[28] Baynes JW, Thorpe SR. Role of oxidative stress in diabetic complications: a new perspective on an old paradigm. *Diabetes* 1999; 48:1-9
[29] Bhawal UK, Ozaki Y, Nishimura M: Association of expression of receptor for advanced glycation end products and invasive activity of oral squamous cell carcinoma. *Oncology* 2005; 69: 246-255
[30] Lorenzi M. Glucose toxicity int he vascular complications of diabetes:The cellular perspective. *Diabets Metab Rev* 1992; 8: 85-103

[31] Boros LG, Cascante M, Lee W-NP. Metabolic profiling of cell growth and death in cancer: Applications in drug discovery. *Drug Discov Today* 2002; 7:18-26

[32] Keku TO, Lund PK, Galanko J, Simmons JG,Woosley JT, Sandler RS. Insulin resistance, apoptosis,and colorectal adenoma risk. *Cancer Epidemiol Biomarkers Prev* 2005; 14:2076-2081

[33] Ujpál M, Barabás J, Kovalszky I, Szabó GY, Németh ZS, Gábris K, Suba ZS. A preliminary comparative study of the prognostic implications of type 2 diabetes mellitus for patients with primary gingival carcinoma treated with surgery and radiation therapy. *J Oral Maxillofac Surg* 2007;65:452-456

[34] Richardson LC, Pollack LA: Therapy insight: Influence of type 2 diabetes on the development, treatment and outcomes of cancer. *Nat Clin Pract Oncol* 2005; 2:48-53

[35] Riu L, Aguirre V, Kim JK. Insulin/IGF-1 and TNF-alpha stimulates phosphorilation of IRS-1 at inhibitory Ser 307 via distinct pathways. *J Clin Invest* 2001;107:181-189

[36] McCall JL, Tuckey JA, Parry BRL. Serum tumor necrosis factor alpha and insulin resistance in gastrointestinal cancer. *Br J Surg* 1992;79:1-5

RESEARCH AND REVIEW STUDIES

In: Progress in Oral Cancer Research
Editor: Frederik L. Nielsen, pp 13-58

ISBN 978-1-60021-865-1

Chapter I

RECENT PROGRESS IN MOLECULAR TARGETS AND ONCOLOGY THERAPEUTICS

Jun Murakami[1,*], Jun-ichi Asaumi[1], Hidetsugu Tsujigiwa[2], Hitoshi Nagatsuka[3], Masahiro Kuroda[4], You-Jin Lee[5] and Susumu Kokeguchi[6]

[1]Department of Oral and Maxillofacial Radiology, [2]Virology, [3]Oral Pathology, [4]Radiology, [6]Oral Microbiology, Graduate Schools of Medicine and Dentistry, Okayama University, Okayama, Japan;
[5]Department of Oral Pathology −BK21, College of Dentistry, Chosun University, Gwangju, Korea.

ABSTRACT

Oral cancer is one of the most widely prevalent cancer types in developing countries, and tobacco use and/or alcohol consumption are known to be risk factors [1,2]. Significant improvement in the survival rates of oral cancer patients has not been reported in years [3]. A major reason for the lack of progress is the high incidence of regional and/or distant metastases, recurrence of the primary cancer, and development of a second primary cancer after treatment of the primary cancer [4]. Although recent research has provided deeper insights into oral cancer, the molecular mechanisms underlying oral carcinogenesis remain largely unknown. More molecular-based studies are needed to provide a better understanding of susceptibility to oral cancer. It is therefore essential to identify the key targets for the diagnosis and therapy of oral cancer. In this chapter, we focus on the new candidate molecular targets for oral cancer, which will allow clinicians to identify the patients most likely to benefit from adjuvant treatment and potentially spare many patients from unnecessary therapy.

---

* Correspondence concerning this article should be addressed to: Jun Murakami, Department of Oral and Maxillofacial Radiology, Field of Tumor Biology, Graduate School of Medicine and Dentistry, Okayama

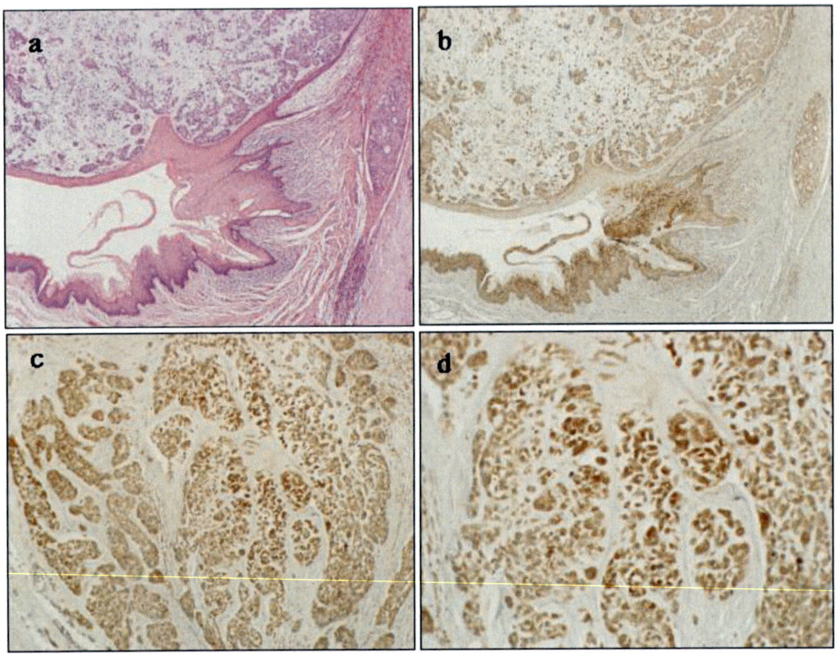

Figure 1. Pathological features. Tissue sample embedded in paraffin wax block was obtained from a patient with oral SCC who underwent curative surgery at the Okayama University Hospital, Okayama, Japan. (a) Haematoxylin and eosin (H&E) staining. Serial sections were cut from each paraffin wax block, and H&E staining was carried out for histopathological diagnosis. Original magnification, x4. (b) Immunohistochemistry of MGMT in oral SCC patient. The sample was probed with monoclonal antibody MT 3.1 specific for human MGMT (NeoMarkers, Fremont CA, USA). MGMT was stained in the tumor cells and corresponding normal epithelium. Original magnification, x4. (c) Immunohistochemistry of MGMT in oral SCC patient. Original magnification, x10. (d) Immunohistochemistry of MGMT in oral SCC patient. Original magnification, x20.

1. New Target in Oral Cancer: O^6-Methylguanine-DNA Methyltransferase (MGMT)

Our research has mainly been focused on the O^6-methylguanine-DNA methyltransferase (MGMT) levels in oral cancer cells as a candidate for a marker to assess the effects of anti-tumor agents. The effectiveness of a given chemotherapeutic agent on tumors of a given histological type varies from patient to patient. Unfortunately, many of the tests that have been devised to screen patients for their sensitivity to specific antineoplastic agents are still not practical for use in the clinic. MGMT is known as a DNA repair enzyme that repairs DNA adducts at the O^6-position of guanine [5-12]. The *MGMT* gene is expressed in virtually all normal tissues [13]. From the results of the immunohistochemistry of MGMT in oral squamous cell carcinoma (SCC) patients (Figure 1), MGMT protein is expressed in the cancer cells and corresponding normal epithelium. Several human cancer-derived cell lines

University, 2-5-1, Shikata-cho, Okayama 700-8525, Japan. E-mail: jun-m@md.okayama-u.ac.jp; Telephone number: +81-86-235-6621; Fax number: +81-86-235-6709.

have little or no methyltransferase activity and are hypersensitive to alkylating agents; these are the so-called Mer- or Mex- cell lines [14-17]. Alkylating agents, one of the most commonly used anti-tumor agents, may generate DNA adducts (such as O^6-methylguanine) and MGMT rapidly repairs those adducts. *N*-methyl-*N*-nitrosourea (MNU), for example, generate adducts at the O^6-position of guanine, and is likely to induce mutations if the adducts are not quickly repaired by MGMT. MGMT activity is likely to be an important marker of the sensitivity to alkylating agents, and similarly may be a predictor of the success of chemotherapeutic regimens using such alkylating agents.

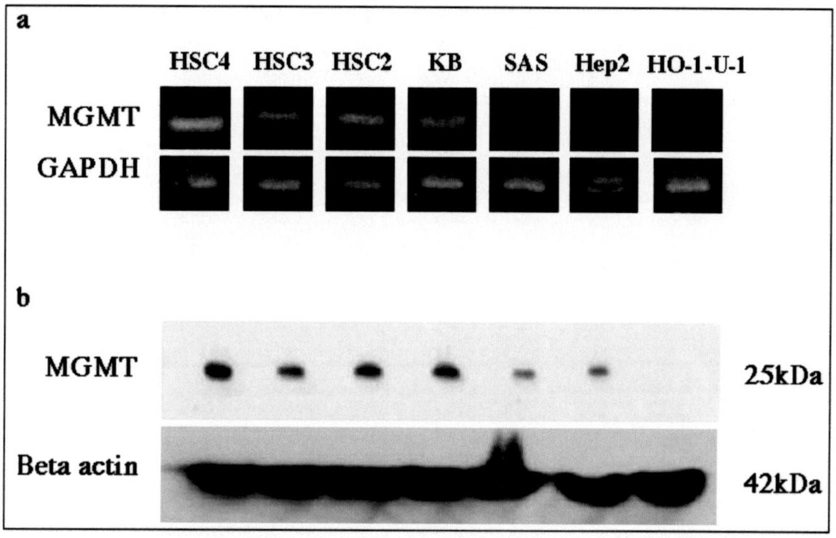

Figure 2. Expressions of MGMT in oral cancer cell lines. (a) Reverse transcription-PCR analysis for *MGMT* mRNA. Total RNA was extracted from cells using the Trizol reaent. RNA samples were treated with RNase-free DNase I and then RNA was reverse-transcribed with a Superscript First-strand synthesis system for RT-PCR kit (Invitrogen Corp., Carlsbad, CA). Amplification of cDNAs was performed under the following a PCR conditions: 7 min at 94°C for 1 cycle; then 26 cycles at 94°C for 30 s, 59°C for 30 s, 72°C for 30 s; and a final elongation step at 72°C for 10 min. The primers used for the amplification were as follows: *MGMT*; sense: 5'-GCCGGCTCTTCACCATCCCG-3', antisense: 5'-GCTGCAGACCACTCTGTGGCACG-3', *GAPDH*; sense: 5'-GAAGGTGAAGGTCGGAGTC-3', antisense: 5'-CAAAGTTGTCATGGATGACC-3'. *MGMT* primers were used to amplify a 211-bp product spanning the sequence 339-527 from GenBank accession number M29971. The amplified *GAPDH* fragment was used as a positive control. The RT-PCR products were separated by electrophoresis on a 2% agarose gel, stained with ethidium bromide, and viewed by UV. (b) Western blot analysis for MGMT protein. Whole cell lysates from the indicated cell lines were loaded onto a 10% SDS-PAGE gel and electrophoresed. Proteins were electroblotted onto a PVDF membrane which was probed with monoclonal antibody specific for human MGMT. Each of the blots shown was demonstrated to have equal protein loading by reprobing with the monoclonal antibody for beta-actin (beta actin AC-15-ab6276, Abcam Limited, Cambridge, UK). Representative results. SAS and Hep2 cell lines appeared to contain only trace amounts of MGMT, whereas little if any expression could be detected in the cell line, HO-1-u-1. On the contrary, the other cell lines (HSC2, HSC3, HSC4, and KB) appeared to be producing uniformly large amounts of MGMT. The protein levels we detected were consistent with the mRNA expression levels. From [Murakami J *et al.* (2004) Oncol Rep. 12(2):339-345.], with permission.

We performed RT-PCR and western blotting to detect the expression levels of MGMT among oral cancer cell lines (Figure 2). SAS and Hep2 cell lines appeared to contain only trace amounts of *MGMT* mRNA, whereas little if any mRNA could be detected in the cell line HO-1-u-1. In contrast, the other cell lines (HSC2, HSC3, HSC4, and KB) appeared to be producing a uniformly large amount of the *MGMT* mRNA, as shown by the very dense bands that appeared in the relevant lanes (Figure 2a). We further examined the MGMT protein levels by western blotting (Figure 2b), and found that the levels we detected were consistent with the mRNA expression levels that we had previously detected, i.e., low levels in the SAS and Hep2 cells, almost none in the HO-1-u-1 cells, and relatively large amounts in the HSC2, HSC3, HSC4 and KB cells. To confirm the location of the MGMT protein expression, we examined the immunocytochemistry of MGMT in HSC3 and HSC4 cells (Figure 3). Both cell lines ubiquitously expressed MGMT protein localized in the nucleus and cytoplasm.

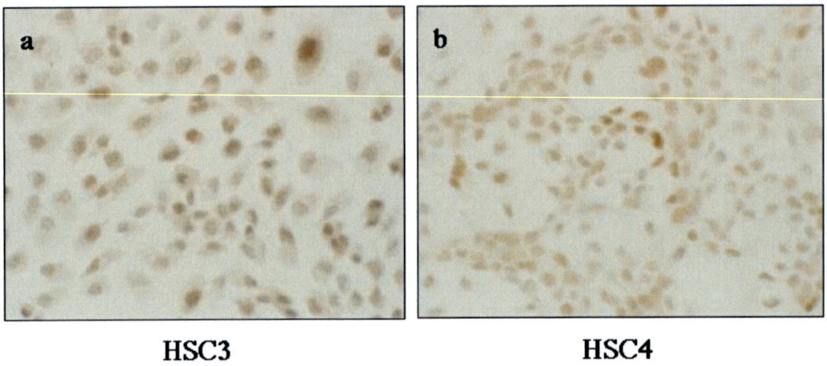

Figure 3. Immunocytochemistry of MGMT in HSC3 and HSC4 cells with rich expression of MGMT. The protein expressions of MGMT were monitored with mouse anti-MGMT monoclonal antibody. The cells were fixed with 10% formaldehyde and processed with the standard avidin-biotin peroxidase complex. DAB was used as chromogen. (a) HSC3 (b) HSC4. Original magnification, x40. Both cell lines expressed MGMT ubiquitously. MGMT protein localized in the nucleus and cytoplasm.

In order to confirm the contribution of the MGMT expression status to cellular sensitivity to the alkylating agents *N*-methyl-*N'*-nitro-*N* nitrosoguanidine (MNNG), we treated each of the oral cancer cell lines with varying concentrations of MNNG (Figure 4). All four cell lines with high MGMT expression (HSC2, HSC3, HSC4 and KB) appeared to be fully resistant to the lethal effects of MNNG at the concentrations used (~10μM), whereas the three cell lines with low MGMT expression (SAS, Hep2 and HO-1-u-1) proved to be much more sensitive.

In addition to alkylating agents, a favorable response to the platinum agent, *cis*-diaminedichloroplatinum(II) (CDDP), has also been reported among cancer cells with promoter methylation of *MGMT* [18]. This response could be explained by the possibility that CDDP abrogates MGMT activity [19,20]. This CDDP-induced attenuation of MGMT renders novel chemotherapeutic approaches such as temozolamide plus CDDP particularly attractive in the treatment of a number of cancers [19]. Previously, we revealed that CDDP could induce the MGMT depletion effect, and that the MGMT expression status could correlate with the clinical cellular response to CDDP in four oral cancer cell lines [21]. Therefore, given that CDDP is more widely used than alkylating agents in the clinical setting for the treatment of oral, colon, and other solid epithelial tumors, it would clearly be a major step forward in cancer chemotherapy if the MGMT expression could also enhance the potential effectiveness of CDDP.

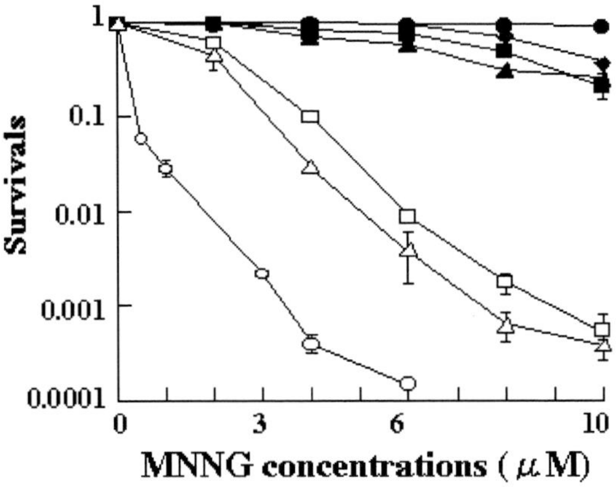

Figure 4. Cellular sensitivity to the alkylating agent *N*-methyl-*N'*-nitro-*N* nitrosoguanidine (MNNG) in oral cancer cell lines. Cell survival rates were assayed by measuring the colony-forming ability of the cells in triplicate samples. Flasks containing 5 ml DMEM were each seeded with 5×10^5 cells. After 24 h, the medium was replaced by one containing MNNG and the flasks were immersed in a 37°C water bath. After treatment for 1 h, the cells were rinsed three times in drug-free medium and the survival rates determined. Only colonies containing more than 50 cells were counted. HSC4, HSC3, HSC2 and KB cells with high MGMT expression were resistant to the lethal effects of MNNG, whereas SAS, Hep2 and HO-1-u-1 cells with low MGMT expression showed sensitivity. The cell-survival rates in groups with high MGMT expression were significantly different ($p<0.01$) from those with low MGMT expression by a Student's *t*-test. Symbols: HO-1-u-1, ○; HSC2, ●; HSC3, ▲; HSC4, ◆; SAS, □; KB, ■; Hep2, Δ. Standard errors are shown for each concentration.

Because MGMT activity has been recognized as an important marker of sensitivity to alkylating agents, many attempts have been made to deplete MGMT by using the specific inhibitor of MGMT to enhance the anti-cancer effects of alkylating agents [22]. O^6-benzylguanine (O^6-BG) is one such specific, rationally designed MGMT inhibitor that produces suicidal inactivation of MGMT with a restoration of sensitivity to chloroethylators or methylators [22-24]. A single administration of O^6-BG to the cells has been known to be non-toxic [25]. O^6-BG treatment has been approved as a phase I study [26], and is currently being administered in combination with BCNU, an O^6-alkylating agent, for the treatment of glioblastoma. In 2005, we reported that the addition of O^6-BG invariably enhanced CDDP sensitivity in human oral cancer cell lines [21]. O^6-BG could be a promising modulating agent for CDDP in oral cancer chemotherapy. However, we could not exclude the involvement of different pathways, other than the apparent one in which MGMT is involved in the control of the combined regimen with O^6-BG and CDDP. Fishel *et al.* also reported that O^6-BG treatment resulted in an additive effect on CDDP- and carboplatin-induced cytotoxicity, but its enhancement seems to be independent of its MGMT status [27]. We also investigated the effects of O^6-BG on 5-FU sensitivity [28]. The pretreatment of O^6-BG exhibited an enhancement of the anti-tumor effect of 5-FU in oral cancer cell lines. As such, the depletion of MGMT in cancer cells could become an important therapeutic target for sensitizing cells to chemotherapy.

Interestingly, Liu *et al.* [29] reported the inhibition of MGMT activity *in vitro* by complex mixtures present in the saliva of tobacco and betel nut chewers. Unquestionably, the use of tobacco products, along with alcohol consumption, is the major cause of oral cancer. Especially in a majority of Indian oral cancer patients, smokeless tobacco use is strongly linked to oral cancer and precancerous lesions to oral cancer. The exposure of buccal cell cultures to various organic and water-based extracts of products related to the use of tobacco and betel nut quid was shown to decrease MGMT activity [29]. Smokeless tobacco products contain tobacco-specific nitrosamines such as *N*-nitrosonornicotine, 4-(methylnitrosamino)-1-(3-pyridyl)-1-butanone, alkaloids and precursors of reactive oxygen species. Tobacco-specific nitrosamines are the most prevalent strong carcinogens in smokeless tobacco products that could be causally associated with the development of oral cancer [30,31]. Tobacco-specific nitrosamines are known to produce O^6-alkylguanine adducts in DNA [32,33]. Sawhney *et al.* evaluated the clinical significance of alteration in the MGMT protein expression in 78 oral precancerous stages (58 hyperplasias and 20 dysplasias) and 107 oral SCCs and determined their correlation with the tobacco consumption habits of these patients and disease prognosis [34]. Reduced MGMT expression was observed in the hyperplasia stage as compared to normal oral tissues obtained from subjects with no evidence of precancerous lesions or SCCs. The decrease in MGMT expression seems to be an early event in the development of smokeless tobacco-associated oral cancer, occurring as early as in hyperplasia [34]. To study the *in vitro* effects of smokeless tobacco (khaini) on modulation of the expression of genes, Rohatgi *et al.* established an oral epithelial cell culture (AMOL-III) from an oral leukoplakia with histological evidence of hyperplasia with hyperkeratosis from the gingivo-buccal sulcus of a smokeless tobacco (khaini) consumer [35]. The smokeless tobacco-extract treatment of these cells resulted in the loss of pRb, RAR, p21 waf1/cip1 and MGMT expressions while the expression of cyclin D1 was increased. They speculated that smokeless tobacco-carcinogens might have induced early changes, which may lead the oral epithelial cells down the carcinogenic pathway in these cells.

In summary, careful examination of the expression status of MGMT may be valuable in future attempts to assess the potential utility of particular anti-cancer agents in oral cancer therapy. Because the majority of oral cancer patients are considered to either chew or smoke tobacco, it seems reasonable to predict that the use of chemotherapeutic agents will enhance their anti-tumor effects by MGMT depletion in these oral cancer patients.

References

[1] Blot WJ, McLaughlin JK, Winn DM, Austin DF, Greenberg RS, Preston-Martin S, Bernstein L, Schoenberg JB, Stemhagen A, Fraumeni JF Jr. Smoking and drinking in relation to oral and pharyngeal cancer. (1988) *Cancer Res. 48 (11)*: 3282-3287.

[2] Rosas SL, Koch W, da Costa Carvalho MG, Wu L, Califano J, Westra W, Jen J, Sidransky D. Promoter hypermethylation patterns of p16, O6-methylguanine-DNA-

methyltransferase, and death-associated protein kinase in tumors and saliva of head and neck cancer patients. (2001) *Cancer Res. 61(3)*: 939-942.

[3] Boffetta P, Merletti F, Magnani C, Terracini B. A population-based study of prognostic factors in oral and oropharyngeal cancer. (1994) *Eur J Cancer B Oral Oncol. 30B* (6): 369-373.

[4] Rafferty MA, O'Dwyer TP. Second primary malignancies in head and neck squamous cell carcinoma. (2001) *J Laryngol Otol. 115(12)*:988-991.

[5] Brent TP. Suppression of cross-link formation in chloroethylnitrosourea-treated DNA by an activity in extracts of human leukemic lymphoblasts. (1984) *Cancer Res. 44(5)*:1887-1892.

[6] Dunn WC, Tano K, Horesovsky GJ, Preston RJ, Mitra S. The role of O6 alkylguanine in cell killing and mutagenesis in Chinese hamster ovary cells. (1991) *Carcinogenesis (Lond.). 12(1)*: 83-89.

[7] Marathi UK, Kroes RA, Dolan ME, Erickson LC. Prolonged depletion of O6-methylguanine DNA methyltransferase activity following exposure to O6-benzylguanine with or without streptozotocin enhances 1, 3-bis (2-chloroethyl) -1-nitrosourea sensitivity in vitro. (1993) *Cancer Res. 53(18)*: 4281-4286.

[8] Chen J, Zhang Y, Moschel RC, Ikenaga M. Depletion of O6-methylguanine DNA methyltransferase and potentiation of 1, -bis (2-chloroethyl)-1-nitrosourea antitumor activity by O6-benzylguanine in vitro. (1993) *Carcinogenesis (Lond.). 14(5)*: 1057-1060.

[9] Egyhazi S, Bergh J, Hansson J, Karran P, Ringborg U. Carmustine-induced toxicity, DNA crosslinking and O^6-methylguanine-DNA methyltransferase activity in two human lung cancer cell lines. (1991) *Eur J Cancer. 27(12)*: 1658-1662.

[10] Pegg AE. Mammalian O^6-alkylguanine-DNA alkyltransferase: regulation and importance in response to alkylating carcinogenic and therapeutic agents. (1990) *Cancer Res. 50(19)*: 6119-6129.

[11] Pegg AE, Dolan ME, Moschel RC. Structure, function and inhibition of O6 alkylguanine-DNA alkyltransferase. (1995) *Prog Nucleic Acid Res Mol Biol. 51*: 167-223.

[12] Brent TP, Lestrud SO, Smith DG, Remack JS. Formation of DNA interstrand crosslinks by the novel chloroethylating agents 2-chloroethyl (methylsulfonyl) methylanesulphonate: suppression by O^6-alkylguanine-DNA-alkyltransferase purified from human leukemic lymphoblasts. (1987) *Cancer Res. 47(13)*: 3384-3387.

[13] Citron M, Decker R, Chen S, Schneider S, Graver M, Kleynerman L, Kahn LB, White A, Schoenhaus M, Yarosh D. O6-methylguanine-DNA methyltransferase in human normal and tumor tissue from brain, lung, and ovary. (1991) *Cancer Res. 51(16)*: 4131-4134.

[14] Day RSIII, Ziolkowski CHJ, Scudiero DA, Meyer SA, Mattern MR. Human tumor cell strains defective in the repair of alkylation damage. (1980) *Carcinogenesis (Lond.). 1*: 21-32.

[15] Day RSIII, Ziolkowski CH, Scudiero DA, Meyer SA, Lubiniecki AS, Girardi AJ, Galloway SM, Bynum GD. Defective repair of alkylated DNA by human tumor and SV40-transformed human cell strains. (1980) *Nature. 288(5792)*: 724-727.

[16] Sklar R, Strauss B. Removal of O6-methylguanine from DNA of normal and xeroderma pigmentosum-derived lymphoblastoid lines. (1981) *Nature. 289(5796)*: 417-420.

[17] Tsujimura T, Zhang YP, Fujio C, Chang HR, Watatani M, Ishizaki K, Kitamura H, Ikenaga M. *O*^{6}-methylguanine methyltransferase activity and sensitiveity of Japanese tumor cell strains to 1- (4-amino-2-methyl-5-pyrimidinyl) methyl-3- (2 chloroethyl) - 3-nitrosourea hydrochloricde. (1987) *Jpn J Cancer Res. 78(11)*: 1207-1215.

[18] Koul S, McKiernan JM, Narayan G, Houldsworth J, Bacik J, Dobrzynski DL, Assaad AM, Mansukhani M, Reuter VE, Bosl GJ, Chaganti RS, Murty VV. Role of promoter hypermethylation in Cisplatin treatment response of male germ cell tumors. (2004) *Mol Cancer. 3*:16.

[19] Wang LG, Setlow RB. Inactivation of O6-alkylguanine-DNA alkyltransferase in HeLa cells by cisplatin. (1989) *Carcinogenesis (Lond.). 10(9)*: 1681-1684.

[20] D'Atri S, Graziani G, Lacal PM, Nistico V, Gilberti S, Faraoni I, Watson AJ, Bonmassar E and Margison GP. Attenuation of O^6-methylguanine-DNA methyltransferase activity and mRNA levels by cisplatin and temozolomide in Jurkat cells. (2000) *J Pharmacol Exp Ther. 294(2)*: 664-671.

[21] Maki Y, Murakami J, Asaumi J, Tsujigiwa H, Nagatsuka H, Kokeguchi S, Fukui K, Kawai N, Yanagi Y, Kuroda M, Tanaka N, Matsubara N, Kishi K. Role of O^6-methylguanine-DNA methyltransferase and effect of O6-benzylguanine on the anti-tumor activity of cis-diaminedichloroplatinum(II) in oral cancer cell lines. (2005) *Oral Oncol. 41(10)*:984-993.

[22] Dolan ME, Pegg AE. *O*^{6}-Benzylguanine and its role in chemotherapy. (1997) *Clin Cancer Res. 3(6)*:837-847.

[23] Dolan ME, Stine L, Mitchell RB, Moschel RC, Pegg AE. Modulation of mammalian *O*6-alkylguanine–DNA alkyltransferase in vivo by *O*^{6}-benzylguanine and its effect on the sensitivity of a human glioma tumor to 1-(2-chloroethyl)-3-(4-methylcyclohexyl)-1-nitrosourea. (1990) *Cancer Commun. 2(11)*: 371-377.

[24] Dolan ME, Moschel RC, Pegg AE. Depletion of mammalian *O*^{6}-alkylguanine-DNA alkyltransferase activity by *O*^{6}-benzylguanine provides a means to evaluate the role of this protein in protection against carcinogenic and therapeutic alkylating agents. (1990) *Proc Natl Acad Sci USA. 87(14)*: 5368-5372.

[25] Pegg AE, Boosalis M, Samson L, Moschel RC, Byers TL, Swenn K, Dolan ME. Mechanism of inactivation of human O^6-alkylguanine–DNA alkyltransferase by O6-benzylguanine, (1993) *Biochemistry 32(45):* 11998-12006.

[26] Friedman HS, Kokkinakis DM, Pluda J, Friedman AH, Cokgor I, Haglund MM, Ashley DM, Rich J, Dolan ME, Pegg AE, Moschel RC, McLendon RE, Kerby T, Herndon JE, Bigner DD, Schold SC Jr. Phase I trial of O6-benzylguanine for patients undergoing surgery for malignant glioma. (1998) *J Clin Oncol. 16(11)*: 3570-3575.

[27] Fishel ML, Delaney SM, Friesen LD, Hansen RJ, Zuhowski EG, Moschel RC, Egorin MJ, Dolan ME. Enhancement of platinum-induced cytotoxicity by O6-benzylguanine. (2003) *Mol Cancer Ther. 2(7)*: 633-640.

[28] Murakami J, Lee Y-J, Kokeguchi S, Tsujigiwa H, Asaumi J, Nagatsuka H, Fukui K, Kuroda M, Tanaka N, Matsubara N. Depletion of O6-methylguanine-DNA

methyltransferase by O6-benzylguanine enhances 5-FU cytotoxicity in colon and oral cancer cell lines. *Oncol Rep. in press*

[29] Liu Y, Egyhazi S, Hansson J, Bhide SV, Kulkarni PS, Grafstrom RC. O6-methylguanine-DNA methyltransferase activity in human buccal mucosal tissue and cell cultures. Complex mixtures related to habitual use of tobacco and betel quid inhibit the activity in vitro. (1997) *Carcinogenesis. 18(10)*: 1889-1895.

[30] Rodu B, Jansson C. Smokeless tobacco and oral cancer: a review of the risks and determinants. (2004) *Crit Rev Oral Biol Med. 15(5)*: 252-263.

[31] Hecht SS. Tobacco carcinogens, their biomarkers and tobacco-induced cancer. (2003) *Nat Rev Cancer. 3(10)*: 733-744.

[32] Saffhill R, Margison GP, O'Connor PJ. Mechanisms of carcinogenesis induced by alkylating agents. (1985) *Biochim Biophys Acta. 823(2)*: 111-145.

[33] Singer B. Alkylation of the O^6 of guanine is only one of many chemical events that may initiate carcinogenesis. (1984) *Cancer Invest. 2(3)*: 233-238.

[34] Sawhney M, Rohatgi N, Kaur J, Gupta SD, Deo SV, Shukla NK, Ralhan R. MGMT expression in oral precancerous and cancerous lesions: Correlation with progression, nodal metastasis and poor prognosis. (2007) *Oral Oncol. 43(5)*: 515-522.

[35] Rohatgi N, Kaur J, Srivastava A, Ralhan R. Smokeless tobacco (khaini) extracts modulate gene expression in epithelial cell culture from an oral hyperplasia. (2005) *Oral Oncol. 41(8)*: 806-820.

2. New Target: Epigenetics

Clinically, oral SCC is preceded by multiple premalignant lesions such as leukoplakia, dysplasia, erythroplakia, lichen planus and oral submucous fibrosis. A potential mechanism for the development of multiple oral premalignant lesions has been explained by the field cancerization theory [1]. This theory was introduced by Slaughter *et al.* over 50 years ago. Exposure to carcinogens such as tobacco and alcohol can cause simultaneous molecular defects on the epithelium of the upper aerodigestive tract, thus increasing the risk of development of multiple cancers. According to the field cancerization theory, the multiple lesions arise from separate molecular events and are considered to be independent of each other. Identification of the additional early molecular alterations needed for neoplastic transformation should be explored further.

From our understanding of carcinogenesis, oral carcinogenesis is believed to be a multi-step process, involving the accumulation of genetic and epigenetic alterations in key regulatory genes [2,3]. In a modification of Knudson's double hit hypothesis [4,5], one allele of a tumor suppressor gene may be inactivated by epigenetic alterations and the other by genetic means.

Representative epigenetic alterations include DNA methylation and histone modifications, both of which may play an important role in carcinogenesis. The DNA methylation of cancer-associated genes leads to their inactivation, and is now known to be involved in the cancer development and progression. Furthermore, DNA methylation in the promoter region of cancer-related genes is a common event in many cancer types, and is observed as an early alteration in the development of cancer [6]. The epigenetic mechanisms may also play an important role in the genesis of oral SCC, and extensive knowledge has been obtained regarding DNA methylation in the promoter region of multiple genes in oral cancers [7,8]. In head and neck SCC, the hypermethylation of *p16INK4a*, *p14ARF*, *p15*, *MGMT*, *DAP-K*, *E-Cadherin*, *GST-P*, *hMLH1*, and *RASSF1A* has been reported [7,9-13].

Technological Advances in Determination of DNA Methylation

A number of approaches are currently being considered in the determination of promoter methylation, including the use of restriction enzymes [14], genomic bisulphite sequencing [15], pyrosequencing [16,17] and various array techniques [18]. Before the mid-90's, attempts at analysis using methylation-specific restriction enzymes were unsuccessful in identifying the precise methylation pattern. The reason is the exceptionally high density of CpGs doublets in the gene promoter sequences and the correspondingly large number of restriction sites. In 1996, Herman *et al.* explored methylation-specific PCR following bisulfite treatment [19]. Since sodium bisulfite treatment exclusively converts unmethylated cytosine to uracil under appropriate conditions, subsequent analysis to differentiate unconverted cytosine from converted uracil has enabled us to pinpoint the primary methylation status [20]. Methylation-specific PCR has been used in the majority of published data, mainly due to its increased sensitivity. However, methylation-specific PCR evaluates only several CpG sites at the 3'-end of the primers, and false positives caused by mis-priming or by the inadequacy of bisulfite treatment may be a problem, especially when high numbers of PCR cycles are used. Furthermore, methylation-specific PCR does not fulfill the need to quantify the level of methylation relating to the gene silencing. Methylation density in promoter CpG islands has been indicated to be important for gene silencing rather than the methylation that occurred at a limited number of CpG islands in the promoter [21]. Conversely, bisulfite DNA sequencing provides the precise methylation status over an amplified region, but requires large-scale sequencing of multiple plasmid clones [15,22,23]. In 2000-2003, several groups showed that the methylation status can be precisely achieved by microarray-based technologies [24-27]. In 2005, our group also established a precise system to identify DNA methylation patterns based on an oligonucleotide microarray technology. This simple signal detection system depended on an avidin–biotinylated peroxidase complex and provided reproducible and precise measurement of methylated CpGs [18].

The pyrosequencing methylation assay is one of many methods that have been developed in an attempt to overcome the shortcomings (*i.e.* false positives) of other methods and to gain quantitative methylation data [17,28]. This assay is a semiquantitative, high throughput and reliable method [17,28,29]. However, the primers used for the pyrosequencing methylation assay are designed to avoid CpG dinucleotides in their sequence, and the assay thus does not have as high a sensitivity and specificity as methylation-specific PCR. In 2006, Shaw *et al.* developed a methylation enrichment pyrosequencing technique, which benefits from the high sensitivity and specificity of methylation-specific PCR but has a second, confirmatory pyrosequencing step [16]. The PCR primers used in this method are specific for methylated CpG sites as in methylation-specific PCR (but unlike the standard pyrosequencing methylation assay). They used the methylation enrichment pyrosequencing technique and gained quantitative data for a series of oral SCCs.

DNA Methylation in Leukoplakia as a Precancerous Lesion

Leukoplakia, a clinically distinct white patch in the oral mucosa that will not rub off and is not attributable to any other known disease, is the most frequent oral precancerous lesion. It is considered to be potentially malignant, but not all leukoplakias undergo malignant transformation. Ten to fifteen percent of leukoplakias will develop into cancer over a period of time [30-32]. The management of oral precancerous lesions varies from watchful waiting to complete resection. However, complete local excision of dysplastic oral leukoplakia does not prevent oral cancer [33-35]. The clinical relevance of field cancerization lies in the development of SCCs that originate from multiple premalignant lesions [36]. Within this context, the study of precancerous tissue is contributory and clinically relevant. Attempts to monitor and prognosticate on the malignant transformation of oral precancerous lesions using methylation status have been reported [37-40].

López *et al.* evaluated *p16INK4a*, *p14ARF* and *MGMT* promoter hypermethylation in the oral rinse of patients with clinically-benign homogeneous leukoplakia [40]. In their report, DNA hypermethylation was observed in almost all of the leukoplakia patients, and thus the methylation of *p16INK4a* and *MGMT* was observed in 44 and 56% of the oral samples, respectively. Only 12% of the cases showed *p14ARF* methylation. The levels of *p16INK4a* and *MGMT* promoter hypermethylation identified in the oral rinses from their leukoplakia cases were similar or higher than those previously observed in cancers from head and neck and oral SCC patients [9,10]. They suggested that *p16INK4a* and *MGMT* promoter hypermethylation might be an early event in oral carcinogenesis. In 2006, Shaw *et al.* determined the methylation status of five genes including *p16INK4a, cytoglobin, cyclin A1, RAR* and *E-cadherin* in primary oral cancer samples by methylation enrichment pyrosequencing [16]. From their results, *p16INK4a* methylation was found in 28% of tumours but in only 4% of the normal tissues. In contrast to some previously published reports, *p16INK4a* promoter methylation was highly tumour specific. However, promoter methylation of the promoters of *E-cadherin* and *RAR* was also seen in surrounding normal tissues as well as in tumours, and is, perhaps, an early event in carcinogenesis.

Tobacco-Associated DNA Methylation in Oral Cancer

As mentioned before, the use of tobacco products, along with alcohol consumption, is unquestionably the major cause of oral cancer. Smokeless tobacco-associated oral cancer may often be preceded by leukoplakia as a precancerous lesion [41]. In lung cancer, several studies have reported an association between smoking and gene promoter methylation [42-44]. In oral SCCs, Ishida *et al.* investigated the promotor hypermethylation status of multiple genes (*p16INK4a*, *p14ARF*, *RB1*, *p21Waf1*, *p27Kip1*, *PTEN*, *p73*, *MGMT*, and *GST-P*) [45]. From their results, DNA methylation was detected in 46.9% (23/49) of samples and was closely correlated with tobacco use and/or alcohol consumption. *p16INK4a*, *p14ARF*,

MGMT, *RB1*, *PTEN* and *p27Kip1* were found to be methylated in 34.7%, 20.4%, 12.2%, 10.2%, 6.1%, and 4.1% of these 49 tumors, respectively, but the methylation of *p21Waf1*, *p73* and *GST-P* was not detected at all. In comparison with the smoking form of tobacco consumption, there have also been many reports about DNA methylation in smokeless tobacco-associated oral cancer. Kulkarni *et al.* observed a high frequency of promoter region hypermethylation in *p16INK4a*, *DAPK* and *MGMT* genes in 60 smokeless tobacco-associated oral cancer tissues as well as in corresponding adjacent normal mucosa [46]. The incidence of hypermethylation in oral cancer and adjacent mucosa for the *p16INK4a* gene was 66.7 and 50%, for *DAPK* was 68.3 and 60%, and for the *MGMT* gene was 51.7 and 26.7%, respectively. The absence of aberrant methylation in the four genes was noted in buccal scrapings from normal healthy individuals with no tobacco habits. Among those previous studies, the DNA methylation of *MGMT* is mainly focused on the tobacco-associated oral carcinogenesis [12,46,47]. These studies also suggested that the DNA methylation of *MGMT* occurs in the early stages in the tobacco-induced carcinogenesis of oral cancer. Interestingly, there are differences in the frequency of hypermethylation of the *MGMT* gene between Western (18.2%) and Indian populations (51.7%) [46,48]. We suspect this difference may be due to the different forms of tobacco consumption. In India, the chewing forms of tobacco are predominantly used, in comparison with smoking in Western countries. In summary, the epigenetic alteration of these genes is a frequent event in oral cancer and is an early event observed in the normal oral mucosa of the patients, indicating the critical importance of the epigenetic alteration in tobacco-associated oral carcinogenesis.

DNA Methylation in Salivary Gland Adenoid Cystic Carcinomas

Salivary gland carcinomas are relatively uncommon malignancies with widely variable histopathologic and biologic characteristics [49]. Adenoid cystic carcinoma (ACC) accounts for 7-20% of all epithelial salivary gland malignancies. ACC is characterized by relentless growth, perineural invasion, a high incidence of recurrence, and distant metastasis primarily to the lungs and bone. However, little is known about the epigenetic alterations in the development of salivary gland carcinogenesis. Therefore, it is possible that DNA methylation may influence the development of salivary gland ACC. Maruya *et al.* reported the promoter methylation in the *E-cadherin* gene in 16 of 23 salivary gland ACC cases (70%) [50]. Nishimine *et al.* found that 3 of 20 salivary gland ACCs (15%) had *p16INK4a* promoter methylation [44]. Kishi *et al.* analyzed 36 salivary gland ACCs, and the *RB1* gene was found to be the most frequently methylated (41.7% of cases), while the methylation of *p27Kip1* or *MGMT* was less frequent (8.3% and 5.6%, respectively) [51]. Li *et al.* reported that the promoter methylation of *p16INK4a*, *RASSF1A*, and *DAPK* was common in salivary gland ACCs, while the DNA methylation of the *MGMT* promoter was infrequent [52]. Of the 60 tumors, DNA methylation of the *p16INK4a* promoter was detected in 28 tumors (47%); the respective values of the DNA methylation of the *RASSF1A*, *DAPK*, and *MGMT* promoters were 25 tumors (42%), 16 tumors (27%), and 4 tumors (7%), respectively. Interestingly, the DNA methylation of *MGMT* seems to be an infrequent event in salivary gland ACCs, in contrast to oral SCCs, where the DNA methylation of *MGMT* occurs frequently.

The Methylation Status: in Relation with Genetic Alterations

The promoter CpG island in normal tissues is generally protected from aberrant hypermethylation, but this protection may be lost in the early phase of tumorigenesis. In 2007, our group studied the extent of promoter methylation in normal epithelium from patients without cancer and in the oesophageal epithelium, ranging from the background non-neoplastic epithelium to oesophageal SCC, and compared the results with the *p53* mutational status [53]. The number of gene promoters with DNA methylation increased gradually from the normal healthy epithelium, through oesophageal SCC-background non-neoplastic epithelium and intraepithelial neoplasia identified in the epithelium of oesophageal SCC, to the main advanced form of oesophageal SCC. By contrast, *p53* mutations were almost exclusively observed in the intraepithelial neoplasia and oesophageal SCC samples and rarely in the background epithelium. Interestingly, within samples of intraepithelial neoplasia or oesophageal SCC samples, a significantly higher number of loci showed methylation in samples with the *p53* mutation, compared with the samples without the mutation. These results suggest that epigenetic changes in a wide epithelial field appear to increase the probability of acquiring changes in genes such as *p53*, and that DNA methylation contributes to the progression of the dysplasia to the carcinoma sequence in oesophageal SCC carcinogenesis.

MGMT Methylation Status: As a Prognostic Marker

The detection of aberrant hypermethylation patterns of tumor-related genes is a suitable diagnostic molecular tool in individuals at a high risk for oral SCC. Moreover, since many DNA repair enzymes have been regulated via the epigenetic pathway, it is conceivable that the impaired DNA repair mechanisms resulting from epigenetic alterations in relevant genes could affect the efficacy of the therapeutic modalities designed to damage tumor DNA, including chemotherapy.

The 5'-upstream region of the human *MGMT* gene includes an extremely GC-rich CpG island that spans approximately 500 bp. Hypermethylation of the *MGMT* promoter has already proven to be of considerable prognostic value for certain colorectal cancer patients [21], and there is no doubt that a method permitting the rapid and efficient determination of the methylation status of the *MGMT* promoter region will soon prove to be of some value in the clinic. Esteller *et al.* also reported that the differential methylation of the *MGMT* promoter might be responsible for the marked differences in prognosis among glioma patients following carmustine treatment [54]. We believe that every effort should be made to use such a method in all future attempts to evaluate the usual range of chemotherapeutic alkylating agents prior to their administration.

We therefore decided to use bisulfite sequencing to examine the CpG island methylation status of the *MGMT* promoter region, plus neighboring sequences in seven oral cancer cell lines (Figure 5). We were able to classify the cell lines into two distinct groups because of their somewhat different methylation patterns. The first group consisted of the SAS, Hep2, and HO-1-u-1 cell lines, all of which were hypermethylated in the *MGMT* promoter region, and a second group consisted of the HSC3, HSC4, HSC2, and KB cell lines for which there was little or no evidence of hypermethylation. Three oral cancer cell lines with fully methylated sequences of the *MGMT* gene (SAS, Hep2 and HO-1-u-1) produced significantly reduced levels of *MGMT* mRNA and protein, whereas copious amounts of *MGMT* mRNA and protein were produced by the four cell lines with poorly methylated sequences (HSC4, HSC3, HSC2 and KB) (Figures 2 and 5). In the addition, the methylation status of the cell lines we tested closely correlated with their differing sensitivities to the alkylating agent MNNG, such that the methylation-silenced oral cancer cell lines are a great deal more sensitive to the lethal effects of these agents than their counterpart unmethylated (and hence MGMT protein expressing) cell lines (Figures 4 and 5). Our results indicate that the methylation patterns of specific regions of the *MGMT* gene might affect the relative sensitivities to alkylating agents of tumor cells from seven different oral cancer cell lines. Careful examination of the methylation status of the promoter of the *MGMT* may therefore be valuable in future attempts to assess the potential utility of particular alkylating agents in oral cancer therapy.

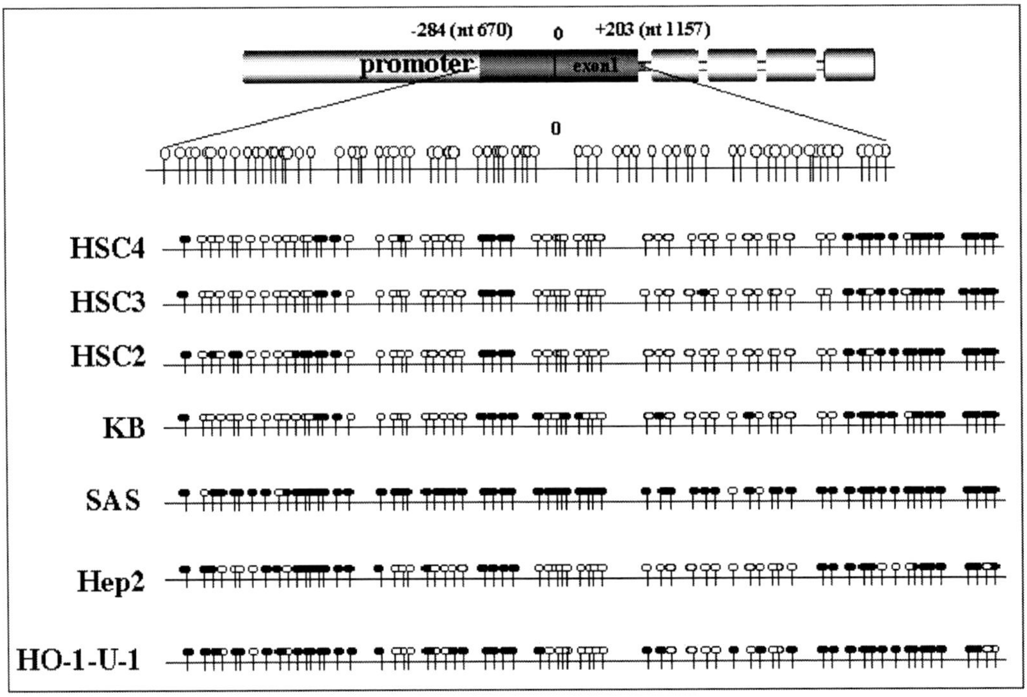

Figure 5. Methylation map of the CpG island in the 5' region of the *MGMT* gene (-284 to +203) CpGs. | bars represent CpG dinucleotides in the *MGMT* promoter. Closed circles on the bars represent methylated cytosine. Bars with open circles show no methylation of the CpG cytosine. From [Murakami J *et al.* (2004) Oncol Rep. 12(2):339-345.], with permission.

References

[1] Slaughter DP, Southwick HW, Smejkal W. Field cancerization in oral stratified squamous epithelium. (1953) *Cancer. 6(5)*: 963-968.

[2] Bishop JM. The molecular genetics of cancer. (1987) *Science (Washington DC). 235(4786):* 305-311.

[3] Califano J, Van der Riet P, Westra W, Nawroz H, Clayman G, Piantadosi S, Corio R, Lee D, Greenberg B, Koch W, Sidransky D. Genetic progression model for head and neck cancer: implications for field cancerization. (1996) *Cancer Res. 56(11)*: 2488-2492.

[4] Esteller M, Fraga MF, Paz MF, Campo E, Colomer D, Novo FJ, Calasanz MJ, Galm O, Guo M, Benitez J, Herman JG. Cancer epigenetics and methylation. (2002) *Science. 297(5588)*: 1807-1808.

[5] Momparler RL, Bovenzi V. DNA methylation and cancer. (2000) *J Cell Physiol. 183(2)*: 145-154.

[6] Baylin SB, Herman JG. DNA hypermethylation in tumorigenesis: epigenetics joins genetics. (2000) *Trends Genet. 16(4)*:168-174.

[7] Rosas SL, Koch W, da Costa Carvalho MG, Wu L, Califano J, Westra W, Jen J, Sidransky D. Promoter hypermethylation patterns of p16, O6-methylguanine-DNA-methyltransferase, and death-associated protein kinase in tumors and saliva of head and neck cancer patients. (2001) *Cancer Res. 61(3)*: 939-942.

[8] Dong SM, Sun DI, Benoit NE, Kuzmin I, Lerman MI, Sidransky D. Epigenetic inactivation of RASSF1A in head and neck cancer. (2003) *Clin Cancer Res. 9*(10 Pt 1): 3635-3640.

[9] Shintani S, Nakahara Y, Mihara M, Ueyama Y, Matsumura T. Inactivation of the p14(ARF), p15(INK4B) and p16(INK4A) genes is a frequent event in human oral squamous cell carcinomas. (2001) *Oral Oncol. 37(6)*: 498-504.

[10] Sanchez-Cespedes M, Esteller M, Wu L, Nawroz-Danish H, Yoo GH, Koch WM, Jen J, Herman JG, Sidransky D. Gene promoter hypermethylation in tumors and serum of head and neck cancer patients. (2000) *Cancer Res. 60(4)*: 892-895.

[11] Hasegawa M, Nelson HH, Peters E, Ringstrom E, Posner M, Kelsey KT. Patterns of gene promoter methylation in squamous cell cancer of the head and neck. (2002) *Oncogene. 21(27)*: 4231-4236.

[12] Viswanathan M, Tsuchida N, Shanmugam G. Promoter hypermethylation profile of tumor-associated genes p16, p15, hMLH1, MGMT and E-cadherin in oral squamous cell carcinoma. (2003*) Int J Cancer. 105(1)*:41-46.

[13] Weber A, Bellmann U, Bootz F, Wittekind C, Tannapfel A. INK4a-ARF alterations and p53 mutations in primary and consecutive squamous cell carcinoma of the head and neck. (2002) *Virchows Arch 441(2)*: 133-142.

[14] Singer-Sam J, LeBon JM, Tanguay RL, Riggs AD. A quantitative HpaII-PCR assay to measure methylation of DNA from a small number of cells. (1990) *Nucleic Acids Res. 18(3)*: 687.

[15] Frommer M, McDonald LE, Millar DS, Collis CM, Watt F, Grigg GW, Molloy PL, Paul CL. A genomic sequencing protocol that yields a positive display of 5-

methylcytosine residues in individual DNA strands. (1992) *Proc Natl Acad Sci USA. 89(5)*: 1827-1831.

[16] Shaw RJ, Liloglou T, Rogers SN, Brown JS, Vaughan ED, Lowe D, Field JK, Risk JM. Promoter methylation of P16, RARbeta, E-cadherin, cyclin A1 and cytoglobin in oral cancer: quantitative evaluation using pyrosequencing. (2006) *Br J Cancer. 94(4)*:561-568.

[17] Colella S, Shen L, Baggerly KA, Issa JP, Krahe R. Sensitive and quantitative universal Pyrosequencing methylation analysis of CpG sites. (2003) *Biotechniques. 35(1)*: 146-150.

[18] Kimura N, Nagasaka T, Murakami J, Sasamoto H, Murakami M, Tanaka N, Matsubara N. Methylation profiles of genes utilising newly developed CpG island microarray on colorectal cancer patients. (2005) *Nucl Acids Res. 33(5)*: e46.

[19] Herman JG, Graff JR, Myohanen S, Nelkin BD, Baylin SB. Methylation-specific PCR: a novel PCR assay for methylation status of CpG islands. (1996) *Proc Natl Acad Sci USA. 93(18)*: 9821-9826.

[20] Hayatsu H, Wataya Y, Kai K, Iida S. Reaction of sodium bisulfite with uracil, cytosine, and their derivatives. (1970) *Biochemistry. 9(14)*:2858-2865.

[21] Nagasaka T, Sharp G.B, Notohara K, Kambara T, Sasamoto H, Isozaki H, MacPhee DG, Jass JR, Tanaka N, Matsubara N. Hypermethylation of O6-methylguanine-DNA methyltransferase promoter may predict nonrecurrence after chemotherapy in colorectal cancer cases. (2003) *Clin Cancer Res. 9(14)*:5306-5312.

[22] Melki JR, Vincent PC, Clark SJ. Concurrent DNA hypermethylation of multiple genes in acute myeloid leukemia. (1999) *Cancer Res. 59(15)*:3730-3740.

[23] Rice JC, Massey-Brown KS, Futscher BW. Aberrant methylation of the BRCA1 CpG island promoter is associated with decreased BRCA1 mRNA in sporadic breast cancer cells. (1998) *Oncogene. 17(14)*:1807-1812.

[24] Yan PS, Perry MR, Laux DE, Asare AL, Caldwell CW, Huang TH. CpG island arrays: an application toward deciphering epigenetic signatures of breast cancer. (2000) *Clin Cancer Res. 6(4)*:1432-1438.

[25] Yan PS, Chen CM, Shi H, Rahmatpanah F, Wei SH, Caldwell CW, Huang TH. Dissecting complex epigenetic alterations in breast cancer using CpG island microarrays. (2001) *Cancer Res. 61(23)*:8375-8380.

[26] Adorjan P, Distler J, Lipscher E, Model F, Muller J, Pelet C, Braun A, Florl AR, Gutig D, Grabs G, Howe A, Kursar M, Lesche R, Leu E, Lewin A, Maier S, Muller V, Otto T, Scholz C, Schulz WA, Seifert HH, Schwope I, Ziebarth H, Berlin K, Piepenbrock C, Olek A. Tumour class prediction and discovery by microarray-based DNA methylation analysis. (2002) *Nucleic Acids Res. 30(5)*:e21.

[27] Chen CM, Chen HL, Hsiau TH, Hsiau AH, Shi H, Brock GJ, Wei SH, Caldwell CW, Yan PS, Huang TH. Methylation target array for rapid analysis of CpG island hypermethylation in multiple tissue genomes. (2003) *Am J Pathol. 163(1)*:37-45.

[28] Tost J, Dunker J, Gut IG. Analysis and quantification of multiple methylation variable positions in CpG islands by pyrosequencing. (2003) *Biotechniques. 35(1)*: 152-156.

[29] Dupont JM, Tost J, Jammes H, Gut IG. De novo quantitative bisulfite sequencing using the pyrosequencing technology. (2004) *Anal Biochem. 333(1)*: 119-127.

[30] Gupta PC, Mehta FS, Pindborg JJ, Bhonsle RB, Murti PR, Daftary DK, Aghi MB. Primary prevention trial of oral cancer in India: a 10-year follow-up study. (1992) *J Oral Pathol Med. 21(10)*:433-439.

[31] Tradati N, Grigolat R, Calabrese L, Costa L, Giugliano G, Morelli F, Scully C, Boyle P, Chiesa F. Oral leukoplakias: to treat or not? (1997) *Oral Oncol. 33(5)*:317-321.

[32] Gupta PC, Mehta FS, Daftary DK, Pindborg JJ, Bhonsle RB, Jalnawalla PN, Sinor PN, Pitkar VK, Murti PR, Irani RR, Shah HT, Kadam PM, Iyer KS, Iyer HM, Hegde AK, Chandrashekar GK, Shiroff BC, Sahiar BE, Mehta MN. Incidence rates of oral cancer and natural history of oral precancerous lesions in a 10-year follow-up study of Indian villagers. (1980) *Community Dent Oral Epidemiol. 8(6)*:283-333.

[33] Sudbø J, Lippman SM, Lee JJ, Mao L, Kildal W, Sudbo A, Sagen S, Bryne M, El-Naggar A, Risberg B, Evensen JF, Reith A. The influence of resection and aneuploidy on mortality in oral leukoplakia. (2004) *N Engl J Med. 350(14)*:1405-1413.

[34] Zhang L, Poh CF, Lam WL, Epstein JB, Cheng X, Zhang X, Priddy R, Lovas J, Le ND, Rosin MP. Impact of localized treatment in reducing risk of progression of low-grade oral dysplasia: Molecular evidence of incomplete resection. (2001) *Oral Oncol. 37(6)*:505-512.

[35] Sudbø J, Reith A, Lippman SM: Dysplastic leukoplakia. (2004) *N Engl J Med. 350*:2718-2719.

[36] Braakhuis BJM, Tabor MP, Kummer JA, Leemans CR, Brakenhoff RH. A genetic explanation of Slaughter's concept of field cancerization. (2003) *Cancer Res. 63(8)*:1727-1730.

[37] Kresty LA, Mallery SR, Knobloch TJ, Song H, Lloyd M, Casto BC, Weghorst CM. Alterations of p16(INK4a) and p14(ARF) in patients with severe oral epithelial dysplasia. (2002) *Cancer Res. 62(18)*: 5295-5300.

[38] McGregor F, Muntoni A, Fleming J, Brown J, Felix DH, MacDonald DG, Parkinson EK, Harrison PR. Molecular changes associated with oral dysplasia progression and acquisition of immortality: potential for its reversal by 5-azacytidine. (2002) *Cancer Res. 62(16)*: 4757-4766.

[39] Yeh KT, Shih MC, Lin TH, Chen JC, Chang JY, Kao CF, Lin KL, Chang JG. The correlation between CpG methylation on promoter and protein expression of E-cadherin in oral squamous cell carcinoma. (2002) *Anticancer Res. 22(6C)*: 3971-3975.

[40] Lopez M, Aguirre JM, Cuevas N, Anzola M, Videgain J, Aguirregaviria J, Martinez de Pancorbo M. Gene promoter hypermethylation in oral rinses of leukoplakia patients--a diagnostic and/or prognostic tool? (2003) *Eur J Cancer. 39(16)*: 2306-2309.

[41] Greenspan D, Jordan RC. The white lesion that kills--aneuploid dysplastic oral leukoplakia. (2004) *N Engl J Med. 350(14)*:1382-1384.

[42] Zochbauer- Muller S, Fong KM, Virmani AK, Geradts J, Gazdar AF, Minna JD. Aberrant Promoter Methylation of Multiple Genes in Non-Small Cell Lung Cancers. (2001) *Cancer Res. 61(1)*:249-255.

[43] Zochbauer-Muller S, Lam S, Toyooka S, Virmani AK, Toyooka KO, Seidl S, Minna JD, Gazdar AF. Aberrant methylation of multiple genes in the upper aerodigestive tract epithelium of heavy smokers. (2003) *Int J Cancer. 107(4)*: 612-616.

[44] Nishimine M, Nakamura M, Kishi M, Okamoto M, Shimada K, Ishida E, Kirita T, Konishi N. Alteration of p14ARF and p16INK4a genes in salivary gland carcinomas. (2003) *Oncol Rep. 10(3)*: 555-560.

[45] Ishida E, Nakamura M, Ikuta M, Shimada K, Matsuyoshi S, Kirita T, Konishi N. Promotor hypermethylation of *p14ARF* is a key alteration for progression of oral squamous cell carcinoma. (2005) *Oral Oncol. 41(6)*: 614-622.

[46] Kulkarni V, Saranath D. Concurrent hypermethylation of multiple regulatory genes in chewing tobacco associated oral squamous cell carcinomas and adjacent normal tissues. (2004) *Oral Oncol. 40(2)*: 145-153.

[47] Guo W, Liu X, Lee S, Park NH. High O6-methylguanine methyl transferase activity is frequently found in human oral cancer cells with p53 inactivation. (1999) *Int J Oncol. 15(4)*: 817-821.

[48] Zuo C, Ai L, Ratliff P, Suen JY, Hanna E, Brent TP, Fan CY. O6-methylguanine-DNA methyltransferase gene: epigenetic silencing and prognostic value in head and neck squamous cell carcinoma. (2004) *Cancer Epidemiol Biomarkers Prev. 13(6)*:967-975.

[49] Johns ME, Goldsmith MM. Incidence, diagnosis, and classification of salivary gland tumors. Part 1. (1989) *Oncology (Huntingt). 3(2)*: 47-56.

[50] Maruya S, Kurotaki H, Wada R, Saku T, Shinkawa H, Yagihashi S. Promoter methylation and protein expression of the E-cadherin gene in the clinicopathologic assessment of adenoid cystic carcinoma. (2004) *Mod Pathol. 17(6)*: 637-645.

[51] Kishi M, Nakamura M, Nishimine M, Ikuta M, Kirita T, Konishi N. Genetic and epigenetic alteration profiles for multiple genes in salivary gland carcinomas. (2005) *Oral Oncol. 41(2)*: 161-169.

[52] Li J, El-Naggar A, Mao L. Promoter methylation of p16INK4a, RASSF1A, and DAPK is frequent in salivary adenoid cystic carcinoma. (2005) *Cancer. 104(4)*: 771-776.

[53] Ishii T, Murakami J, Notohara K, Cullings HM, Sasamoto H, Kambara T, Shirakawa Y, Naomoto Y, Ouchida M, Shimizu K, Tanaka N, Jass JR, Matsubara N. Oesophageal squamous cell carcinoma may develop within a background of accumulating DNA methylation in normal and dysplastic mucosa. (2007) *Gut. 56(1)*:13-19.

[54] Esteller M, Garcia-Foncillas J, Andion E, Goodman SN, Hidalgo OF, Vanaclocha V, Baylin SB, Herman JG. Inactivation of the DNA-repair gene MGMT and the clinical response of gliomas to alkylating agents. (2000) *N Engl J Med. 343(19)*:1350-1354.

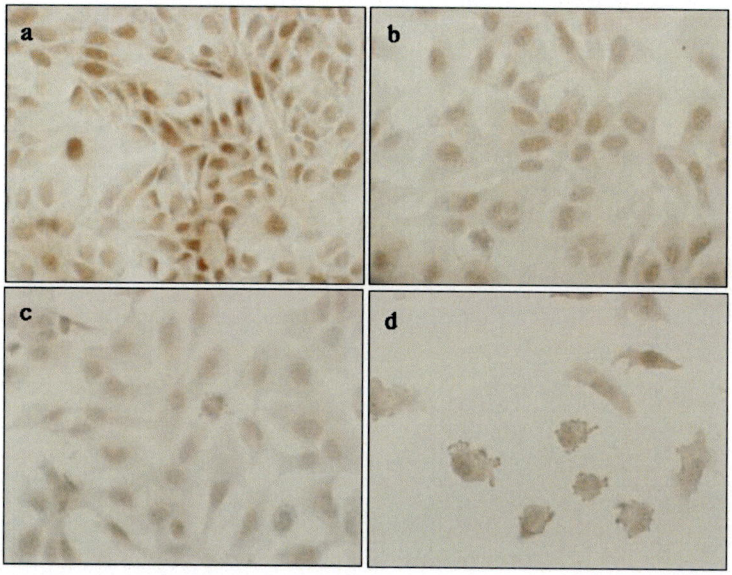

Figure 6. Immunocytochemistry of Histone deacetylase 1 (HDAC1) in HSC4 cells treated with varying concentrations of TSA for 24 h. The inhibition of HDAC1 by TSA was monitored with specific antibodies recognizing HDAC1 (Cell Signaling Technology, Beverly, MA). Cells were fixed with 10% formaldehyde and processed with the standard avidin-biotin peroxidase complex. DAB was used as a chromogen. (a) HSC4; non-treated, (b) HSC4; TSA treated (800 nM), (c) HSC4; TSA treated (1.6 microM), (d) (c) HSC4; TSA treated (2.4 microM). Original magnification, x40. HDAC1 was highly expressed in TSA untreated HSC4 cells, and was downregulated after TSA treatment in a concentration-dependent manner.

3. New Target in Chemotherapeutics: Histone Deacetylase

The presence of histone acetylation/deacetylation might be a useful therapeutic target in oral SCC patients.

Histone Acetylation/Deacetylation

Transcriptional regulation largely depends on epigenetic mechanisms. The alteration of gene expression due to epigenetic modification seems to play a role in carcinogenesis [1,2]. The most important epigenetic mechanisms in transcription control are both DNA methylation and chromatin remodeling. Modifications of core histone tails play an important role in the regulation of chromatin architecture. The acetylation and deacetylation of N-terminal lysine residues in nuclear histones are particularly important among modifications of core histone tails, and the balance between the two processes may result in changes in the regulation of patterns of gene expression by modulating the chromatin structure [3,4]. The acetylation of histones alters the nucleosome structure and results in a more open, transcriptionally active chromatin structure [5,6]. Histone acetylation is regulated by a group of enzymes known as histone acetyltransferases. In contrast, the deacetylation of histones works synergistically with promoter DNA methyltransferases and results in a close, transcriptionally inactive heterochromatin [7,8]. Histone deacetylation is regulated by the histone deacetylases (HDACs) [9].

New Chemotherapeutic Agent: HDAC Inhibitors

The inhibition of HDACs is a novel strategy for the treatment of cancer, and HDAC inhibitors are thus a promising new class of chemotherapeutic agents against a broad range of hematologic and solid tumors (10-12). A variety of HDAC inhibitors have been developed and structurally classified into (1) short-chain fatty acids (e.g. sodium butyrate), (2) hydroxamic acids [e.g. suberoylanilide hydroxamic acid, oxamflatin, and trichostatin A (TSA), (3) cyclic tetrapeptide (e.g. trapoxin A), (4) cyclic peptides [e.g. depsipeptide (FR901228, FK228) and apicidin], and (5) benzamides (e.g. MS-275). Some of the HDAC inhibitors, including suberoylanilide hydroxamic acid [13,14], MS-275 [15], phenylbutyrate [16,17], and depsipeptide (FR901228, FK228, NSC630176)[18-20], are currently in Phase I and II clinical trials for the treatment of both solid and liquid tumors [21]. Phase II trials with FK228 have been initiated in cutaneous T-cell lymphoma, peripheral T-cell lymphoma, and recurrent or metastatic SCC of the head and neck [18,22,23]. Promising results are being reported which support the development of these compounds for clinical use. HDAC inhibitors have been shown to inhibit the proliferation and survival of cells and to induce differentiation as anti-tumor agents for the treatment of human cancers [24,25]. HDAC inhibitors regulate the transcription of genes by altering chromatin structure, and they activate the transcription of selected genes related to the differentiation, cell-cycle arrest or apoptosis in a variety of cancer cells [29-33]. The induction of gene expression by HDAC inhibitors is mediated primarily through the inhibition of HDAC and the relative activation of histone acetyltransferase. Despite numerous studies demonstrating these activities in cancer cell lines and animal models, the mechanisms underlying their action have not been fully delineated.

To confirm the inhibition of HDAC activity by HDAC inhibitors, we performed immunocytochemical staining against HDAC1 for TSA-treated oral cancer cell line HSC4 cells (Figure 6). HSC4 cells were treated with varying concentrations of TSA for 24 h. HDAC1-positive cells disappeared after TSA treatment in a concentration-dependent manner, whereas HDAC1 was highly expressed in TSA untreated HSC4 cells (Figure 6). We also examined whether the administration of TSA induced histone H3 acetylation in oral cancer cells (Figures 7 and 8). TSA-induced hyperacetylation of histone H3 were monitored with specific antibodies recognizing acetylated N-terminal lysine residues (Lys9) of histones H3. As shown in Figure 7, the HSC4 cells were treated with varying concentrations of TSA for 24 h and analyzed by immunocytochemistry. TSA mediated an increase in the acetyl histone H3 (Lys9) levels in HSC4 cells after the onset of drug exposure. Acetyl histone H3 (Lys9) - positive HSC4 cells appeared after TSA treatment in a concentration-dependent manner. The histone acetylation was further determined by western blot analysis. HSC4 and KB cells were treated with TSA (800nM) for up to 24h (Figure 8). In a time course experiment, treatment with TSA led to a marked increase in acetyl histone H3 (Lys9) in 4h, whereas little acetylated histone H3 expression was detected in non-treated cells. The accumulation of acetylated histone remained elevated to 8h.

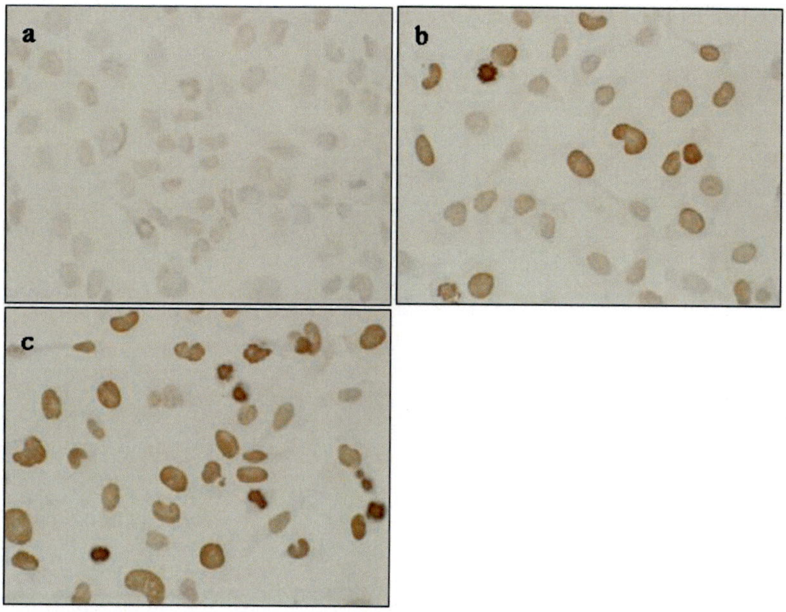

Figure 7. Immunocytochemistry of acetyl-histone H3 (Lys9) in HSC4 cells treated with varying concentrations of TSA for 24 h. The TSA-induced hyperacetylation of histone H3 were monitored with specific antibodies recognizing acetyl-histone H3 (Lys9) (Cell Signaling Technology, Beverley, MA). The cells were fixed with 10% formaldehyde and processed with the standard avidin-biotin peroxidase complex. DAB was used as a chromogen. (a) non-treated; (b) TSA treated (500 nM); (c) TSA treated (800 nM). Original magnification, x40. Acetylation of histone tails in HSC4 cells was upregulated after TSA treatment in a concentration-dependent manner.

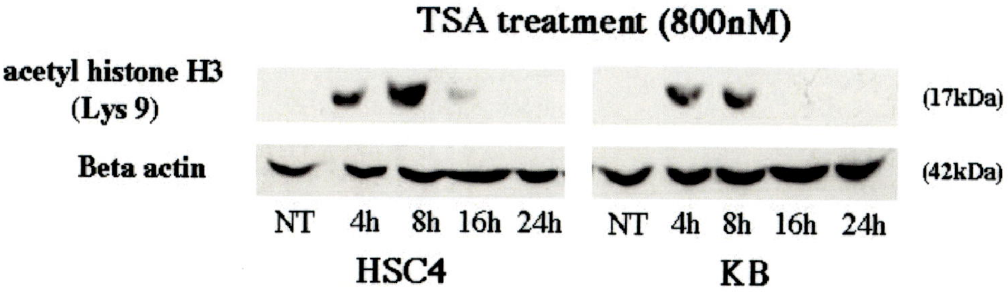

Figure 8. Effect of TSA on histone acetylation. To confirm the upregulation of histone acetylation by HDAC inhibitors, we carried out western blotting using HSC4 and KB cell lines. The histone acetylation was further determined by western blot analysis using a specific antibody against acetyl histone H3 (Lys9). The total cell lysate from untreated HSC4, KB cells, and cells treated with TSA (800 nM) for up to 24 hours was electrophoretically separated and transferred to a polyvinylidene difluoride membrane. The membrane was then subsequently probed with specific antibodies recognizing histones acetylated at the following site: lysine 9 of histone H3 (H3-K9). Westernblotting was carried out according to the standard method. Representative results. Whereas little acetyl histone H3 (Lys9) expression was detected in non-treated cells, in a time course experiment, the acetylation of the histone tail became evident 4 to 8 hours after treatment with TSA.

Many Aspects of Actions

In addition to the cytotoxic action, HDAC inhibitors are able to block the cell cycle [26] and angiogenesis [27], and induce apoptosis [28] in human cancer cells.

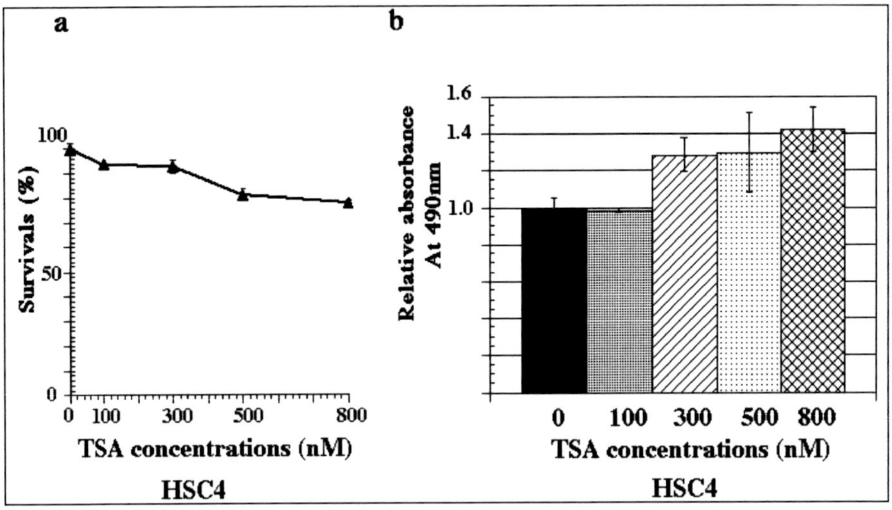

Figure 9. Effect of TSA on the proliferation and apoptosis of HSC4 cells. HSC4 cells were cultured in the presence or absence of varying concentrations of TSA for 24h. (a) Cellular sensitivity to TSA. The cell survival rates were assayed by an MTT (3-(4,5-dimethylthiazol-2-yl)-2,5-diphenyl tetrasodium bromide) assay. Eight replicate wells/assay conditions were seeded into 96-well plates at a density of 1.5 x 104 cells in 0.1 ml of medium and incubated at 37°C for 24h. The cells were incubated with several concentrations of TSA ranging from 100-800 nM for an additional 24h. At the end of the TSA exposure, an MTT assay was carried out using an MTT Cell Growth Kit (Chemicon International, Inc. Temecula, CA) according to the manufacturer's instructions. The percentage of cell-growth inhibition was calculated by comparison of the absorbance reading from treated versus untreated control cells. The concentration-dependent inhibition of cell proliferation was observed. (b) Apoptotic effects of TSA. We assessed TSA-induced apoptosis by an "Apoptosis Screening Kit" using the manufacturer's protocol (Wako Pure Chemical Industries, Ltd. Osaka, Japan). The cells were seeded in 96 well plates, as described above. The cells were then treated with varying doses of TSA ranging from 100-800 nM for 24h. After drug treatment, the cells were fixed with 10% formaldehyde and assayed for apoptosis. The percentage of apoptosis was calculated by comparison of the absorbance at a 490nm reading from treated versus untreated control cells. The treatment of HSC4 cells for 24 h with the TSA induced apoptosis of cells in a dose-dependent manner.

We determined the cytotoxicity of HDAC inhibitor TSA in HSC4 (Figure 9a). HSC4 cells were cultured in the presence or absence of varying concentrations of TSA for 24h. We found that the treatment of HSC4 cells for 24 h with TSA induced the death of cells in a dose-dependent manner. Consistent with the result of cytotoxicity for TSA, the treatment with TSA induced the apoptosis of cells in a dose-dependent manner (Figure 9b). TSA treatment induced morphologic changes and cell death in oral cancer cells (Figure 10). HSC4 and KB cells were treated with varying concentrations of TSA for 24h. Reduced cell density was observed in cultures treated with TSA and dead cells were floating in the medium. HSC4 and KB cells are normally oval or polygonal (Figures 10a and d). Compared with the controls, many TSA-treated cells became enlarged and formed long processes (Figures 10b, c, e and f). As shown in Figure 11, to confirm the induction of apoptosis by the HDAC inhibitor, we performed TUNEL staining for TSA-treated HSC4 cells. HSC4 cells were cultured in the presence or absence of 800 nM of TSA for 24 h, and then the cells were stained with the TUNEL method. TUNEL-positive cells appeared after 24 h of TSA treatment, indicating that TSA causes apoptosis in HSC4. To examine the pathway of TSA stimulated apoptosis, we carried out western blotting of proteins involved in the apoptosis including caspase-7, caspase-9, PARP and cytochrome c (Figure 12). The effectiveness of TSA in activating apoptosis was assessed by the cleavage of the caspases and PARP. As shown in Figure 12, the activation of caspases became evident 16 hours after treatment with TSA in a time course experiment. Furthermore, TSA treatment induced proteolytic PARP, which is a caspase-3 substrate, indicating that the caspases were really activated in TSA-treated cells. These results indicated that TSA induces apoptosis by facilitating the cleavage of caspases. Given that the acetylation of the histone tail became evident 4 to 8 hours after treatment with TSA (Figure 8), TSA induced the apoptosis of HSC4 or KB cells in a time-dependent manner, preceded by the accumulation of acetylated histones H3. The activation of the mitochondrial apoptotic pathway by TSA was assessed by analysis of the expression level of cytochrome *c*. We used whole cell lysates in western blotting, and did not assess the release of cytochrome *c* from the mitochondria into the cytosol. However, TSA treatment had no effects on the levels of cytochrome c in the KB cells, and only a trace amount of expressions were observed and unchanged in the HSC4 cells. The mitochondrial pathway might not be required mainly in the activation of apoptosis by TSA in oral cancer cells.

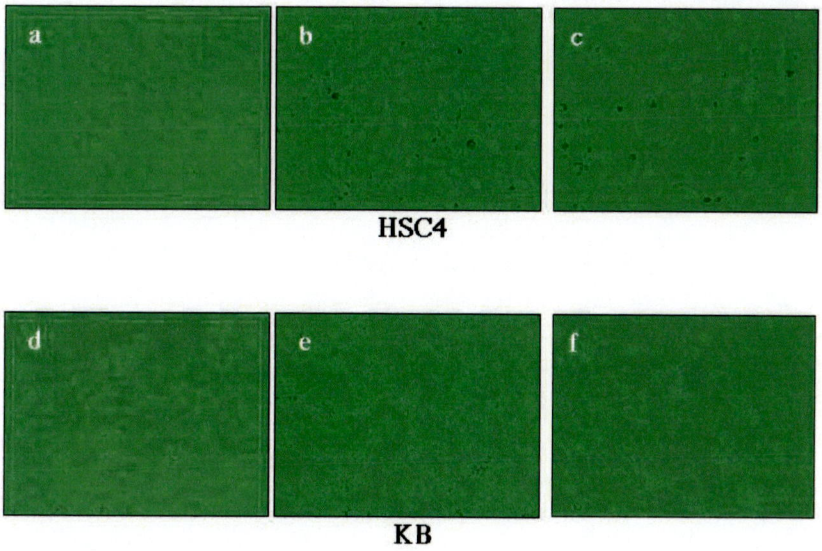

Figure 10. Morphologic changes and cell death induced by TSA. HSC4 and KB cells were treated with varying concentrations of TSA for 24h. Exponentially growing cells were used. (a) HSC4; non-treated, (b) HSC4; TSA treated (500nM), (c) HSC4; TSA treated (800nM), (d) KB; non-treated, (e) KB; TSA treated (500nM), (f) KB; TSA treated (800nM). Reduced cell density was observed in the cultures treated with TSA and dead cells were floating in the medium. HSC4 and KB cells are normally oval or polygonal. Compared with the controls, many TSA-treated cells became enlarged and formed long processes. Original magnification x40.

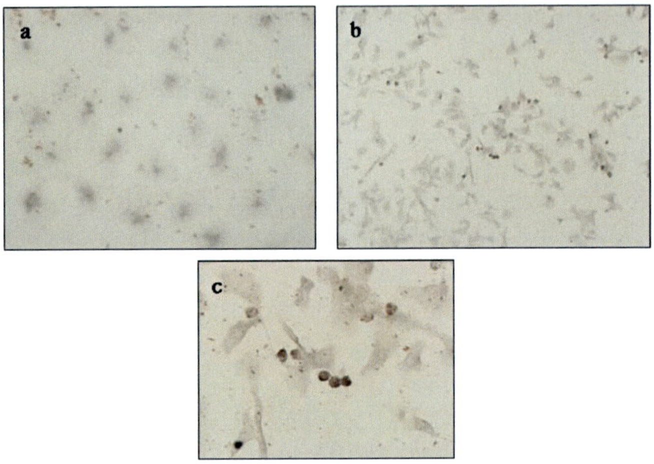

Figure 11. TUNEL detection of apoptosis in HSC4 cells following TSA treatment. TSA-induced apoptosis was assessed by an "Apoptosis *in situ* Detection Kit" using the manufacturer's protocol (Wako Pure Chemical Industries, Ltd. Osaka, Japan). HSC4 cells were cultured in the presence or absence of 800nM of TSA for 24 h. The cells were fixed with 10% formaldehyde and stained with the TUNEL method. (a) non-treated; original magnification x40, (b) TSA treated; original magnification x10, (c) TSA treated; original magnification x40. TUNEL-positive cells appeared after 24 h of culture, indicating that TSA causes apoptosis in HSC4. Apoptotic cells stained dark brown.

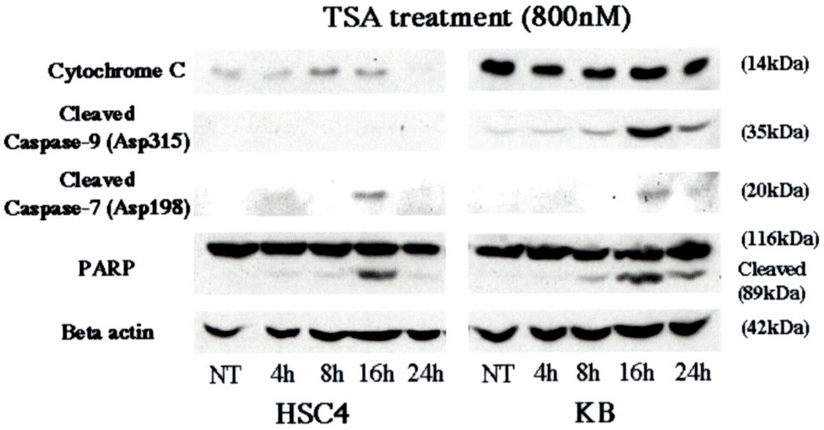

Figure 12. Effect of TSA on the expression level of proteins involved in apoptosis. To confirm the activation of apoptosis by HDAC inhibitors, we carried out western blotting using HSC4 and KB cell lines. Westernblotting was carried out using the following antibodies: anti-cleaved caspase-7, anti-cleaved caspase-9, anti-PARP, anti-cytochrome c (all purchased from Cell Signaling Technology, Beverly, MA). The effectiveness of TSA in activating caspase activity was assessed by analysis of the cleavage of the caspases and PARP. The activation of the mitochondrial apoptotic pathway by TSA was assessed by analysis of the expression level of cytochrome c. The total cell lysates were separated from cells untreated and treated with TSA (800nM) for the indicated time. TSA administration caused cleavage of either PARP or caspase-9. In a time course experiment, the activation of caspases became evident 16 hours after treatment with TSA. The cleaved caspases-7, and -9 appeared in cells after 16 h of culture with TSA, whereas no such changes were detected in the cytochrome c expression. Furthermore, TSA treatment induced proteolytic PARP, which is a caspase-3 substrate, indicating that caspases were really activated in TSA-treated cells. These results indicate that TSA induces apoptosis by facilitating the cleavage of caspases.

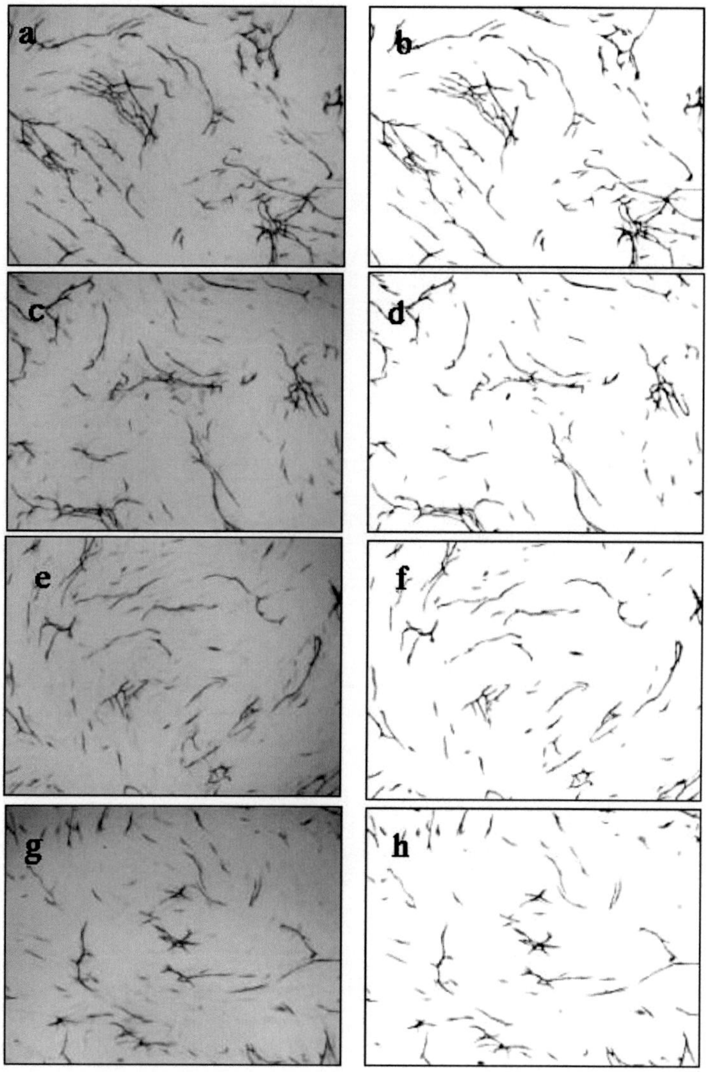

Figure 13. TSA inhibited *in vitro* angiogenesis. To explore the in vitro antiangiogenic activity of TSA, HUVECs were co-cultured with human fibroblasts and incubated for 11 days with 10 ng/mL VEGF with or without various concentrations of TSA. Tubule formation was examined by immunochemical staining with anti-CD31 (PECAM-1) antibody according to the protocol by the manufacturer. Left panel; microscopic pictures of tubules stained with CD31. Right panel; images graphically analyzed by KURABO angiogenesis Image Analyzer Ver.2 (KURABO Inc., Osaka, Japan). (a) non-treated; microscopic picture, (b) non-treated; analyzed image, (c) TSA treated (1.0nM); microscopic picture, (d) TSA treated (1.0nM); analyzed image, (e) TSA treated (10nM); microscopic picture, (f) TSA treated (10nM); analyzed image, (g) TSA treated (100nM); microscopic picture, (h) TSA treated (100nM); analyzed image. TSA treated Day 11 culture of TSA-untreated HUVECs in which VEGF (10ng/ml) was present from day 0, showed increased capillary-like structures. In contrast, the formation of capillary-like structures in the TSA-treated HUVECs was less than that of the TSA-untreated control. Representative micrographs of capillary structures formed by HUVECs. Original magnification, x4.

Next, we investigated the inhibitory effect of an HDAC inhibitor on angiogenesis. A co-culture tubule formation assay was set up (Figure 13). An "angiogenesis assay kit" comprised of co-cultures of human umbilical vein endothelial cells (HUVEC) and human dermal fibroblasts was purchased from KURABO Inc. (Osaka, Japan) and used according to the manufacturer's instructions. Cells were seeded onto 24-well plate and cultivated in the basal medium with 10ng/ml vascular endothelial growth factor (VEGF). Various concentrations of TSA were added to the medium of the HUVEC/fibroblast co-culture. The medium was changed every 3 days, and the HUVECs were cultured in the presence or absence of TSA for 11 days. At the end of the assay, the cells were then fixed with 70% ethanol and incubated with diluted anti-human PECAM-1 (CD31) antibody (Kurabo Inc., Osaka, Japan) for 1 hour followed by a 1-hour incubation with a goat anti-mouse IgG alkaline phosphatase-conjugated secondary antibody. Visualization of the tube-like structures formed by HUVECs was achieved with 5-bromo-4-chloro-3-indolyl phosphate/nitro blue tetrazolium (BCIP/NBT), and tubeule formation was measured. In Figures 13 and 14, the TSA treatment (100nM) reduced tubule formations and inhibited in vitro angiogenesis. Day 11 culture of the TSA-untreated HUVECs, in which VEGF was present from day 0, showed increased capillary-like structures. In contrast, the formation of capillary-like structures in the TSA-treated HUVECs was less than that of the TSA-untreated control.

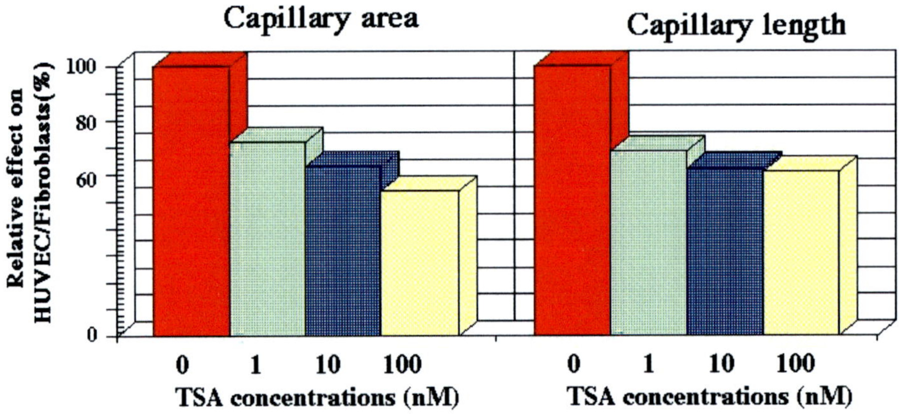

Figure 14. TSA inhibited *in vitro* angiogenesis. As described in Figure13, the microscopic pictures were graphically analyzed, and those results (capillary area and capillary length) were quantified by a KURABO angiogenesis Image Analyzer. The capillary area and length of the capillary-like structures in the TSA-treated HUVECs were less than those of the TSA-untreated control.

Profiling of the HDAC Inhibitors-Related Genes

Recently, array studies have focused on the gene expression profiles of cancer cells treated with HDAC inhibitors. From those reports, interestingly, only a small number of genes were reported to be affected by HDAC inhibitors [13,16,34]. For example, Glaser *et al.* studied the gene profiles of HDAC inhibitors (SAHA, TSA, and MS-27-275)-treated bladder and breast cancer cell lines [35]. Among 6,800 genes tested, they identified a common set of 13 genes modulated by several HDAC inhibitors in various cancer cells. Those genes were regulated positively or negatively. Eight genes were found to be upregulated and 5 genes were found to be downregulated. Suzuki *et al.* reported that TSA upregulated 23 genes in the colorectal cancer cell line RKO among 10,814 genes tested [36].

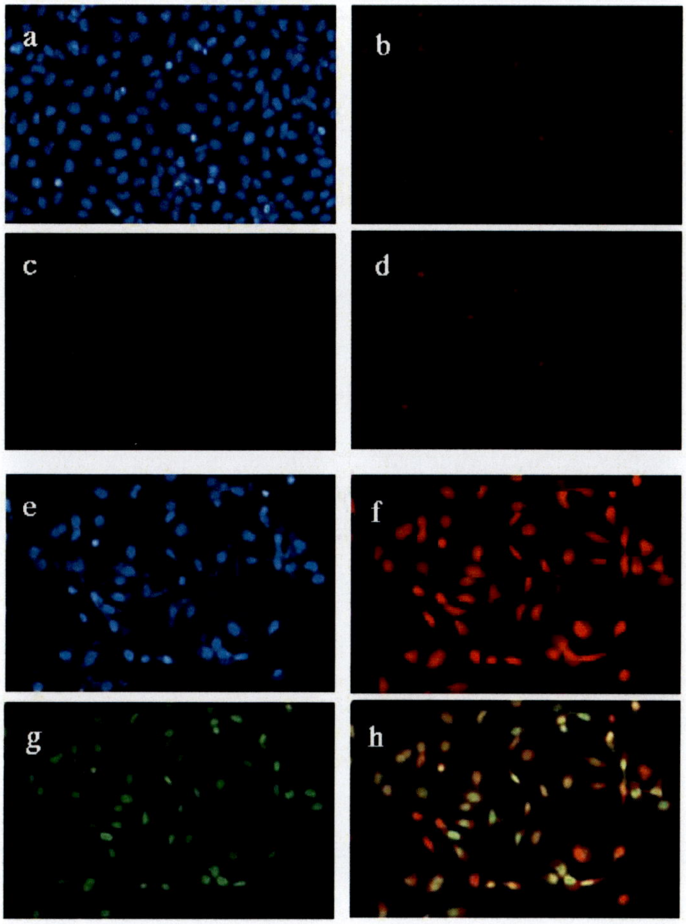

Figure 15. The induction of $p21^{WAF1}$ by HDAC inhibitors might occur via histone acetylation. HSC4 cells were cultured 24h in the absence or the presence of 800nM TSA. After TSA treatment, immunofluorescence microscopy was carried out. Briefly, the cells were fixed with 4% formaldehyde in PBS for 10 min at RT and followed by 70% to 100% ethanol. Non-specific binding was blocked with normal goat and swine serum in PBS for 30 min at RT. The cells were probed with rabbit polyclonal anti-acetyl-histone H3 (Lys9) antibody and mouse monoclonal anti-$p21^{WAF1}$ Ab-3 (DCS-60.2) antibody (NeoMarkers, Fremont, CA, USA) overnight at 4°C. The cells were then washed with PBS three times, followed by incubation with tetramethylrhodamine isomer R (TRITC)-conjugated swine anti-rabbit IgG (Dakocytomation, Denmark) and fluorescein-isothiocyanate isomer 1(FITC)- conjugated goat anti-mouse IgG (Dakocytomation, Denmark) in PBS for 30min. After the cells were washed with PBS three times, the cells were counterstained with 4,6-diamidine-2-phenylindole, dihydrochloride (DAPI) and then mounted with GEL/MOUNT (Biomeda Corp., Foster City, CA, USA). They were then examined with a confocal laser scanning microscope (LSM Pascal; Zeiss, Oberkochen, Germany). The panels show representative data of HSC4 cells in the absence (a, b, c, d) or presence of TSA (e, f, g, h). (a) non-treated; indicating DAPI (blue), (b) non-treated; indicating acetyl-histone H3 (Lys9) (red), (c) non-treated; indicating $p21^{WAF1}$ (green), (d) non-treated; merge of green and red, (e) TSA-treated; indicating DAPI (blue), (f) TSA-treated; indicating acetyl-histone H3 (Lys9) (red), (g) TSA-treated; indicating $p21^{WAF1}$ (green), (h) TSA-treated; merge of green and red. TSA strongly induced the expressions of acetyl-histone H3 (Lys9) (f) and $p21^{WAF1}$ (g). From the merged image (h), the induction of both proteins was observed in the nucleus of the same cell.

Among the HDAC inhibitors-related genes, a number of studies have demonstrated that the cell cycle inhibitor p21^{WAF1} is commonly upregulated in response to HDAC inhibitors [37,38]. Induction of p21^{WAF1} is tightly associated with HDAC inhibitor antiproliferative action via the G_1 cell cycle arrest of many cancer cells. We also confirmed the effect of the HDAC inhibitor on p21^{WAF1} expression (Figure 15). HSC4 cells were treated with TSA and the induction of p21^{WAF1} proteins was detected using immunofluorescence. The panels show representative data of the HSC4 cells treated with or without TSA 800 nM for 24h, indicating DNA (blue), acetyl-histone H3 (Lys9) (red), p21^{WAF1} (green), and a merger of both images. TSA strongly induced the expressions of acetyl-histone H3 (Lys9) (Figure 15f) and p21^{WAF1} (Figure 15g). From the merged image (Figure 15h), the induction of both proteins was observed in the nucleus of the same cell. The induction of p21^{WAF1} by HDAC inhibitors might occur via histone acetylation.

As for apoptosis, the transcriptional modulation of proapoptotic genes by HDAC inhibitors has been suggested to mediate HDAC inhibitors-induced apoptosis. In the HDAC inhibitor-induced upregulation of death receptor-mediated apoptosis, Fas and FasL have been reported in promyelocytic leukemia [39] and in uveal melanoma [40]. Previously, the HDAC inhibitors CBHA, FK228 and MS-275 were reported to increase a proapoptotic BH3-only Bim in gastrointestinal adenocarcinoma MKN45 and DLD-1 cells [41]. In HDAC inhibitor-induced downregulation, the expressions of the anti-apoptotic molecules Bcl-2, Bcl-XL and MCl-1 were inhibited by FK228 [42]. The expression of the FLIP-L protein was also downregulated by FK228 and MS-275 in chronic lymphocytic leukemia cells [43,44].

Synergistic Actions by HDAC Inhibitors

There has been strong interest in HDAC inhibitors due to their synergistic activities in combination with other existing cancer treatments such as chemotherapy, ionizing radiation therapy and gene therapy. The synergistic activities of HDAC inhibitors have been reported with other anticancer agents, including retinoic acids [45], vitamin D analogues [46], and peroxisome proliferator-activated receptor ligands [47]. When combined with radiation therapy, the radiation-sensitizing effects of HDAC inhibitors have been reported. Arundel *et al.* and others reported that butyrate enhanced radiation injury in human colon tumor cells and increased the radiation sensitivity of V79 Chinese hamster lung fibroblasts [48,49]. When combined with gene therapy, the addition of HDAC inhibitors after adenovirus infection increased viral protein and transgene expression [50,51]. Lee *et al.* has reported that the addition of sodium butyrate increased the transduction of adenovirus [52].

FK228: a Promising new HDAC Inhibitor

FK228 (formally called FR901228) is a bi-cyclic depsipeptide isolated from the fermentation broth of *Chromobacterium violaceum* [53] and inhibits HDAC activity at nanomolar concentrations [54]. Among HDAC inhibitors, FK228 is an especially promising new anticancer agent, because this agent is reported to be effective *in vitro* and *in vivo* against various malignancies including breast cancer [55], B-cell chronic lymphocytic leukemia [56], and malignant lymphoid cells [57]. FK228 is currently being evaluated in phase I/II clinical trials with solid and hematologic malignancies [18,20]. Phase I clinical trials have revealed that FK228 can be safely administered for advanced cancer as well as leukemia without any life-threatening toxicities or cardiac toxicities [19,58]. Recently, the development of resistance may become a problem with FK228 therapy in a clinical setting. The National Cancer Institute Drug Screen database indicated that FK228 is a substrate for multidrug resistance protein (MDR1, P-glycoprotein, ABCB1) [59]. Previous studies have demonstrated that P-glycoprotein (P-gp)-expressing cancer cells are more resistant to the anticancer activities of FK228 [33,59-61]. Furthermore, the P-gp system is highly susceptible to be the predominant mechanism of FK228 resistance in cancer cells [23,33,62,63]. It has been demonstrated that continued exposure to FK228 results in the induction of P-gp and that FK228 is removed from cancer cells by P-gp [23,33,59,62,63]. It was assumed that FK228 might upregulate its own drug resistance.

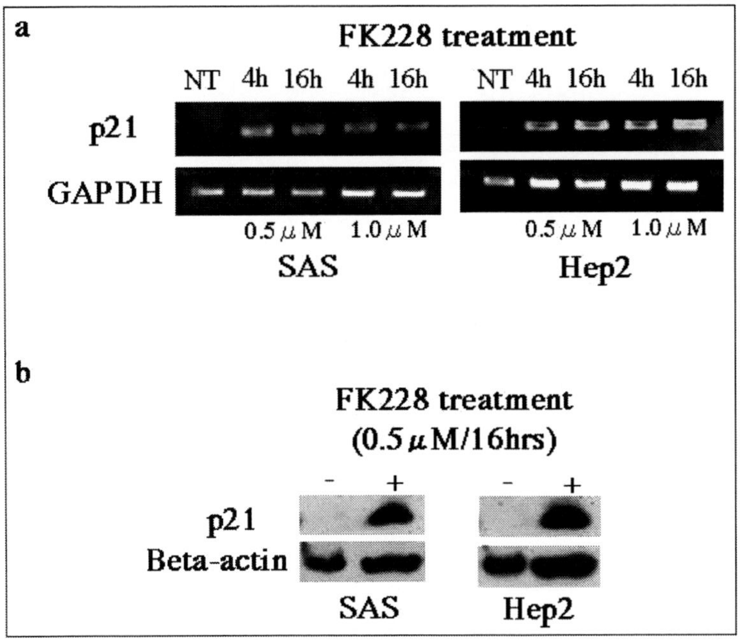

Figure 16. FK228 is a potent inducer of $p21^{WAF1}$ expression in oral cancer cells. SAS and Hep2 cells were treated with FK228 for up to 16 hours. The samples were collected at indicated time points; and assessed by RT-PCR and western blotting. (a) Reverse transcription-PCR analysis for $p21^{WAF1}$ mRNA. Amplification of cDNAs was performed under the following PCR conditions: 7 min at 94°C for 1 cycle; then repeated cycles at 94°C for 30 s, 59°C for 30 s, 72°C for 30 s; and a final elongation step at 72°C for 10 min. The primers used for the amplification were as follows: $p21^{WAF1}$; sense: 5'-CCTCTTCGGCCCGGTGGAC -3', antisense: 5'-CCGTTTTCGACCCTGAGAG -3'. The amplified *GAPDH* fragment was used as a positive control. (b) Western blot analysis for $p21^{WAF1}$ protein. The cells were cultured either continuously in medium containing FK228 or in FK228-free medium for 16h. Whole cell lysates were prepared and subjected to immunoblot analysis with mouse monoclonal antibody $p21^{WAF1}$. Representative results. Each of the blots shown was demonstrated to have equal protein loading by reprobing with the monoclonal antibody for beta-actin. The amounts of $p21^{WAF1}$ readily increased in the cells after 16h of culture with FK228.

To find out whether FK228 upregulates its own existence, we examined the effect of FK228 in oral cancer cell lines. Because the precise mechanism underlying its apoptotic activity has not been fully understood, we have been attempting to identify a novel FK228-related target and pathway [64,65]. In 2004, we reported the regulatory effects of FK228 on the transcription of the *maspin* gene, whose expression has been implicated in apoptosis pathways as another possible candidate gene, in favor of its epigenetic regulation through a process such as histone acetylation in oral cancer cells [64]. *Maspin* expression was induced after 4-16 h of treatment with FK228 in the maspin downregulated cell lines, while the *maspin* transcriptional levels were not altered after treatment with FK228 in the *maspin*-expressed cell lines. In 2005, we analyzed the epigenetic effects of FK228 on *hTERT* transcription in oral cancer cell lines [65]. The mRNA expression of *hTERT* was upregulated after exposure to FK228 in *hTERT*-negative Hep2 cells, and even in SAS and KB cells expressing high levels of *hTERT*. This induction of *hTERT* by FK228 requires de novo protein synthesis to some extent and is more likely a direct than an indirect effect on epigenetic changes such as histone acetylation/deacetylation. In this study, similar to other HDAC inhibitors, we demonstrated by RT-PCR and western blotting that FK228 is a potent inducer of $p21^{WAF1}$ expression in oral cancer cells (SAS, Hep2) (Figures 16). Cells were cultured either continuously in medium containing FK228 or in FK228-free medium for up to 16h. Western blotting and RT-PCR experiments revealed that FK228 mediated an increased $p21^{WAF1}$ not only at mRNA levels, but also at the protein level in cells 16h after the onset of drug exposure.

REFERENCES

[1] Cress WD, Seto E. Histone deacetylases, transcriptional control and cancer. (2000) *J Cell Physiol. 184(1)*:1-16.

[2] Lund AH, van Lohuizen M. Epigenetics and cancer. (2004) *Genes Dev. 18(19)*:2315-2335.

[3] Bjorklund S, Almouzni G, Davidson I, Nightingale K, Weiss K. Global transcription regulators of eukaryotes. (1999) *Cell. 96(6)*:759-767.

[4] Jenuwein T, Allis CD. Translating the histone code. (2001) *Science. 293*(5532): 1074-1080.

[5] Schubeler D, MacAlpine DM, Scalzo D, Wirbelauer C, Kooperberg C, van Leeuwen F, Gottschling DE, O'Neill LP, Turner BM, Delrow J, Bell SP, Groudine M. The histone modification pattern of active genes revealed through genome-wide chromatin analysis of a higher eukaryote. (2004) *Genes Dev. 18(11)*: 1263-1271.

[6] Kurdistani SK, Tavazoie S, Grunstein M. Mapping global histone acetylation patterns to gene expression. (2004) *Cell. 117(6)*:721-733.

[7] Nakayama J, Rice JC, Strahl BD, Allis CD, Grewal SI. Role of histone H3 lysine 9 methylation in epigenetic control of heterochromatin assembly. (2001) *Science. 292*(5514): 110-113.

[8] Zhu WG, Lakshmanan RR, Beal MD, Otterson GA. DNA methyltransferase inhibition enhances apoptosis induced by histone deacetylase inhibitors. (2001) *Cancer Res. 61(4)*: 1327-1333.

[9] Khochbin S, Verdel A, Lemercier C, Seigneurin-Berny D. Functional significance of histone deacetylase diversity. (2001) *Curr Opin Genet Dev. 11(2)*: 162-166.

[10] Vigushin DM, Coombes RC. Histone deacetylase inhibitors in cancer treatment. (2002) *Anticancer Drugs. 13(1)*: 1-13.

[11] Piekarz R, Bates S. A review of depsipeptide and other histone deacetylase inhibitors in clinical trials. (2004) *Curr Pharm Des. 10(19)*:2289-2298.

[12] Marks PA, Richon VM, Breslow R, Rifkind RA. Histone deacetylase inhibitors as new cancer drugs. (2001) *Curr Opin Oncol. 13(6)*:477-483.

[13] Munster PN, Troso-Sandoval T, Rosen N, Rifkind R, Marks PA, Richon VM. The histone deacetylase inhibitor suberoylanilide hydroxamic acid induces differentiation of human breast cancer cells. (2001) *Cancer Res. 61(23)*:8492-8497.

[14] Lee BI, Park SH, Kim JW, Sausville EA, Kim HT, Nakanishi O, Trepel JB, Kim SJ. MS-275, a histone deacetylase inhibitor, selectively induces transforming growth factor beta type II receptor expression in human breast cancer cells. (2001) *Cancer Res. 61(3)*:931-934

[15] Kelly WK, O'Connor OA, Krug LM, Chiao JH, Heaney M, Curley T, MacGregore-Cortelli B, Tong W, Secrist JP, Schwartz L, Richardson S, Chu E, Olgac S, Marks PA, Scher H, Richon VM. Phase I study of an oral histone deacetylase inhibitor, suberoylanilide hydroxamic acid, in patients with advanced cancer. (2005) *J Clin Oncol. 23(17)*:3923-3931.

[16] Ryan QC, Headlee D, Acharya M, Sparreboom A, Trepel JB, Ye J, Figg WD, Hwang K, Chung EJ, Murgo A, Melillo G, Elsayed Y, Monga M, Kalnitskiy M, Zwiebel J, Sausville EA. Phase I and pharmacokinetic study of MS-275, a histone deacetylase inhibitor, in patients with advanced and refractory solid tumors or lymphoma. (2005) *J Clin Oncol. 23(17)*:3912-3922.

[17] Carducci MA, Gilbert J, Bowling MK, Noe D, Eisenberger MA, Sinibaldi V, Zabelina Y, Chen TL, Grochow LB, Donehower RC. A phase I clinical and pharmacological evaluation of sodium phenylbutyrate on an 120-h infusion schedule. (2001) *Clin Cancer Res. 7(10)*:3047-3055.

[18] Sandor V, Bakke S, Robey RW, Kang MH, Blagosklonny MV, Bender J, Brooks R, Piekarz RL, Tucker E, Figg WD, Chan KK, Goldspiel B, Fojo AT, Balcerzak SP, Bates SE. Phase I trial of the histone deacetylase inhibitor, depsipeptide (FR901228, NSC 630176), in patients with refractory neoplasms. (2002) *Clin Cancer Res. 8(3)*:718-728.

[19] Byrd JC, Marcucci G, Parthun MR, Xiao JJ, Klisovic RB, Moran M, Lin TS, Liu S, Sklenar AR, Davis ME, Lucas DM, Fischer B, Shank R, Tejaswi SL, Binkley P, Wright J, Chan KK, Grever MR. A phase 1 and pharmacodynamic study of depsipeptide (FK228) in chronic lymphocytic leukemia and acute myeloid leukemia. (2005) *Blood. 105(3)*:959-967.

[20] Piekarz RL, Robey R, Sandor V, Bakke S, Wilson WH, Dahmoush L, Kingma DM, Turner ML, Altemus R, Bates SE. Inhibitor of histone deacetylation, depsipeptide

(FR901228), in the treatment of peripheral and cutaneous T-cell lymphoma: a case report. (2001) *Blood. 98(9)*:2865-2868.

[21] Dokmanovic M, Marks PA. Prospects: histone deacetylase inhibitors. (2005) *J Cell Biochem. 96(2)*:293-304.

[22] Furumai R, Matsuyama A, Kobashi N, Lee KH, Nishiyama M, Nakajima H, Tanaka A, Komatsu Y, Nishino N, Yoshida M, Horinouchi S. FK228 (depsipeptide) as a natural prodrug that inhibits class I histone deacetylases. (2002) *Cancer Res. 62(17)*: 4916-4921.

[23] Piekarz RL, Robey RW, Zhan Z, Kayastha G, Sayah A, Abdeldaim AH, Torrico S, Bates SE. T-cell lymphoma as a model for the use of histone deacetylase inhibitors in cancer therapy: impact of depsipeptide on molecular markers, therapeutic targets, and mechanisms of resistance. (2004) *Blood. 103(12)*: 4636-4643.

[24] Marks PA, Richon VM, Miller T, Kelly WK. Histone deacetylase inhibitors. (2004) *Adv Cancer Res. 91*: 137-168.

[25] Villar-Garea A, Esteller M. Histone deacetylase inhibitors: understanding a new wave of anticancer agents. (2004) *Int J Cancer. 112(2)*: 171-178.

[26] Qiu L, Burgess A, Fairlie DP, Leonard H, Parsons PG, Gabrielli BG. Histone deacetylase inhibitors trigger a G2 checkpoint in normal cells that is defective in tumor cells. (2000) *Mol Biol Cell. 11(6)*: 2069-2083.

[27] Kim MS, Kwon HJ, Lee YM, Baek JH, Jang JE, Lee SW, Moon EJ, Kim HS, Lee SK, Chung HY, Kim CW, Kim KW. Histone deacetylases induce angiogenesis by negative regulation of tumor suppressor genes. (2001) *Nat Med. 7(4)*: 437-443.

[28] Bernhard D, Ausserlechner MJ, Tonko M, Loffler M, Hartmann BL, Csordas A, Kofler R. Apoptosis induced by the histone deacetylase inhibitor sodium butyrate in human leukemic lymphoblasts. (1999) *FASEB J. 13(14)*: 1991-2001.

[29] Yoshida M, Horinouchi S. Trichostatin and leptomycin. Inhibition of histone deacetylation and signal-dependent nuclear export. (1999) *Ann NY Acad Sci. 886*: 23-36.

[30] Marks PA, Richon VM, Rifkind RA. Histone deacetylase inhibitors: inducers of differentiation or apoptosis of transformed cells. (2000) *J Natl Cancer Inst. 92(15)*: 1210-1216.

[31] Nervi C, Borello U, Fazi F, Buffa V, Pelicci PG, Cossu G. Inhibition of histone deacetylase activity by trichostatin A modulates gene expression during mouse embryogenesis without apparent toxicity. (2001) *Cancer Res. 61(4)*: 1247-1249.

[32] Goldsmith ME, Kitazono M, Fok P, Aikou T, Bates S, Fojo T. The histone deacetylase inhibitor FK228 preferentially enhances adenovirus transgene expression in malignant cells. (2003) *Clin Cancer Res. 9(14)*: 5394-5401.

[33] Peart MJ, Tainton KM, Ruefli AA, Dear AE, Sedelies KA, O'Reilly LA, Waterhouse NJ, Trapani JA, Johnstone RW. Novel mechanisms of apoptosis induced by histone deacetylase inhibitors. (2003) *Cancer Res. 63(15)*: 4460-4471.

[34] Marks P, Rifkind RA, Richon VM, Breslow R, Miller T, Kelly WK. Histone deacetylases and cancer: causes and therapies. (2001) *Nat Rev Cancer. 1(3)*:194-202.

[35] Glaser KB, Staver MJ, Waring JF, Stender J, Ulrich RG, Davidsen SK. Gene expression profiling of multiple histone deacetylase (HDAC) inhibitors: Defining a

common set produced by HDAC inhibition in T24 and MDA carcinoma cell lines. (2003) *Mol Cancer Ther. 2(2)*: 151-163.

[36] Suzuki H, Gabrielson E, Chen W, Anbazhagan R, van Engeland M, Weijenberg MP, Herman JG, Baylin SB. A genomic screen for genes upregulated by demethylation and histone deacetylase inhibition in human colorectal cancer. (2002) *Nat Genet. 31(2)*: 141-149.

[37] Archer SY, Meng S, Shei A, Hodin RA. p21WAF1 is required for butyrate-mediated growth inhibition of human colon cancer cells. (1998) *Proc Natl Acad Sci USA. 95(12)*: 6791-6796.

[38] Richon VM, Sandhoff TW, Rifkind RA, Marks PA. Histone deacetylase inhibitor selectively induces p21WAF1 expression and gene-associated histone acetylation. (2000) *Proc Natl Acad Sci USA. 97(18)*: 10014-10019.

[39] Kwon SH, Ahn SH, Kim YK, Bae GU, Yoon JW, Hong S, Lee HY, Lee YW, Lee HW, Han JW. Apicidin, a histone deacetylase inhibitor, induces apoptosis and Fas/Fas ligand expression in human acute promyelocytic leukemia cells. (2002) *J Biol Chem. 277(3)*: 2073-2080.

[40] Klisovic DD, Katz SE, Effron D, Klisovic MI, Wickham J, Parthun MR, Guimond M, Marcucci G. Depsipeptide (FR901228) inhibits proliferation and induces apoptosis in primary and metastatic human uveal melanoma cell lines. (2003) *Invest Ophthalmol Vis Sci. 44(6)*: 2390-2398.

[41] Zhang Y, Adachi M, Zhao X, Kawamura R, Imai K. Histone deacetylase inhibitors FK228, *N*-(2-aminophenyl)-4-[*N*-(pyridin-3-yl- methoxycarbonyl) amino- methyl] benzamide and m-carboxycinnamic acid bis-hydroxamide augment radiation-induced cell death in gastrointestinal adenocarcinoma cells. (2004) *Int J Cancer. 110(2)*: 301-308.

[42] Khan SB, Maududi T, Barton K, Ayers J, Alkan S. Analysis of histone deacetylase inhibitor, depsipeptide (FR901228), effect on multiple myeloma. (2004) *Br J Haematol. 125(2)*: 156-161.

[43] Aron JL, Parthun MR, Marcucci G, Kitada S, Mone AP, Davis ME, Shen T, Murphy T, Wickham J, Kanakry C, Lucas DM, Reed JC, Grever MR, Byrd JC. Depsipeptide (FR901228) induces histone acetylation and inhibition of histone deacetylase in chronic lymphocytic leukemia cells concurrent with activation of caspase 8-mediated apoptosis and down-regulation of c-FLIP protein. (2003) *Blood. 102(2)*: 652-658.

[44] Lucas DM, Davis ME, Parthun MR, Mone AP, Kitada S, Cunningham KD, Flax EL, Wickham J, Reed JC, Byrd JC, Grever MR. The histone deacetylase inhibitor MS-275 induces caspase-dependent apoptosis in B-cell chronic lymphocytic leukemia cells. (2004) *Leukemia. 18(7)*: 1207-1214.

[45] Kitamura K, Hoshi S, Koike M, Kiyoi H, Saito H, Naoe T. Histone deacetylase inhibitor but not arsenic trioxide differentiates acute promyelocytic leukaemia cells with t(11;17) in combination with all-*trans* retinoic acid. (2000) *Br J Haematol. 108(4)*: 696-702.

[46] Rashid SF, Moore JS, Walker E, Driver PM, Engel J, Edwards CE, Brown G, Uskokovic MR, Campbell MJ. Synergistic growth inhibition of prostate cancer cells

by 1,25 dihydroxyvitamin D3 and its 19-nor-hexafluoride analogs in combination with either sodium butyrate or trichostatin A. (2001) *Oncogene. 20(15)*: 1860-1872.

[47] Chang TH, Szabo E. Enhanced growth inhibition by combination differentiation therapy with ligands of peroxisome proliferator-activated receptor- and inhibitors of histone deacetylase in adenocarcinoma of the lung. (2002) *Clin Cancer Res. 8(4)*: 1206-1212.

[48] Arundel CM, Glicksman AS, Leith JT. Enhancement of radiation injury in human colon tumor cells by the maturational agent sodium butyrate (NaB). (1985) *Radiat Res. 104(3)*:443-448.

[49] Heussen C, Nackerdien Z, Smit BJ, Bohm L. Irradiation damage in chromatin isolated from V-79 Chinese hamster lung fibroblasts. (1987) *Radiat Res. 110(1)*:84-94.

[50] Dion LD, Goldsmith KT, Tang DC, Engler JA, Yoshida M, Garver RI Jr. Amplification of recombinant adenoviral transgene products occurs by inhibition of histone deacetylase. (1997) *Virology. 231(2)*: 201-209.

[51] Gaetano C, Catalano A, Palumbo R, Illi B, Orlando G, Ventoruzzo G, Serino F, Capogrossi MC. Transcriptionally active drugs improve adenovirus vector performance in vitro and in vivo. (2000) *Gene Ther. 7(19)*: 1624-1630.

[52] Lee CT, Seol JY, Park KH, Yoo CG, Kim YW, Ahn C, Song YW, Han SK, Han JS, Kim S, Lee JS, Shim YS. Differential effects of adenovirus-p16 on bladder cancer cell lines can be overcome by the addition of butyrate. (2001) *Clin Cancer Res. 7(1)*: 210-214.

[53] Ueda H, Nakajima H, Hori Y, Goto T, Okuhara M. Action of FR901228, a novel antitumor bicyclic depsipeptide produced by Chromobacterium violaceum no. 968, on Ha-ras transformed NIH3T3 cells. (1994) *Biosci Biotechnol Biochem. 58(9)*:1579-1583.

[54] de Ruijter AJ, van Gennip AH, Caron HN, Kemp S, van Kuilenburg AB. Histone deacetylases (HDACs): Characterization of the classical HDAC family. (2003) *Biochem J. 370(3)*:737-749.

[55] Rajgolikar G, Chan KK, Wang HC. Effects of a novel antitumor depsipeptide, FR901228, on human breast cancer cells. (1998) *Breast Cancer Res Treat. 51(1)*:29-38.

[56] Byrd JC, Shinn C, Ravi R, Willis CR, Waselenko JK, Flinn IW, Dawson NA, Grever MR. Depsipeptide (FR901228): a novel therapeutic agent with selective, in vitro activity against human B-cell chronic lymphocytic leukemia cells. (1999) *Blood. 94(4)*:1401-1408.

[57] Murata M, Towatari M, Kosugi H, Tanimoto M, Ueda R, Saito H, Naoe T. Apoptotic cytotoxic effects of a histone deacetylase inhibitor, FK228, on malignant lymphoid cells. (2000) *Jpn J Cancer Res. 91(11)*:1154-1160.

[58] Marshall JL, Rizvi N, Kauh J, Dahut W, Figuera M, Kang MH, Figg WD, Wainer I, Chaissang C, Li MZ, Hawkins MJ. A phase I trial of depsipeptide (FR901228) in patients with advanced cancer. (2002) *J Exp Ther Oncol. 2(6)*: 325-332.

[59] Scala S, Akhmed N, Rao US, Paull K, Lan LB, Dickstein B, Lee JS, Elgemeie GH, Stein WD, Bates SE. P-Glycoprotein substrates and antagonists cluster into two distinct groups. (1997) *Mol Pharmacol. 51(6)*: 1024-1033.

[60] Ueda H, Manda T, Matsumoto S, Mukumoto S, Nishigaki F, Kawamura I, Shimomura K. FR901228, a novel antitumor bicyclic depsipeptide produced by Chromobacterium violaceum No. 968. III. Antitumor activities on experimental tumors in mice. (1994) *J Antibiot. 47(3)*: 315-323.

[61] Lee JS, Paull K, Alvarez M, Hose C, Monks A, Grever M, Fojo AT, Bates SE. Rhodamine efflux patterns predict P-glycoprotein substrates in the National Cancer Institute drug screen. (1994) *Mol Pharmacol. 46(4)*: 627-638.

[62] Xiao JJ, Huang Y, Dai Z, Sadee W, Chen J, Liu S, Marcucci G, Byrd J, Covey JM, Wright J, Grever M, Chan KK. Chemoresistance to depsipeptide FK228 [(*E*)-(1*S*,4*S*,10*S*,21*R*)-7-[(*Z*)-Ethylidene]- 4,21-diisopropyl-2-oxa-12,13-dithia-5,8,20,23-tetraazabicyclo[8,7,6]-tricos-16-ene-3,6,9,22-pentanone] is mediated by reversible MDR1 induction in human cancer cell lines. (2005) *J Pharmacol Exp Ther. 314(1)*:467-475.

[63] Xiao JJ, Foraker AB, Swaan PW, Liu S, Huang Y, Dai Z, Chen J, Sadee W, Byrd J, Marcucci G, Chan KK. Efflux of depsipeptide FK228 (FR901228, NSC-630176) is mediated by P-glycoprotein and multidrug resistance-associated protein 1. (2005) *J Pharmacol Exp Ther. 313(1)*:268-276.

[64] Murakami J, Asaumi J, Maki Y, Tsujigiwa H, Kuroda M, Nagai N, Yanagi Y, Inoue T, Kawasaki S, Tanaka N, Matsubara N, Kishi K. Effects of demethylating agent 5-aza-2(')-deoxycytidine and histone deacetylase inhibitor FR901228 on maspin gene expression in oral cancer cell lines. (2004) *Oral Oncol. 40(6):*597-603.

[65] Murakami J, Asaumi J, Kawai N, Tsujigiwa H, Yanagi Y, Nagatsuka H, Inoue T, Kokeguchi S, Kawasaki S, Kuroda M, Tanaka N, Matsubara N, Kishi K. Effects of histone deacetylase inhibitor FR901228 on the expression level of telomerase reverse transcriptase in oral cancer. (2005) *Cancer Chemother Pharmacol. 56(1)*:22-28.

4. Future Target for Cancer Therapies: Cancer Stem Cells

Most cancers are comprised of a heterogenous population of cells with respect to proliferation and differentiation. A great deal of cancer research is still focused on the molecular and cellular analysis of the bulk tumor mass. Within the past decade, there is increasing evidence that a rare population of undifferentiated cells drives the formation and growth of tumors [1-3]. In solid tumors, it has been demonstrated that only a minority of cancer cells have the capacity to form colonies in an *in vitro* clonogenic assay [4-8]. Those cells have been referred to as cancer stem cells, tumorigenic cells, or cancer-initiating cells, because they consistently formed tumors, whereas other cancer cell populations were depleted of cells capable of tumor formation. Although cancer stem cells represent a small fraction of cancer cells, those cells have the ability to self-renew, giving rise to another malignant stem cell as well as undergoing differentiation to give rise to the phenotypically diverse non-tumorigenic cancer cells. The existence of cancer stem cells has been established in malignancies such as leukemia [1,9,10], multiple myeloma [11], breast cancer [12], brain [3,13-16] and colon cancer [17,18]. However, a cancer stem cell has not been identified for oral cancer. As in other cancer types, cancer stem cells seem to be the target of oncogenic transformation in oral cancer. Thus, this cancer stem cell model may establish a new cellular target for more effective cancer therapies.

Cancer Stem (Cancer Initiating) Cells in Breast Cancer

Al-Hajj *et al.* prospectively identified and isolated the tumorigenic (cancer initiating) human breast cancer cells as the $CD44^{+}CD24^{-/lowLineage-}$ phenotype [12]. This tumorigenic subpopulation was only a small subset of cells within human breast cancer, but as few as 100 cells with this phenotype were able to proliferate and form new tumors after transplantation into NOD/SCID mice. The tumorigenic subpopulation could be serially passaged: each time cell within this population generated new tumors containing additional $CD44^{+}CD24^{-/lowLineage-}$ tumorigenic cells as well as the phenotypically diverse mixed populations of nontumorigenic cells present in the initial tumor.

Cancer Stem (Cancer Initiating) Cells in Colon Cancer

O'Brien *et al.* have identified and characterized colon cancer initiating cells on the basis of their ability to initiate human colon cancer after transplantation into NOD/SCID mice [17]. Purification experiments established that all cancer initiating cells were CD133+; the CD133- cells that comprised the majority of the tumor were unable to initiate tumor growth. Those cancer initiating cells were able to maintain themselves as well as differentiate and re-establish tumor heterogeneity upon serial transplantation. Ricci-Vitiani *et al.* also reported that subcutaneous injection of colon cancer CD133+ cells readily reproduced the original tumor in SCID mice, whereas CD133- cells did not form tumors [18]. CD133+ colon cancer cells were serially transplanted for several generations, in each of which we observed progressively faster tumor growth without significant phenotypic alterations. *In vitro,* CD133+ colon cancer cells grew exponentially for more than one year as undifferentiated tumor spheres in serum-free medium, maintaining the ability to reproduce the same phenotypic pattern of the original tumor.

Cancer Stem (Cancer Initiating) Cells in Brain Cancer

In brain cancer, Singh *et al* identified human brain cancer initiating cells that initiate tumors *in vitro* and *in vivo* [3,19]. The brain cancer initiating cells were also exclusively isolated with the cell fraction expressing the neural stem cell surface marker CD133. In a xenograft model, only the CD133+ brain tumor fraction contains cells that are capable of tumor initiation in NOD-SCID mouse brains. The injection of as few as 100 CD133+ cells produced a tumor that could be serially transplanted and was a phenocopy of the patient's original tumor, whereas the injection of 10^5 CD133- cells engrafted but did not cause a tumor [3]. Recent studies imply that cancer stem cells contribute to therapeutic responses in brain cancers. Interestingly, Hirschmann-Jax *et al.* also reported that cancer stem cells were detected as a subpopulation in brain tumors [20]. The subpopulation was capable of sustained expansion *ex vivo* and showed evidence for asymmetric division, generating both subpopulation and non- subpopulation progeny. The cells in the subpopulation also expressed high levels of *ABCG2* and *ABCA3* transporter genes and had a greater capacity to expel cytotoxic drugs, such as mitoxantrone, resulting in better survival. This suggested that cancer stem cells tend to be highly resistant to chemotherapeutic agents that should be targeted during the treatment of malignant disease. Bao *et al.* reported that CD133+ cancer stem cells contribute to glioma radioresistance through preferential checkpoint response and DNA repair after radiation in glioblastoma [21]. From their results, CD133+ glioma cells survive ionizing radiation in increased proportions relative to most CD133- cells in the immunocompromised mice-xenograft model and *in vitro* model. CD133+ glioma cells preferentially activate the DNA damage checkpoint in response to radiation, and repair radiation-induced DNA damage more effectively than CD133- tumor cells. Recently, Piccirillo *et al.* reported that BMP4 triggers a significant reduction in the stem-like, cancer initiating cells of human glioblastomas [22]. Their findings suggested that the BMP–BMPR signaling system might act as a key inhibitory regulator of stem-like, cancer initiating cells from glioblastomas and as a novel therapeutic effector.

CD133: A Candidate as a Cancer Stem Cell-Marker?

These tumorigenic, or cancer initiating cells have been identified and enriched on the basis of their expression of markers that distinguish these cells from other nontumorigenic cells. The expression of CD133 has been proposed as one of the candidates for cancer stem cell-markers. CD133 is a 120-kDa five-transmembrane-domain glycoprotein expressed on normal primitive haematopoietic, endothelial, neural and epithelial cells [23-25]. CD133 originally was identified in mouse neuroepithelium and was termed *prominin* [26]. This antigen is expressed at the microvilli of various epithelial cells and is enriched in plasma membrane protrusions of nonepithelial cells. Notably, CD133+ was also detected in some types of tumor tissues, especially in some cancer stem cells within AML, brain tumor, ependymoma and prostate cancer [3,16,19,24,27,28]. The CD133+ cell subpopulation was separated from human brain tumors. For the purification of the cancer stem cells from brain tumors, as a novel approach, cell sorting for CD133 expression was applied using CD133 antibody. Glioma subpopulations expressing CD133 exhibited greater tumorigenic potential and stem cell properties [3,14,19]. However, this has not been explored for oral cancer. Thus, the identification of CD133 expression in oral cancer provides strong support for the cancer stem cell hypothesis as the basis for oral cancer. In the present study, we investigated CD133+ cells in several human oral cancer cell lines. The expression levels of *CD133* mRNA in 5 oral cancer cell lines were examined by RT-PCR. The gels clearly showed that the HSC4, HSC3, HSC2 and HO-1-u-1 cell lines contained only trace amounts of *CD133* mRNA (Figure 17). Interestingly, Ca9-22 cells produced uniformly large amounts of the CD133 mRNA, as indicated by the very dense bands that appear in the relevant lanes. Immunocytochemical staining was also used to detect the expression of CD133 (Figure 18). Only a small proportion of cells in the cell lines expressed CD133. In most instances, these

CD133+ cells were distributed in a scattered pattern. These CD133+ oral cancer cells were an oval or cubical in shape, and were much larger than other cancer cells. The representative features are illustrated in Figure 18. We further examined the expression level of CD133 by immunohistochemical staining within tissue sections of an *in vivo* mouse xenograft (Figure 19). The human oral cancer cell line Hep2 was transplanted in a nude-mouse. Consistent with the results of the *in vitro* study, only a small proportion of cancer cells expressed CD133.

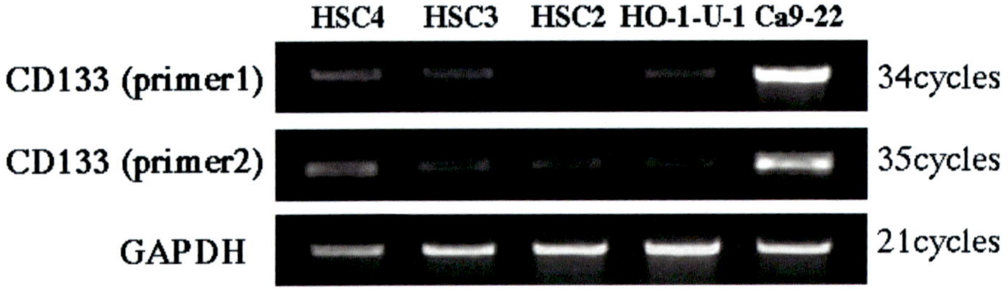

Figure 17. Reverse transcription-PCR analysis for *CD133* mRNA in oral cancer cell lines. Amplification of cDNAs was performed under the following PCR conditions: 7 min at 94°C for 1 cycle; then repeated cycles at 94°C for 30 s, 59°C for 30 s, 72°C for 30 s; and a final elongation step at 72°C for 10 min. The primers used for the amplification were as follows: *CD133* (primer1); sense: 5'-TACCAAGGACAAGGCGTTCAC-3', antisens: 5'-CAGTCGTGGTTTGGCGTTGTA-3'. *CD133* (primer2); sense: 5'-TCTCTATGTGGTACAGCC G-3', antisense: 5'-TGATCCGGGTTCTTACCTG-3'. The amplified *GAPDH* fragment was used as a positive control.

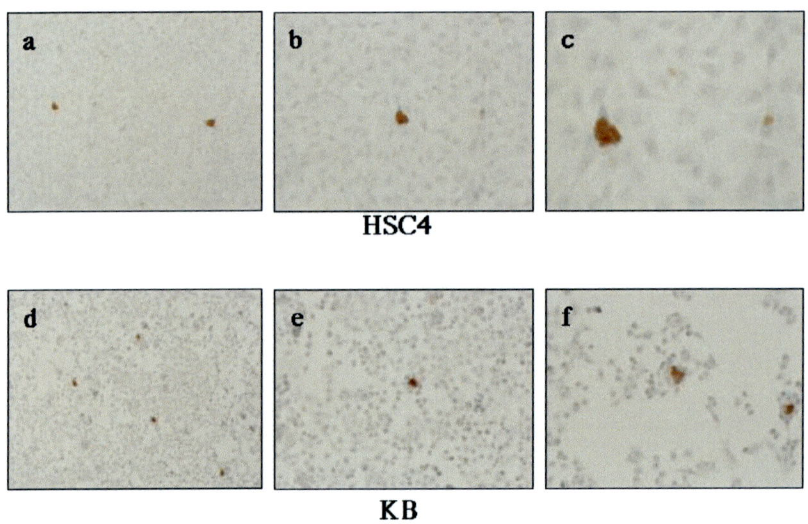

Figure 18. Immunocytochemistry of CD133 in HSC4 and KB cells. The CD133 expressions were monitored with specific antibodies recognizing CD133; CD133/1 (AC133) antibody (Miltenyi Biotec Inc. Auburn CA, USA). The cells were fixed with 10% formaldehyde and processed with the standard avidin-biotin peroxidase complex. DAB was used as chromogen. (a) HSC4; original magnification x10, (b) HSC4; original magnification x20, (c) HSC4; original magnification x40, (d) KB; original magnification x10, (e) KB; original magnification x20, (f) KB; original magnification x40, These CD133+ cells represented an extremely small subpopulation.

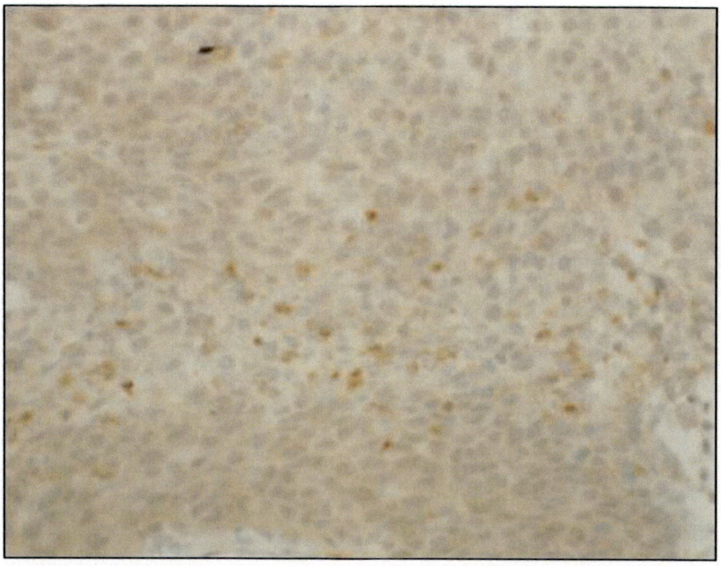

Figure 19. Immunohistochemistry of CD133+ cells within tissue sections of *in vivo* mouse xenograft. Human oral cancer cell line Hep2 was transplanted in a nude-mouse. The tumors were dissected, weighed, and examined immunohistochemically. Original magnification, x40.

Implications for the new Therapies that Target Cancer Stem Cells

A great deal of cancer research is still focused on the identification of therapies that target essential genes critical to the development of cancer. However, the cancer stem cell model has important implications for the way we study and treat cancer. This new model for cancer predicts that therapies that target the cancer stem cells would have a greater chance of success, because only a rare subset of cancer stem cells drives tumor formation (Figure 20). To date, only a few studies have addressed the differential sensitivity to treatment between the tumorigenic and non-tumorigenic populations. In 2007, Zhou *et al.* reported that CD133 cells in human laryngeal tumor, the Hep-2 cell line, possess a marked capacity for self renewal, extensive proliferation, and mutilineal differentiation potency [29]. Our findings might provide some insights into cancer stem cells in oral cancer development. In a forthcoming study, we will attempt to examine the CD133 expression in human primary oral cancer. Furthermore, we will attempt to isolate CD133+ cells from oral cancer and investigate whether these cells play a role in the clonogenicity and tumorigenicity.

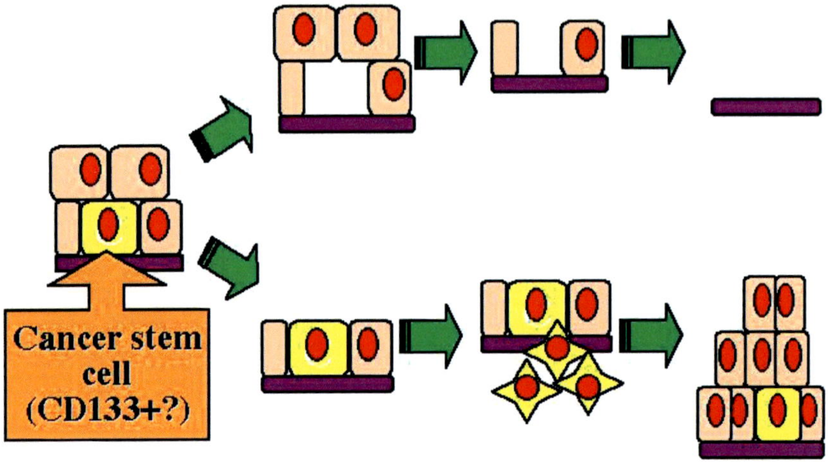

Figure 20. The cancer stem cell theory provides several new insights into strategies for cancer therapy. It has been suggested that novel strategies for successful cancer therapy should focus on the elimination of cancer stem cells, because only a rare subset of cancer stem cells drives tumor formation. We attempted to investigate whether oral cancer cell lines contain a subpopulation of putative stem cells that can be targeted for anti-cancer therapy.

References

[1] Bonnet D, Dick JE. Human acute myeloid leukemia is organized as a hierarchy that originates from a primitive hematopoietic cell. (1997) *Nat Med. 3(7)*: 730-737.

[2] Pardal R, Clarke MF, Morrison SJ. Applying the principles of stem-cell biology to cancer. (2003) *Nat Rev Cancer. 3(12)*: 895-902.

[3] Singh SK, Hawkins C, Clarke ID, Squire JA, Bayani J, Hide T, Henkelman RM, Cusimano MD, Dirks PB. Identification of human brain tumour initiating cells. (2004) *Nature. 432*(7015): 396-401.

[4] Heppner GH. Tumor heterogeneity. (1984) *Cancer Res. 44(6)*:2259-2265.

[5] Hamburger AW, Salmon SE. Primary bioassay of human tumor stem cells. (1977) *Science. 197*(4302): 461-463.

[6] Fialkow PJ. Human tumors studied with genetic markers. (1976) *Birth Defects Orig Artic Ser. 12(1)*: 123-132.

[7] Bergsagel DE, Valeriote FA. Growth characteristics of a mouse plasma cell tumor. (1968) *Cancer Res. 28(11)*: 2187-2196.

[8] Weisenthal L, Lippman ME. Clonogenic and nonclonogenic in vitro chemosensitivity assays. (1985) *Cancer Treat Rep. 69(6)*: 615-632.

[9] Reya T, Morrison SJ, Clarke MF, Weissman IL. Stem cells, cancer, and cancer stem cells. (2001) *Nature. 414*(6859): 105-111.

[10] Lapidot T, Sirard C, Vormoor J, Murdoch B, Hoang T, Caceres-Cortes J, Minden M, Paterson B, Caligiuri MA, Dick JE. A cell initiating human acute myeloid leukaemia after transplantation into SCID mice. (1994) *Nature. 367*(6464): 645-648.

[11] Park CH, Bergsagel DE, McCulloch EA. Mouse myeloma tumour stem cells: a primary cell culture assay. (1971) *J Natl Cancer Inst. 46(2)*: 411-422.

[12] Al-Hajj M, Wicha MS, Benito-Hernandez A, Morrison SJ, Clarke MF. Prospective isolation of tumorigenic breast cancer cells. (2003) *Proc Natl Acad Sci USA. 100(7)*: 3983-3988.

[13] Ignatova TN, Kukekov VG, Laywell ED, Suslov ON, Vrionis FD, Steindler DA. Human cortical glial tumors contain neural stem-like cells expressing astroglial and neuronal markers *in vitro.* (2002) *Glia. 39(3)*: 193-206.

[14] Hemmati HD, Nakano I, Lazareff JA, Masterman-Smith M, Geschwind DH, Bronner-Fraser M, Kornblum HI. Cancerous stem cells can arise from pediatric brain tumors. (2003) *Proc Natl Acad Sci USA. 100(25)*: 15178-15183.

[15] Galli R, Binda E, Orfanelli U, Cipelletti B, Gritti A, De Vitis S, Fiocco R, Foroni C, Dimeco F, Vescovi A. Isolation and characterization of tumorigenic, stem-like neural precursors from human glioblastoma. (2004) *Cancer Res. 64(19):* 7011-7021.

[16] Taylor MD, Poppleton H, Fuller C, Su X, Liu Y, Jensen P, Magdaleno S, Dalton J, Calabrese C, Board J, Macdonald T, Rutka J, Guha A, Gajjar A, Curran T, Gilbertson RJ. Radial glia cells are candidate stem cells of ependymoma. (2005) *Cancer Cell. 8(4)*: 323-335.

[17] O'Brien CA, Pollett A, Gallinger S, Dick JE. A human colon cancer cell capable of initiating tumour growth in immunodeficient mice. (2007) *Nature. 445*(7123): 106-110.

[18] Ricci-Vitiani L, Lombardi DG, Pilozzi E, Biffoni M, Todaro M, Peschle C, De Maria R. Identification and expansion of human colon-cancer-initiating cells. (2007) *Nature. 445*(7123): 111-115.

[19] Singh SK, Clarke ID, Terasaki M, Bonn VE, Hawkins C, Squire J, Dirks PB. Identification of a cancer stem cell in human brain tumors. (2003) *Cancer Res. 63(18)*: 5821-5828.

[20] Hirschmann-Jax C, Foster AE, Wulf GG, Nuchtern JG, Jax TW, Gobel U, Goodell MA, Brenner MK. A distinct "side population" of cells with high drug efflux capacity in human tumor cells. (2004) *Proc Natl Acad Sci U S A. 101(39)*: 14228-14233.

[21] Bao S, Wu Q, McLendon RE, Hao Y, Shi Q, Hjelmeland AB, Dewhirst MW, Bigner DD, Rich JN. Glioma stem cells promote radioresistance by preferential activation of the DNA damage response. (2006) *Nature. 444*(7120): 756-760.

[22] Piccirillo SG, Reynolds BA, Zanetti N, Lamorte G, Binda E, Broggi G, Brem H, Olivi A, Dimeco F, Vescovi AL. Bone morphogenetic proteins inhibit the tumorigenic potential of human brain tumour-initiating cells. (2006) *Nature. 444*(7120): 761-765.

[23] Uchida N, Buck DW, He D, Reitsma MJ, Masek M, Phan TV, Tsukamoto AS, Gage FH, Weissman IL. Direct isolation of human central nervous system stem cells. (2000) *Proc Natl Acad Sci USA. 97(26)*: 14720-14725.

[24] Yin AH, Miraglia S, Zanjani ED, Almeida-Porada G, Ogawa M, Leary AG, Olweus J, Kearney J, Buck DW. AC133, a novel marker for human hematopoietic stem and progenitor cells. (1997) *Blood. 90(12)*: 5002-5012.

[25] Salven P, Mustjoki S, Alitalo R, Alitalo K, Rafii S. VEGFR-3 and CD133 identify a population of CD34+ lymphatic/vascular endothelial precursor cells. (2003) *Blood. 101(1)*: 168-172.

[26] Weigmann A, Corbeil D, Hellwig A, Huttner WB. Prominin, a novel microvilli-specific polytopic membrane protein of the apical surface of epithelial cells, is targeted to plasmalemmal protrusions of non-epithelial cells. (1997) *Proc Natl Acad Sci USA. 94(23)*: 12425-12430.

[27] Collins AT, Berry PA, Hyde C, Stower MJ, Maitland NJ. Prospective identification of tumorigenic prostate cancer stem cells. (2005) *Cancer Res. 65(23)*: 10946-10951.

[28] Horn PA, Tesch H, Staib P, Kube D, Diehl V, Voliotis D. Expression of AC133, a novel hematopoietic precursor antigen, on acute myeloid leukemia cells. (1999) *Blood. 93(4)*: 1435-1437.

[29] Zhou L, Wei X, Cheng L, Tian J, Jiang JJ. CD133, One of the Markers of Cancer Stem Cells in Hep-2 Cell Line. (2007) *Laryngoscope. 117(3)*:455-460.

In: Progress in Oral Cancer Research
Editor: Frederik L. Nielsen, pp 55-72
ISBN 978-1-60021-865-1

Chapter II

Current Therapies and Future Treatment Modalities for Oral Cavity Cancer

***Constance Q. Zhou*[1,*]*, Robert J. DeFatta*[1] *and Yadranko Ducic*[1,2]
[1]Department of Otolaryngology-Head and Neck Surgery, University of Texas Southwestern Medical Center in Dallas, Texas, USA;
[2]Division of Otolaryngology and Facial Plastic and Reconstruction Surgery, John Peter Smith Hospital in Fort Worth, Texas, USA.

Abstract

Oral cancer is an increasingly prevalent disease in the United States. Although it accounts for only about 3% of all malignancies in this country, it encompasses approximately 30 percent of all head and neck neoplasms. It is estimated that 34,360 Americans will be diagnosed with oral cancer in 2007 and of these, 7,550 individuals will eventually succumb to their disease. Despite recent advances in surgery, radiation, chemotherapy, and the shift toward multi-modality treatment, the overall 5-year survival rates have not improved from the 1970s (50-55%).

Oral cancers often begin as premalignant lesions, such as leukoplakia, erythroplakia, and, less commonly, lichen planus. Because clinical evidence of such lesions may be visible with a thorough physical exam, dentists, oral surgeons and otolaryngologists all play an integral role in early detection and prevention of cancers of the oral cavity. Ongoing technological advances have facilitated radiological detection of primary tumors and surveillance for the early detection of recurrences. While computed tomography (CT) and magnetic resonant imaging (MRI) have become the mainstay imaging tools for surgeons, the widespread availability of positron emission tomorgraphy (PET) has allowed for whole body surveillance where applicable, and has brought new hope for cancer detection. On the surgical front, the utility of sentinel lymph node biopsy (SLNB) for staging malignant melanoma and breast cancer has served as an impetus for its early experimental use as a potential procedure of choice for staging oral cavity cancers.

* Correspondence concerning this article should be addressed to: Dr. Yadro Ducic, 1500 south main street, suite 303 Fort Woth, Texas 76104. Email: yducic@sbcglobal.net.

However, the effectiveness of SLNB for oral cancer staging has yet to be proven. While radiation therapy continues to evolve in its precision in the treatment of oral cavity cancers, chemotherapy adjuncts have remained largely unchanged in the agents administered, but the duration and timing of chemotherapy regimes continues to be investigated and evolving. One of the main drawbacks from the use of radiation therapy, and to a lesser extent, chemotherapy are the unique treatment-related sequelae of the oral cavity.

In this chapter, we will review current practices and investigate some future directions for the diagnosis and treatment of oral cancers.

INTRODUCTION

Squamous cell carcinoma, by far, is the most common cancer of the oral cavity. In fact, it is the sixth most common malignancy worldwide [1,2]. It accounts for 4% of all cancers and 2% of all cancer-related deaths worldwide each year [3]. In some of the areas of the world, the prevalence of oral cavity cancer is even more significant, as evidenced in India, where this disease process is the most common malignancy, accounting for 30% to 50% of all cancers [4,5].

This is a disease of older individuals, with the mean age at diagnosis of 60 years of age [6-8]. This fact is realized once one understands that the incidence in patients younger than forty years of age ranges between 0.4% and 4% [9]. At the turn of the century, a very strong male predilection was seen, however, now, the incidence rates for both men and women are nearly equal, as the rate of tobacco use has equalized between the sexes. The rate of a second primary, *ie* synchronous, tumor in the upper aerodigestive tract is 3.7% per year [10,11].

Of all of the prognostic factors, the cervical lymph node status, is the single most important factor in determining a patient's overall survival. In fact, the presence of regional metastasis to the cervical lymph nodes reduces the 5-year survival rate by 50% [12-14]. The primary treatment of oral cavity cancer is via surgical resection, with adjuvant chemoradiation therapy reserved for more advanced stage disease, nonresectable disease, patients with distant metastatic disease, or patients with significant comorbidities that would preclude surgery. Despite advances in surgical and adjuvant chemoradiation therapy, the diagnosis of oral cavity cancer continues to portend a poor prognosis. This is evidenced by the fact that the overall 5-year survival rate has remained essentially unchanged, at approximately 50%, over the past 30 years [12,15]. The aggressiveness of this disease is emphasized by the fact that the recurrence rate ranges from 25% to 48% despite adequate local control [16-18].

Since the 5-year survival rate for oral cavity cancer is directly related to the stage at the time of diagnosis, prevention and early detection are vital to decreasing the incidence and improving the overall survival rates of individuals diagnosed with this disease. It is important to understand that oral premalignant lesions and early stage malignancies often arise as subtle lesions. A physician should always have a high index of suspicion for any abnormality that presents in the oral cavity of a patient, especially if any risk factors are present.

Invasive squamous cell carcinoma of the oral cavity is often preceded by the presence of a clinically detectable premalignant lesion on the oral mucosa. This is defined as morphologically altered tissue in which cancer is more likely to occur than in its normal counterpart [19]. These lesions frequently present as either a white or red lesion, and as they progress, may ulcerate. It is important to note that even at this stage, these lesions are still normally asymptomatic.

Primary oral cavity lesions are normally noted by the patient, their dentist, or their physician as an ulcer or mass. 90% of all oral cavity lesions arise from three sites: the floor of mouth, the ventrolateral aspect of the tongue, and the soft palate [20]. Therefore, a focused exam in these areas is of the utmost importance. The importance of this is understood once one realizes that it has been estimated that only approximately 20% of Americans receives a thorough, focused oral cavity examination regularly [21].

Initial Evaluation

All patients should be evaluated beginning with a complete history and physical examination, including a thorough exam of the head, neck, and the oral cavity. All mucosal surfaces, skin, scalp, tongue, hard and soft palate, dentition, cervical nodes, and the cranial nerves should be examined. Characteristics of any suspicious lesions should be carefully noted. These include size, appearance, location, texture, color, and fixation to adjacent structures. Some telltale signs of malignancy consist of otalgia, dysphagia, odynophagia, and unexplained bleeding.

Once a suspicious lesion is identified, a simple biopsy may be performed under local anesthesia. However, some patients may require flexible fiberoptic laryngoscopy, direct laryngoscopy, and/or esophagoscopy to better visualization and determine the extent of the masss and ultimately obtain an adequate biopsy for pathological diagnosis.

Premalignant Lesions

Oral squamous cell carcinoma is, by far, the most common type of oral cavity cancer, accounting for greater than 90% of all oral cavity cancers. The risk factors include tobacco, alcohol, and viruses. Tobacco use is well documented in multiple studies as a dose-dependent risk factor in increasing the risk of developing oral cancer. Not only does smoking increase the incidence of developing a first primary carcinoma, but it also increases an individual's risk of recurrence, as well as, developing a second primary carcinoma by as much as 40% [22]. Excessive alcohol consumption, in addition to tobacco use, has been shown to have a synergistic effect in terms of acquiring an oral cavity tumor. One study quotes as much as a 2.5 fold risk increase over the additive risk of these two habits [23]. Evidence suggests human papilloma virus (HPV) may be a precursor in the development of some oral cancers. This is based in the discovery of HPV isolates in both oral squamous cell carcinoma and premalignant lesions of the oral cavity [24].

The 5-year survival rate for oral cancer is directly related to the stage of the disease at the time of diagnosis [25]. Therefore, prevention and early detection of premalignant lesions are essential to improve both morbidity and mortality. A premalignant lesion is defined as any morphologically altered tissue in which cancer is more likely to occur than in its apparently normal counterpart [19]. Three of the most common examples of these lesions in the oral cavity include leukoplakia, erythroplakia, and lichen planus.

Leukoplakia is also known as the "white plaque" due to its physical appearance. Microscopically, it has characteristics of both hyperkeratosis and dysplasia. The rate of malignant transformation from leukoplakia to squamous cell carcinoma has been shown to increase as the percentage of epithelial dysplasia increases. In fact, some studies have quoted transformation rates as high as 39% [26]. Of interest, the rate of transformation for leukoplakia is significantly higher in nonsmokers than that of smokers. Other risk factors for malignant transformation of oral leukoplakia include female gender, longstanding lesions, lesions isolated to the floor-of-mouth and tongue subsites, inhomogeneous leukoplakia, and the presence of Candida albicans within the lesion [27]. Because of the high malignant potential, all lesions require biopsy. Once a diagnosis has been established, the treatment options include surgical excision, cryosurgery, and CO_2 laser excision, all of which have been shown to have similar success in effectively removing the lesion. Nonsurgical therapies, such as the use of Vitamin A and beta carotene, have also shown promise in multifocal lesions, and carry the added benefit of a more favorable side effect profile.

Oral erythroplakia is a red lesion and occurs much less commonly than leukoplakia. Almost all true erythroplakias demonstrate significant epithelial dysplasia, carcinoma *in situ*, or invasive squamous cell carcinoma at the time of diagnosis [28]. Therefore, excisional biopsies are recommended so that the specimen may be assessed microscopically for margin control.

Oral lichen planus is thought to be an immunologically induced degeneration of the basal cell layer of the mucosa [29]. It presents clinically in six histological subtypes: reticular, popular, plaque-like, atrophic, bullous, and erosive. The malignant transformation rate for lichen planus is relatively low, ranging 0.4% to 5.6%. It is important to note that the atrophic and erosive subtypes have the highest rates of malignant transformation [30]. At the present time, there is no definitive cure for lichen planus, however, either topical or systemic corticosteroids are the mainstay therapy. Observation alone is a reasonable alternative.

Radiographic Imaging

Panorex represents an inexpensive readily available modality that is useful in assessing dentition. In addition, patient with gross cortical involvement will have changes noted on a panorex (Figure 1). Computed tomography (CT) is the most common imaging modality used today in the assessment of oral cavity tumors because of its ability to distinguish tumor from fat with intravenous contrast use. CT scans also visibly display bone changes, such as cortical destruction of skull base and mandible (Figures 2,3), and perineural tumor invasion (Figure 4). The recent advent of the DentaScan technology has further enhanced the anatomic details provided by CT with better images of the mandible, maxilla, and teeth [31]. Advantages of CT include availability, lower cost, and good soft tissue discrimination.

The most significant drawback to CT imaging of the oral cavity is beam-hardening artifact attributing to dental amalgam. Due to the prevalence of such artifacts, magnetic resonant imaging (MRI) may be beneficial in the evaluation of oral cavity tumors (Figure 5). MRI has been demonstrated to be superior for delineating tumor margins because of its enhanced soft tissue contrast. In addition, MRI of the face and skull base is more sensitive than CT for evaluation of perineural tumor spread (Figure 6). This point is extremely important, because this finding automatically upgrades a tumor's status to T4. It is also important to note that perineural invasion can be a clinically silent occurrence [32]. While the properties of a MRI scan often allow superior delineation of soft tissue details compared to a CT scan, the same properties of the MRI prevent the acquisition of the same bony detail. Therefore, if bony tumor invasion is suspected or if bone resection is anticipated due to the proximity of a tumor, a CT scan with intravenous contrast should be considered to help assess bone involvement in the surgical planning stage of the patient's work-up. MR angiography is an excellent screen for carotid artery involvement by carcinoma (Figure 7).

In the last few years, positron emission tomography (PET) has emerged as an exciting new imaging modality. Detection of a tumor by PET is based on the differential uptake of the radiolabled glucose (fluoro-deoxy-glucose or FDG) in the malignant tissues compared to the surrounding normal tissues. This is due to the increased metabolic rate of the cancer cells compared to metabolism of normal tissues. Hence, tumors will routinely tend to uptake FDG more readily than normal tissues. Two studies have already demonstrated the superiority of PET over CT or MRI in tumor surveillance and recurrence, although much more investigation is needed to verify these results on a larger scale [33,34]. Currently, PET use is limited by its availability and high cost. Although PET has already proven to be a valuable tool in tumor surveillance, it should be noted that one of the major limitations is during the early postoperative period. PET scanning may remain positive at the resection site for several months. Therefore, it is recommended that the first PET scan following a resection of an oral cavity cancer should be postponed for 12 weeks to avoid a false-positive result.

More recently, combined PET-CT scanners have allowed for the combination of the molecular contrast of PET with the anatomic precision of CT (Figure 7). In concert, they enhance the ability to distinguish abnormal from physiologic FDG uptake, and hence, enhance tumor detection. Moreover, the role of PET-CT has evolved from a cancer detection and surveillance modality to one of cancer treatment. In this capacity, it is used to direct radiation therapy. Further investigation is still warranted to determine the usefulness of PET-CT in the treatment of oral cavity cancer.

STAGING

In 1940, the French surgeon, Pierre Denoix, developed the TNM staging system for classification of malignant tumors. It is still accepted today as the gold standard for tumor staging is due to the foresight and innovative thinking of Dr. Denoix at a time when little was known about cancer principles. The system takes into account all three main components of any malignancy. The first parameter, T, is determined by the surface diameter of the primary tumor. The second parameter, N, is based not only on the presence or absence of regional lymph node metastasis, but also on the actual size of the affected node. While N is based on the regional or cervical lymph node status, M, indicates either the presence or absence of distant metastasis. Table 1 details the TNM staging system for oral cancer [35]. The TNM classification of a patient is the basis of determining the overall stage of a patient. In 1959, the American Joint Committee on Cancer (AJCC) used the basic premise of a patient's TNM classification as the basis of determining the overall stage of a patient's tumor burden. The AJCC published the first edition of the Manual for Staging of Cancer in 1977, and every few years, a new edition is published with updates and new schemes for additional cancer sites. In Table 2, the most recent AJCC staging system for oral cavity malignancies is outlined [36].

Table 1. TNM staging system for tumors of oral cavity

Tumor	
Tx	Primary tumor cannot be assessed
T0	No evidence of primary tumor
Tis	Carcinoma in situ
T1	Tumor ≤ 2cm in greatest dimension
T2	Tumor > 2cm but < 4cm in greatest dimension
T3	Tumor > 4cm in greatest dimension
T4a	Tumor invades through cortical bone, into deep tongue musculature, maxillary sinus, or skin of face
T4b	Tumor involves masticator space, pterygoid plates, or skull base and/or encases internal carotid artery
Node	
Nx	Regional lymph nodes cannot be assessed
N0	No regional lymph node metastasis
N1	Single ipsilateral lymph node, ≤ 3cm in greatest dimension
N2a	Single ipsilateral lymph node > 3cm but < 6cm in greatest dimension
N2b	Multiple ipsilateral lymph nodes, non > 6cm in greatest dimension
N2c	Bilateral or contralateral lymph nodes, non > 6cm in greatest dimension
N3	Any lymph node > 6cm in greatest dimension
Metastasis	
Mx	Distant metastasis cannot be assessed
M0	No distant metastasis
M1	Distant metastasis

Surgical Management of the Neck

Although there are many various factors that will adversely influence the overall survival of a patient diagnosed with oral cavity squamous cell carcinoma, cervical lymph node metastasis has been shown to be the single most reliable prognostic factor in determining the outcome of an individual with this disease. In patients with cervical metastasis at the time of diagnosis, the 5-year overall survival rate is reduced by approximately 50% [37,38].

Therefore, an oncologically sound surgical removal of the cervical lymph nodes and detection of occult nodal metastasis are crucial in the comprehensive management of squamous cell carcinoma of the oral cavity. Occult neck disease is defined as disease that is present microscopically but cannot be palpated clinically and may defy identification by any of the various imaging modalities. These patients are staged as N0 on the basis of their clinical examination and pN+ if pathologically positive nodes are discovered after the neck dissection has been evaluated by the Pathologist. Salvage rates for these patients are unfavorable, and thus, elective surgical removal of the cervical lymph nodes should be executed liberally with curative intent [39].

Table 2. AJCC stage groupings

Stage group	T stage	N stage	M stage
0	Tis	N0	M0
I	T1	N0	M0
II	T2	N0	M0
III	T3	N0	M0
	T1	N1	M0
	T2	N1	M0
	T3	N1	M0
IV A	T4a	N0	M0
	T4a	N1	M0
	T1	N2	M0
	T2	N2	M0
	T3	N2	M0
	T4a	N2	M0
IV B	T4b	Any N	M0
	Any T	N3	M0
IV C	Any T	Any N	M1

Each side of the neck is divided into various levels, and the delineation of each of the levels is explained in Table 3. While each of the levels of the neck have an anatomical basis, they also correlate to the specific regions of the neck that each head and neck primary cancer is most prone to metastasize to in the neck. Therefore, the origin of the primary tumor will determine which type of neck dissection should be performed. Table 4 explains each of the various neck dissections that are routinely performed [40,41].

In oral cavity carcinoma patients with a clinically N0 neck, the first echelon nodes that must be addressed are present in levels I, II, and III. Because a supraomohyoid neck dissection, by definition, removes lymph node levels I-III while preserving the spinal accessory nerve, internal jugular vein, and sternocleidomastoid muscle, it is the best modality for detecting cervical metastasis [42-46]. The supraomohyoid neck dissection has an estimated accuracy in detection of regional metastasis of 98%, a sensitivity of 95%, and specificity of 100% [47]. This selective approach reduces morbidity compared with that of the more traditional modified radical neck dissection. It is now recommended to perform supraomohyoid neck dissection in all T1-T4 lesions with a clinically N0 neck [48,49].

The concept of skip metastases from oral tongue cancers beyond level 3 initially challenged the effectiveness of the supraomohyoid neck dissection. This is because Byers *et al.* showed that stage I and II squamous cell carcinoma of the tongue had a high likelihood of occult level IV metastases, and would therefore not be addressed by the procedure [50]. However, since this study, T1-T3 N0 oral tongue cancers have demonstrated a low rate of metastasis (≤ 2%) to level IV. It has also been shown that when the decision is made intraoperatively to perform a level IV dissection based on the suspicion of metastatic disease in levels II or III, there is no increase in the rate of recurrence in the neck [51].

Table 3. Oncologic lymph node levels of the neck

LN Group		Description
IA	Submental	Within the triangular boundary of the anterior belly of the digastric muscles and the hyoid bone
IB	Submandibular	Within the boundaries of the anterior belly of the digastric muscle and the stylohyoid muscle and the inferior border of the mandible
II	Upper jugular	Around the upper third of the internal jugular vein and the adjacent spinal accessory nerve
IIA		Anterior (medial) to the spinal accessory nerve
IIB		Posterior (lateral) to the spinal accessory nerve
III	Middle jugular	Around the middle third of the internal jugular vein, between the inferior border of the hyoid bone and the inferior border of the cricoid cartilage
IV	Lower jugular	Around the lower third of the internal jugular vein, extend from the inferior border of the cricoid cartilage to the clavicle
V	Posterior triangle	Along the lower half of the spinal accessory nerve and the transverse cervical artery
VI	Central compartment	In the prelaryngeal, pretracheal, paratracheal, and tracheoesophageal groove, bounded by the hyoid bone to the suprasternal notch and between the medial borders of the carotid sheaths (LNs generally not dissected in oral cancer patients)
VII	Superior mediastinal	In the anterior superior mediastinum and tracheoesophageal grooves, extending from the suprasternal notch to the innominate artery (LNs generally not dissected in oral cancer patients)

When patients present with clinically palpable cervical metastasis, *i.e.* the N+ neck, levels I-IV are all at high risk. In this situation, a type I modified radical neck dissection is warranted. In this dissection, all the lymph nodes are removed from these levels without sacrificing the spinal accessory nerve, internal jugular vein, or the sternocleidomastoid muscle, as long as these structures are not involved with the tumor. It is important to note that palpable nodes have a significantly higher incidence of extracapsular spread of disease, which in turn, compromises the aponeurotic planes that are critical in preserving the sternocleidomastoid muscle, cranial nerve XI, and internal jugular vein [52]. Postoperative radiation therapy following type I modified radical neck dissection in an N+ neck results in failure rates of 7%-10% in N1 patients, and 12% in N2 patients [53]. These outcomes are as favorable as the cure rates that result from radical neck dissections in similar patients, and carry much less morbidity due to the preservation of function of these key structures [54].

Thus, a type I modified radical neck dissection is both a safe and appropriate treatment modality in treating N+ patients with oral cavity cancers.

Table 4. Classification of neck dissections

Neck dissection	Description
Selective	
Supraomohyoid	Lymph nodes (LNs) are removed from levels I, II, and III
Anterolateral	LNs are removed from levels II, III, and IV
Posterolateral	LNs are removed from levels II, III, IV, and V
Modified	Excision of LNs from levels I-IV with the preservation of one or more nonlymphatic structures
Type I	Preservation of the spinal accessory nerve, internal jugular vein, and sternocleidomastoid muscle
Type II	Preservation of the spinal accessory nerve and the internal jugular vein
Type III	Preservation of the spinal accessory nerve
Radical	Excision of LNs from levels I-IV, the spinal accessory nerve, the internal jugular vein, the sternocleidomastoid muscle, and the submandibular gland
Extended	Excision of LN groups and/or additional structures not included in the classic neck dissection

Sentinel Lymph Node Biopsy

The theory of sentinel lymph node biopsy (SLNB) relies on the concept that metastasis from a primary tumor occurs by an orderly spread to the first echelon lymph nodes before reaching nodes in the lymphatic basin. SLNB has improved the staging accuracy in melanoma and breast cancers while, at the same time, reducing the morbidity from performing unnecessary lymph node dissections. Therefore, the success of SLNB for staging malignant melanoma and breast cancer has made it the potential procedure of choice for staging oral cavity cancers [55-56]. Hence, it has been hypothesized that if applied to patients diagnosed with oral cavity cancer, this modality could limit both the extent and number of neck dissections that would be otherwise be required for local control in patients with oral cavity cancer.

The Second International Conference on Sentinel Node Biopsy in Mucosal Head and Neck Cancer piloted the study with contributions from twenty centers from around the world. Sentinel lymph nodes were identified in 366 out of 379 patients with N0 disease, for an identification rate of 97% [57]. Of the 366 patients with a positive sentinel lymph node, 103 (29%) were positive for occult metastasis while 263 (71%) were negative. Of the 263 patients, 11 (4%) showed nodal disease that was not revealed by the sentinel lymph node biopsy. Hence, the negative predictive value of a negative sentinel node for the remaining neck was 96% [58]. As one can ascertain, SLNB was felt to be sufficiently validated for early oral cancer with a N0 neck [59].

The original promising results of SLNB have since been validated by other studies. For example, the preliminary results of the 1998 Canniesburn trial, the largest multicenter cohort study on SLNB to date, described an identification rate of 93%. Since then, results from other centers and trials have revealed an overall identification rate of 97.7%.

Once the sentinel lymph node is successfully identified, the possibility of the presence of an occult metastasis must also be determined. This is important because it upstages the clinically N0 neck, which inversely correlates to the overall 5-year survival of patients. The rate of upstaging by SLNB was compared to elective neck dissection in the Canniesburn trial, as well as, another study. From these trials two trials, 34%-60% of patients were upstaged. This is a dramatic improvement compared to the 30% of patients where were upstaged after undergoing a traditional elective neck dissection [60]. It is generally felt that the increased rate in upstaging following sentinel lymph node biopsy may be explained by the increase in identification of micrometastases. Due to this belief, the presence of micrometastatic disease has been given the new classification pNmi, or pathologic nodal micrometastasis. The clinical significance of pNmi has yet to be confirmed, and prospective studies with uniform pathologic evaluations are still warranted to answer this very important question [61].

The accuracy of SLNB must also be validated before it can be accepted as a satisfactory alternative to the elective neck dissection. This may be accomplished by evaluating the sensitivity of sentinel lymph node biopsy, which is defined as the proportion of patients with occult metastasis who are found to have positive sentinel lymph nodes. In published reports, including the Canniesburn trial, the sensitivity of SLNB ranges from 86%-100%. In addition, the Canniesburn trial also reported a negative predictive value of 83%-99% with a 95% confidence interval. The trial also determined the likelihood ratio to be 0.09 for negative SLNB findings [58]. These results strongly suggest that sentinel lymph node biopsy has a low false-negative rate and is sensitive enough to rule out occult metastasis when the result is negative [61].

Despite its high sensitivity and accuracy comparable to that of an elective neck dissection in detecting occult metastases, SLNB must offer advantages over neck dissection in order to become the standard of care. Currently, management of patients staged by sentinel lymph node biopsy has not been compared with that of patients staged by elective neck dissection in prospective studies. Furthermore, additional challenges specific to the oral cavity such as lymphatic mapping in deeply infiltrative primary oral tumors and the phenomenon of skip metastasis from carcinoma of the tongue still need to be investigated. The American College of Surgeons Oncology Group and the European Organization for Research and Treatment of Cancer are presently each performing a trial in an attempt to further elucidate the validity of SLNB [62,63].

Radiation Therapy

It is generally accepted that radiation therapy and surgery are equally successful in controlling early T1 lesions of the oral cavity [64-66]. However, Carvalho and colleagues found that among 1,500 patients with T1 and T2 oral cavity cancer, the highest recurrence rate occurred after treatment by radiation therapy alone (32.8%). When compared to the group of patients who were treated with surgery alone, the recurrence rate was decreased to 13.9% [65]. Therefore, it is clear that these results indicate that one should surgically excise any oral cavity lesions of any T2 or more advanced disease. For T1 disease, the treatment option should be determined by location of the lesion, patient's physical condition, and the experience of the treating physician. Anyone opting for radiation therapy as their treatment should be counseled that this treatment modality usually requires at least six weeks. The patient should also understand that if a cure is not obtained through radiation therapy, then surgery would have to be performed in hopes of curing the disease process. Hence, these facts may very well affect a patient's preference in which therapy they are more amenable to undergoing. Although radiation therapy does offer better functional results, such as, superior speech and swallowing, it also carries substantial side effects. The most common include diminution of taste, xerostomia, and osteoradionecrosis of the mandible. It should be noted that newer technologies, such as intensity-modulated radiation therapy (IMRT), are overcoming some of these challenges through more focused targeting [67] (Figure 9).

For patients with T3 and T4 oral cavity cancer, combined therapy with surgery and postoperative radiation therapy is the standard of care [68]. On the other hand, preoperative radiation therapy has not provided any advantages one would expect. This was concluded from the first and only large randomized trial comparing preoperative and postoperative radiation treatments, which revealed no significant difference between overall survival, disease-free survival, and surgical complications [69]. Robotic radiosurgery as sole treatment of recurrences or given as a boost with primary radiation therapy may play a substantial role in future organ preservation protocols (Figure 9).

Chemotherapy

In the early 1980s, locally advanced head and neck cancer was found to have a high response rate to induction chemotherapy [70]. Naturally, there was great hope that induction chemotherapy would be of benefit before surgical resection for advanced disease by reducing the tumor burden to such an extent that important structures could be spared in the resection due to the response to the induction chemotherapy, and thereby causing less morbidity to the patient. Unfortunately, the initial enthusiasm failed to produce any statistically significant survival advantage. In the same regard, the recent Radiation Therapy Oncology Group (RTOG) trial reported no improvement in survival for adjuvant chemotherapy after surgical resection of head and neck cancer [71]. A number of reasons have been postulated for the relative ineffectiveness of chemotherapy in head and neck cancer. These include low growth fractions in squamous cell carcinomas, insensitivity of squamous cells to chemotherapeutic agents, decreased vascularity to tumor bed secondary to surgery or radiation, and poor patient compliance or tolerance to chemotherapy toxicities [72,73].

Optimism for the role of chemotherapy in the treatment of stage III and IV oral cavity cancer rose again when it was realized that combining chemotherapy with postoperative radiation therapy improved both local regional control, as well as, overall survival. The theory behind these observations is that chemotherapy agents can enhance radiation efficacy by the mechanism of radiosensitization. Hypotheses for this phenomenon favor the belief that chemotherapy may alter the repair of sublethal cell damage, alter the cell cycle kinetics to favor G2/M arrest, and eliminate clonogens responsible for accelerated repopulation. All of these effects would augment the effectiveness of postoperative radiation therapy [74].

There are now several phase III trials supporting the use of concomitant chemotherapy with postoperative radiation therapy over radiation alone in terms of progression-free, disease-free, relapse-free, and overall survival. From the results of these studies, it is recommended that patients who have unresectable disease, as well as those who are at high risk for recurrence, should be strongly considered for concurrent chemoradiation therapy [71,75-87].

RECURRENCE

Recurrence rates for oral squamous cell carcinoma have been reported to be as high as 25-48% despite a sound, oncologic primary resection and treatment of cervical lymph nodes [16,17,88]. Because recurrent cancer most likely occurs at the primary site within the first 24 to 36 months, close follow-up for tumor surveillance is critical. Regularly scheduled imaging with CT, MRI, and PET scan are all important modalities used for tumor surveillance. Physical examination is also very important in this regard. Patients should understand that abstinence from tobacco and alcohol is paramount in an attempt to minimize the risk of developing a second primary lesion.

It has been found that the time interval between the completion of treatment and the local recurrence is critical in determining the overall prognosis and salvageability of the patient. Schwartz *et al* reported that recurrences that occurred within the first 6 months of primary tumor treatment resulted in an average of a 20 month survival time with no overall survivors. On the other hand, recurrences that occurred later than 6 months after initial treatment had a 58 month mean survival time, and 21% of the patients were ultimately salvaged through surgery [89].

Interestingly, several studies have found no correlation between the stage of the recurrence and the survival time. Instead, the stage and histologic grade of the primary tumor were more important in predicting the overall survival time and salvageability [90,91]. Distant recurrence after initial treatment in oral cavity cancer is associated with a very poor prognosis. In fact, these patients have a mean survival time of 4 to 12 months. Although maintenance chemotherapy may be of benefit in these cases, most patients die from local regional failure and other comorbid medical conditions [92].

Among all of the oral cavity cancer patients who present with a recurrence, about half are considered not salvageable through surgery because of the advanced stage of the tumor at presentation, involvement of local vital structures, distant metastatic disease, and poor surgical risk [45,93-95].

It is important to note that the initial treatment a patient receives for the primary tumor is important in determining the options ultimately available for salvage. For instance, location of the recurrence in relation to vital structures, previous reconstructions, and previous adjuvant chemoradiation therapies all need to be considered in evaluation for salvage therapy. Ultimately, surgeons must determine whether salvage surgery for recurrent oral cavity cancer is justified for each patient on an individual basis.

CONCLUSION

As evidenced from this chapter, oral cavity cancer remains an aggressive disease. Although the advent of technology has brought about many advances in both the diagnosis and treatment of this disease, we still have a long road ahead in an attempt to reduce both the morbidity of treatment and the overall mortality.

REFERENCES

[1] Parkin SM, Laara E, Muir CS. Estimates of the worldwide frequency of sixteen major cancers in 1980. *Int J Cancer*. 1988;41:184-97.

[2] Park BZ, Kohn WG, Malvitz DM. Preventing and controlling oral and pharyngeal cancer- recommendations from a national planning conference. *MMWR Morb Mortal Wkly Rep*. 1998;47:1-12.

[3] Johnson NW, Warnakulasuriya KAA. Oral Cancer. Is it more common than cervical? *Br Dent J*. 1991;170:170-171.

[4] Nair UJ, Friesen M, Richard I, et al. Effect of lime composition on the formation of reactive oxygen species from the areca nut extract in vivo. *Carcinogenesis*. 1990;11:2145-2148.

[5] Hindle I, Downer MC, Speight PM. The epidemiology of oral cancer. *Br J Oral Maxillofac Surg*. 1996;34:471-476.

[6] Devesa SS, Silverman DT, Young JL, et al. Cancer incidence and mortality trends among whites in the United States, 1947-1987. *J Natl Cancer Inst*. 1987;79:701-770.

[7] Worrall SF. Oral cancer incidence between 1971 to 1989. *Br J Oral Maxillofac Surg*. 1995;33:195-199.

[8] Zakrzewska JM. Oral cancer and precancer-our responsibility. *Br Dent J*. 1994;176:286-287.

[9] Friedlander PL, Schantz SP, Shaha AR, et al. Squamous cell carcinoma of the tongue in young patients. A matched paired analysis. *Head Neck*. 1988;20:363-368.

[10] Day GL, Blot WJ. Second primary tumors in patients with oral cancer. *Cancer*. 1992;70:14-19.

[11] Foulkes WD, Brunet JS, Sieh W, et al. Familial risks of squamous cell carcinoma of the head and neck, retrospective case controlled study. *Cancer*. 1996;313:716-721.

[12] Moore S, Johnson N, Pierce A. The epidemiology of mouth cancer. *Oral Dis*. 2000;6:65-74.

[13] Woolgar J, Scott J. Prediction of cervical metastasis in squamous cell carcinoma of the tongue and floor of mouth. *Head Neck*. 1995;17:463-472.

[14] Shah J. Cervical lymph node metastasis, its diagnostic, therapeutic, and prognostic implications. *Oncology*. 1990;4:61-69.

[15] Centers for Disease Control and Prevention. Current trends; deaths from oral cavity and pharyngeal cancer- United States 1987. *JAMA*. 1990;264:678-685.
[16] Jones KR, Lodge-Rigal RD, Reddick RL, et al. Prognostic factors in the recurrence of stage 1 and 2 squamous cell carcinoma of the oral cavity. *Arch Otolaryngol Head Neck Surg*. 1992;118:483-485.
[17] Nathanson A, Agren K, Biorklund A. Evaluation of some prognostic factors in small squamous cell carcinoma of the mobile tongue: a multicenter study in Sweden. *Head Neck*. 1989;11:387-392.
[18] Pearlman NW. Treatment outcome in recurrent head and neck cancer. *Arch Surg*. 1979;114:39-42.
[19] World Health Organization. Report from meeting on histological definition of precancerous lesions. 1973. Geneva, Switzerland.
[20] Mashberg A, Barsa P. Screening for oral and oropharyngeal squamous carcinomas. *CA Cancer J Clin*. 1984;34:262-268.
[21] Kerr AR, Changrani JG, Gany FM, et al. An academic dental center grapples with oral cancer disparities: current collaboration and future opportunities. *J Dent Educ*. 2004;68:531-541.
[22] 22. Lewin F, Norell SE, Johansson H, et al. Smoking tobacco, oral snuff, and alcohol in the etiology of squamous cell carcinoma of the head and neck: a population-based case-referent study in Sweden. *Cancer*1998;82:1367-1375.
[23] Baden E. Prevention of cancer of the oral cavity and pharynx. *CA Cancer J Clin* 1987;37:49-62.
[24] Elamin F, Steingrimsdottir H, Wanakulasuriya S, et al. Prevalence of human papillomavirus infection in premalignant and malignant lesions of the oral cavity in U.K. subjects: a novel method of detection. *Oral Oncol* 1998;34:191-197.
[25] Reddi SP, Shafer AT. Oral premalignant lesions: management considerations. *Oral Maxillofac Surg Clin N Am* 2006;18:425-433.
[26] Pindborg JJ, Renstrup G, Poulsen HE, et al. Studies in oral leukoplakia. V. Clinical and histologic signs of malignancy. *Acta Ondont Scand* 1963;21:407-414.
[27] van der Wall I, Schepman KP, vander Meij EH, et al. Oral leukoplakia: a clinicopathologic review. *Oral Oncol* 1997;33:291-301.
[28] Reichart PA, Philipsen HP. Oral erythroplakia – a review. *Oral Oncol* 2005;41:551-561.
[29] Boisnic S, Frances C, Branchet MC, et al. Immunohistochemical study of oral lesions of lichen planus: diagnostic and pathophysiologic aspects. *Oral Surg Oral Med Oral Pathol Oral Radiol Endod* 1990;70:462-465.
[30] Murti PR, Daftary KD, Bhonsle RB, et al. malignant potential of oral lichen planus: observations in 722 patients from India. *J Oral Pathol Med* 1986;15:71-77.
[31] Brockenbrough JM, Petruzzelli GJ, Lomasney L. DentaScan as an accurate method of predicting mandibular invasion in patients with squamous cell carcinoma of the oral cavity. *Arch Otolaryngol Head Neck Surg* 2003;129:113-117.
[32] Aulino JM, Strother MK, Shipman JL. Imaging of oral cavity squamous cell carcinoma. *Oral Maxillofac Surg Clin N Am* 2006;18:445-463.

[33] Teknos TN, Rosenthal EL, lee D, et al. Positron emission tomography in the evaluation of stage III and IV head and neck cancer. *Head Neck* 2001;23:1056-1060.

[34] Schwartz DL, Rajendran J, Yueh B, et al. Staging of head and neck squamous cell cancer with extended-field FDG-PET. *Arch Otolaryngol Head Neck Surg* 2003;129:1173-1178.

[35] Greene FL, Page DL, Fleming ID, et al., eds. *AJCC cancer staging handbook: from the AJCC cancer staging manual,* 6th ed. New York: Springer, 2002:35.

[36] Patel SG, shah JP. TNM staging of cancers of the head and neck: striving for uniformity among diversity. *CA Cancer J Clin* 2005;55:242-258.

[37] Johnson JT, Barnes L, Myers EN, et al. The extracapsular spread of tumors in cervical node metastasis. *Arch Otolaryngol* 1981;107:725-729.

[38] Landis SH, Murray T, Bolden S, et al. Cancer statistics. *CA Cancer J Clin*1999;1999:8-31.

[39] Carlson ER, Miller I. Surgical management of the neck in oral cancer. *Oral Maxilofac Surg Clin N Am* 2006;18:533-546.

[40] Ferlito A, rinaldo A. Errare humanum est, in errore perseverare stultum: this is true also for neck dissection. *Oral Oncol* 2005;41:132-134.

[41] Robbins KT, Clayman G, Levine PA, et al. Neck dissection classification update: revisions proposed by the American Head and Neck Society and the American Academy of Otolaryngology, Head and Neck Surgery. *Arch Otolaryngol Head Neck Surg* 2002;128:751-758.

[42] Henick DH, Silver CE, Heller KS, et al. Supraomohyoid neck dissection as a staging procedure for squamous cell carcinoma of the oral cavity and oropharynx. *Head Neck* 1995;17:119-123.

[43] Medina JE, Byers RM. Supraomohyoid neck dissection: rationale, indications, and surgical technique. *Head Neck* 1989;11:111-122.

[44] Kligerman J, Lima RA, Soares JR. Supraomohyoid neck dissection in the treatment of T1/T2 squamous cell carcinoma of oral cavity. *Am J Surg* 1994;168:391-394.

[45] Kowalski LP, Magrin J, Waksman G, et al. Supraomohyoid neck dissection in the treatment of head and neck tumors. *Arch Otolaryngol Head Neck Surg* 1993;119:958-963.

[46] Spiro JD, Spriro RH, Shah JP, et al. Critical assessment of supraomohyoid neck dissection. *Am J Surg* 1988;156:286-289.

[47] Carlson ER, Miller I. Surgical management of the neck in oral cancer. *Oral Maxillofac Surg Clin N Am* 2006;18:533-546.

[48] Shah JP, Candela FC, Poddar AK. The patterns of cervical lymph node metastases from squamous carcinoma of the oral cavity. *Cancer* 1990;66:109-133.

[49] Robbins, KT, Samant S. Neck dissection. In: Cummings CW, editor. Cummings otolaryngology head and neck surgery. 4th edition. Philadelphia: Mosby; 2005. p. 2614-2645.

[50] Byers RM, Weber RS, Andrew T, et al. Frequency and therapeutic implications of "skip metastases" in the neck from squamous cell carcinoma of the oral tongue. *Head Neck* 1997;19:14-19.

[51] Khafif A, Lopez-Garza JR, Media JE. Is dissection of level IV necessary in patients with T1-T3 N0 tongue cancer? *Laryngoscope* 2001;111:1088-1091.
[52] Snow GB, Annyas AA, Van Slooten EA, et al. Prognostic factors of neck node metastasis. *Clin Otolaryngol* 1982;7:185-192.
[53] Anderson PE, Spiro RH, Cambronero E, et al. The role of comprehensive neck dissection with preservation of the spinal accessory nerve in the clinically positive neck. *Am J Surg* 1994;168:499-502.
[54] Shah JP, Andersen PE. Evolving role of modifications in neck dissection for oral squamous carcinoma. *Br J Oral Maxillofac Surg* 1995;33:3-8.
[55] Morton DL, Thompson JF, Essner R, et al. Validation of the accuracy of intraoperative lymphatic mapping and sentinel lymphadenectomy for early-stage melanoma: a multicenter trial. Multicenter Selective Lymphadenectomy Trial Group. *Ann Surg* 1999;230:453-463.
[56] Veronesi U, Paganelli G, Viale G, et al. A randomized comparison of sentinel-node biopsy with routine axillary dissection in breast cancer. *N Engl J Med* 2003;349:546-553.
[57] Stoeckli SJ, Pfaltz M, Ross GL, et al. The Second International Conference on Sentinel Node Biopsy in Mucosal Head and Neck Cancer. *Ann Surg Oncol* 2005;12:919-924.
[58] Ross GL, Soutar DS, Gordon MD, et al. Sentinel node biopsy in head and neck cancer: preliminary results of a multicenter trial. *Ann Surg Oncol* 2004;11:690-696.
[59] Paleri V, Rees G, Arullendran P, et al. Sentinel node biopsy in squamous cell carcinoma of the oral cavity: a diagnostic meta-analysis. *Head Neck* 2005;27:739-747.
[60] Rigual NR, Douglas W, Lamonica D, et al. Sentinel lymph node biopsy: a rational approach for staging T2N0 oral cancer. *Laryngoscope* 2005;115:2217-2220.
[61] Shellengerger TD. Sentinel lymph node biopsy in the staging of oral cancer. *Oral Maxillofac Surg Clin N Am* 2006;18:547-563.
[62] Civantos F, Zitsch RP, Myers J. A trial of lymphatic mapping and sentinel node lymphadectomy for patients with T1 or T2 clinically N0 oral cavity squamous cell carcinoma. Chicago: American College of Surgeons Oncology Group. Protocol Z0360, activated September, 2002.
[63] Shah JP, Extent of surgical intervention in case of N0 neck in head and neck cancer patients. *Eur Arch Otorhinolaryngol* 2004;261:293-294.
[64] Harrison LB, Fass DE. Radiation therapy for oral cavity cancer. *Dent Clin North Am* 1990;34:205-222.
[65] Carvalho AL, Magrin J, Kowalski LP. Sites of recurrence in oral and oropharyngeal cancers according to the treatment approach. *Oral Dis* 2003;9:112-118.
[66] Brennan CT, Sessions DG, Spitznagel EL, et al. Surgical pathology of cancer o the oral cavity and oropharynx. *Laryngoscope* 1991;101:1175-1197.
[67] Lapeyre M, Bollet MA, Racadot S, et al. Postoperative brachytherapy alone and combined postoperative radiotherapy and brachytherapy boost for squamous cell carcinoma of the oral cavity, with positive or close margins. *Head Neck* 2004;26:216-223.

[68] Woolgar JA. Histological distribution of cervical lymph node metastases from intraoral / oropharyngeal squamous cell carcinomas. *Br J Oral Maxillofac Surg* 1999;37:175-180.

[69] Snow JB, Guber RD, Kramer S, et al. Randomized preoperative and postoperative radiation therapy for patients with carcinoma of the head and neck: preliminary report. *Laryngoscope* 1980;90:930-945.

[70] Kish J, Jacos J. Clinical trial of cisplatin and 5-FU infusion as initial treatment for advanced squamous cell carcinoma of the head and neck. *Cancer Treat Rep* 1982;66:471-476.

[71] Al-Sarraf M, LeBlanc M, Giri PG, et al. Chemoradiotherapy versus radiotherapy in patients with advanced nasopharyngeal cancer: phase III randomized Intergroup study 0099. *J Clin Oncol* 1998;16:1310-1317.

[72] Jacobs C, Makuch R. Efficacy of adjuvant chemotherapy for patients with respectable head and neck cancer: a subset analysis of the head and neck contracts program. *J Clin Oncol* 1990;8:838-847.

[73] Shikani AH, Domb AJ. Polymer chemotherapy for head and neck cancer. *Laryngoscope* 2000;110:907-917.

[74] Murphy BA, Cmelak, A. Chemoradiation therapy: the evolving role in head and neck cancer and its application to oral cavity tumors. *Oral Maxillofac Surg Clin N Am* 2006;18:605-614.

[75] Wendt T, Granbenbauer G, rodel C. simultaneous radiochemotherapy versus radiotherapy alone in advanced head and neck cancer: a randomized multicenter study. *J Clin Oncol* 1998;16:1318-1324.

[76] Lo T, Wiley A, Ansfield F. Combined radiation therapy and 5-fluorouracil for advanced squamous cell carcinoma of the oral cavity and oropharynx: a randomized study. *AJR Am J Roentgenol* 1976;126:229-235.

[77] Shanta V, Krishnamurthi S. Combined bleomycin and radiotherapy in oral cancer. *Clin Radiol* 1980;31:617-620.

[78] SECOG. A randomized trial of combined multidrug chemotherapy and radiotherapy in advanced squamous cell carcinoma of the head and neck. *Eur J Surg Oncol* 1986;12:289-295.

[79] Fu K, Philips T, Silverberg I. combined RT and CT with bleomycin in advanced inoperable head and neck cancer: update of the Northern California Oncology group randomized trial. *J Clin Oncol* 1987;5:1410-1418.

[80] Weissberg J, Son Y, Papac R. Randomized clinical trial of mitomycin C as an adjunct to radiotherapy in head and neck cancer. *Int J Radiat Oncol Biol Phys* 1989;17:3-9.

[81] Adelstein D, Sharan V, Earle A. Simultaneous versus sequential combined technique for head and neck cancer. *Cancer* 1990;65:1685-1691.

[82] Sanichiz R, Milla A, Torner J. Single fraction per day versus two fractions per day versus radiochemotherapy in the treatment of head and neck cancer. *Int J Radiat Oncol Biol Phys* 1990;19:1347-1350.

[83] Merlano M, Vitale V, Rosso R. Treatment of advanced squamous-cell carcinoma of the head and neck. *N Engl J Med* 1992;327:1115-1121.

[84] Adelstein D, Saxton J, Lavertu T. A phase III randomized trial comparing concurrent radiotherapy alone in advanced head and neck cancer. *Head Neck* 1997;19:567-575.

[85] Brizel DM, Fisher SE, Scher RL, et al. Hyperfractionated irradiation with or without concurrent chemotherapy for locally advanced head and neck cancer. *N Engl J Med* 1998;338:1798-1804.

[86] Zakotnik B, Smid L, Budhina M. concomitant radiotherapy with mitomycin C and bleomycin compared with radiotherapy alone in inoperable head and neck cancer: final report. *Int J Radiat Oncol Biol Phys* 1998;41:1121-1127.

[87] Dorbrowsky W, Naude J, Widder J, et al. Continuous hyperfractionated accelerated radiotherapy with/without mitomycin C in head nad neck cancer. *Int J Radiat Oncol Biol Phys* 1998;42:803-806.

[88] Bachaud JM, Altzieu C, David JM, et al. combined postoperative radiotherapy and weekly cisplatin infusion for locally advanced head and neck carcinoma: final report of a randomized trial. *Int J Radiat Oncol Biol Phys* 1996;36:999-1004.

[89] Schwartz GJ, Mehra RM, Wening BL, et al. Salvage treatment of local and regional recurrence. *Semin Oncol* 1993;20:419-429.

[90] Kademani D, Bell RB, Dierks EJ, et al. Prognostic factors in intraoral squamous cell carcinoma: the influence of histologic grade. *J Oral Maxillofac Surg* 2005;63:1599-1605.

[91] Kademani D, Dierks ED. Management of locoregional recurrence in oral squmous cell carcinoma. *Oral Maxillofac Surg Clin N Am* 2006;18:615-625.

[92] Kowalski LP, Carvalho AL, Prinate AVM, et al. Predictive factors for distant metastasis from oral and oropharyngeal squamous cell carcinoma. *Oral Oncol* 2005;41:524-541.

[93] Shah J, et al. Carcinoma of the oral cavity. Factors affecting treatment failure to the primary site and neck. *Am J Surg*1976;132:504-507.

[94] Leemans C, Tiwari R, Nauta JJ, et al. Recurrence at the primary site in head and neck cancer and the significance of neck lymph node metastasis as a prognostic factor. *Cancer* 1994;73:187-190.

[95] Grandi C, Allossio M, Moglia DEA. Prognostic significance of lymphatic spread in head and neck carcinomas: therapeutic implications. *Head Neck Surg* 1985;8:67-73.

In: Progress in Oral Cancer Research
Editor: Frederik L. Nielsen, pp 73-90
ISBN 978-1-60021-865-1

Chapter III

Current Trends in Oral Cavity Cancer Treatment

Alfio Jose Tincani
Head and Neck Division, Dept. of Surgery, Univ. of Campinas, Brazil

Introduction

Oral cavity tumors account for the sixth cause of cancer in the world and rank second in the head and neck, after skin cancer only [1]. In Brazil, the estimate incidence for the year 2006 was 10,060 new cases among men and 3,410 among women [2]. In the United States there are over 21,500 oral carcinomas diagnosed each year, causing 6,000 deaths. About 90% of all oral cavity cancers are squamous cell carcinoma, and its etiology is the well established exposure to carcinogens present in tobacco and the synergistic action of ethanol. Smokers have a 7 fold risk of developing oral cancers; heavy drinkers have a 6 fold risk; and those who abuse both alcohol and tobacco have a 30 fold risk. Other factors involved are chewing tobacco or betel nut, poor oral hygiene and dentition, and poorly fit dental prostheses.

Chronic exposure to tobacco carcinogens results in the field cancerization effect, as proposed by Slaughter in 1953 [4], and there is a higher risk of developing other upper aero digestive mucosal cancers, as pharyngeal, laryngeal and esophageal tumors. The chronically exposed mucosal cells tend to develop genetic abnormalities, activating proto-oncogenes and down regulating tumor-suppressor genes. Cell cycle becomes abnormal and mucosal cell population becomes instable with rapid cell cycling and decreased cell surveillance, with impaired capacity of cell repair and apoptosis, evolving to premalignant and malignant cell clones.

Although not directly related to smoking, there are other mouth neoplasms such as minor salivary gland cancers (mostly adenoid cystic tumors) and soft tissue sarcomas, which are very rare: less than 1% of all head and neck malignancies. Their primary treatment is also surgery, often combined with adjuvant Radiotherapy.

Anatomy

The mouth has its anterior limit in the skin of the vermilion on both upper and lower lips. Its posterior limit is delineated by the junction of the hard and soft palates superiorly, and by the V-shaped line of the circumvallated papillae inferiorly. Laterally, it is bounded by the buccal mucosa. There are seven mouth subsites which are: lips, buccal mucosa, gingiva, hard palate, retromolar trigone, floor of the mouth and oral tongue. All these structures have important functions such as articulation of speech, mastication, facial expression, among others.

The lip region is defined by and upper and a lower folds of fleshy tissues which converge laterally to form the lateral comissures, delimitating the buccal orifice, or the anterior wall of the oral cavity. The upper lip is marked by a medial infra nasal groove or philtrum, which ends at the lips free border as a tubercle. In the lower lip there is a similar groove: the sulcus mentolabialis. The lip is divided in three zones, which are cutaneous, glabrous and villous. The most important muscle of the lip is the orbicularis oris, disposed in an elliptical manner surrounding the oral aperture, forming laterally the oral commissures, where the facial muscles, dilators of the oral cavity, attach. There are multiple minor salivary glands in the lips, most of which are located between the musculature and the mucosa. The blood supply to the lips is made by the labial arteries, branches of the facial artery. The labial veins follow the arteries and commonly drain to the internal jugular vein. The lymphatic vessels are arranged in plexuses and lie within the mucous membrane and the skin. They follow the facial veins and drain in the submental nodes; the mid portion of the lip drains to submental nodes. Innervation is supplied by the by the mandibular branch of the facial nerve.

The inner lining of the mouth is covered by the buccal mucosa of the vestibule. This mucosa begins at lip, continues with the cheeks and ends in the alveolar process of the gingiva. The vestibule communicates with the oral cavity through both interdental spaces and the posterior aspect of the ascending ramus of the mandible. In the upper and posterior aspect of the mucosa, adjacent to the second molar tooth, opens the Stensen's duct or parotid duct.

The alveolar process or gingiva is covered by mucosa and submucosal tissue that firmly adheres to the adjacent mandibular periosteum. The periosteum is contiguous with the tooth sockets or alveolar cavities, a common path to tumor spread.

The hard palate separates the oral cavity from the nasal cavity and nasopharynx. It is a vault-shaped, horizontal plate covered by a dense and firmly adherent mucoperiosteum, important for deglutition and phonation. The hard palate is rich in minor salivary glands, blood vessels and nerves.

The retromolar trigone is a portion of adherent keratinized mucosa that covers the ascending ramus of the mandible from the third mandibular molar below to the maxillary tubercle above. It is the oral cavity site between the buccal mucosa laterally and the anterior tonsillar pillar medially and posteriorly.

The floor of the mouth is a crescent-shaped groove that lies from the mandible to the root of the tongue. Its posterior limit is the glossopalatine arch or anterior tonsil pillar. The muscle floor is formed by the mylohyoid and the hyoglossus muscles covered by oral mucosa. A mid fold, next to the root of the tongue, or frenulum, separates the salivary caruncules, where the submandibular ducts or Wharton's duct open.

The tongue, the most common site of oral carcinoma, is a muscular structure attached to the floor of the mouth, hyoid bone and mandible. It is divided in oral portion, or mobile tongue, and base of tongue, which is an oropharyngeal structure. Posteriorly, the oral tongue is bounded by a V-shaped line of circumvallated papillae, and in the V's vertex by the *foramen caecum.* The oral tongue has ventral and dorsal surfaces and is composed by intrinsic and extrinsic muscles. The intrinsic muscles are arranged in vertical and horizontal fascicles that allow the mobile tongue to change shape and consistency. The three pairs of extrinsic muscles that provide mobility of the tongue are the genioglossus, hyoglossus, and styloglossus, which arise in the mandible, hyoid bone, soft palate and styloid process and fuse in the intrinsic musculature. Its covering mucosa, adherent to the underlying muscles, is simple stratified squamous epithelium with sparse papillae or taste buds of different morphologies: filiform, foliate, fungiform, and circumvallated. The blood is supplied by branches of the lingual arteries, direct branches of the external carotid arteries in each side. The motor supply to the intrinsic and extrinsic tongue muscles is the hypoglossal nerve, which exits the skull through the hypoglossal canal and courses laterally and anteriorly between the external and internal carotid arteries, inferior to the occipital artery. The sensation of the tongue is supplied by the lingual nerve, a branch of the mandibular division of the trigeminal nerve, which also transports parasympathetic fibers from the chorda tympani branch of the facial nerve to the submandibular ganglion. The lymphatic drainage of the tongue begins in a rich submucosal plexus, which may drain bilaterally close to the midline or the tip of the tongue.

Risk Factors

About 75% of all head and neck cancers are attributable to tobacco use and alcohol consumption. Above all others, cigarette smoking is the single most important risk factor, accounting for proximally 90% of oral squamous cell cancers. Tobacco contains more than thirty carcinogens, the majority of which are polycyclic aromatic hydrocarbons and nitrosamines [5]. The risk of developing oral cancer is higher for pipe and cigar smokers than in other sites. Chewing tobacco is associated with a higher risk of alveolar ridge and buccal mucosa tumors.

Although non-smoking alcohol users have a higher risk of pharyngeal cancer [6], its association with smoking has a synergistic effect, exponentially increasing the risk of cancer [7]. In drinkers, the floor of the mouth is at a higher risk for tumor development. Alcohol itself has no carcinogen effect, but acts increasing the cell membrane permeability to other carcinogens, mainly those present in tobacco, and decreasing the activity of DNA-repair enzymes.

Poor oral hygiene is often associated with oral cavity cancer, but a causal relationship is yet to be established. As patients in this condition commonly present edentulous, the chronic use of ill fit oral dentures increase the risk of cancer [8].

Several virus infections have demonstrated an increase in cancer risk, mainly by human papillomavirus (HPV) [9] and herpes simplex virus [10]. The Epstein - Barr virus, although prevalent for nasopharyngeal cancer, is rarely detected in oral tumors [11].

Although smoking and alcohol can increase the risk of lip cancer, exposure to sunlight is a more important factor, since the lip is highly susceptible to actinic changes because there is no layer of pigment for local protection. Cell damage occurs due to ultra-violet types A and B radiation, and affects more often the lower lip in its inferior border.

MOLECULAR BIOLOGY

Oral cavity squamous cell carcinomas (SCC) vary considerably in aggressiveness, metastatic potential and sensitivity to radiotherapy and chemotherapy. Histological and clinical parameters alone can not predict the potential aggressiveness or the outcome of these tumors after standard treatment.

In the past years, an effort to study biological markers for head and neck squamous cell carcinoma was performed in several cancer centers around the world. Although many studies on the subject were published, data are still controversial and a reliable tumor marker is still a utopia.

The most commonly studied marker is the p53. This protein, when mutated, plays a crucial role in carcinogenesis, acting as a tumor suppressor gene. p53 is more frequently mutated in areas of SCC of the oral cavity than in other upper aerodigestive mucosal sites [12]. In this same study, Parise et al. reported that the presence of p53 and absence of Epidermal grow factor receptor (EGFR), a type 1 transmembrane receptor of the mucosal epithelium, in oral SCC might indicate a group of patients with better prognosis. EGFR hyperexpression is often observed in other human cancers.

Other analyzed marker in this study was the c-erbB-2, also a type 1 transmembrane receptor. The loss of its expression, especially when associated with increased EGFR activity, is involved in SCC carcinogenesis and worse prognosis. Xia et al. found that c-erbB-2 overexpression correlated with shorter overall survival [13].

Geisler et al. studied somatic mutations in the p16 and p53 tumor suppressor gene showed that patients whose tumors showed increased p53 protein expression had three times the risk of dying from cancer-specific causes after adjustment for age, therapy, and stage [14].

Several other biological markers have been studied and suggested to yield additional prognostic information. In a study that compared different ratios of expression among cyclin-dependent kinases, showed that *CCND1* and/or *c-MYC* amplification, when combined with *CDKN2A* deletion, yield additional prognostic information of tumor behavior, since *c-MYC*:*CDKN2A* and *CCND1*:*CDKN2A* ratios correlated with disease-specific survival enhancement and of *c-MYC*:*CDKN2A* was associated with a shorter disease-free interval as marked by the development of recurrences or metastases [15].

Markers related to tumor neovascularization also predict outcome in head and neck patients. Both primary tumors and their micrometastases must initiate angiogenesis. Vascular endothelial growth factor (VEGF), under hypoxic conditions, promotes tumor angiogenesis in head and neck SCC and many other tumor types by stimulating endothelial-cell proliferation and promoting vascular permeability [16]. In a study by Smith et al. [17], showed that patients with VEGF-positive tumors were more likely to recur locally and distantly and that

VEGF positivity was the most significant predictor of poor disease-free survival and overall survival.

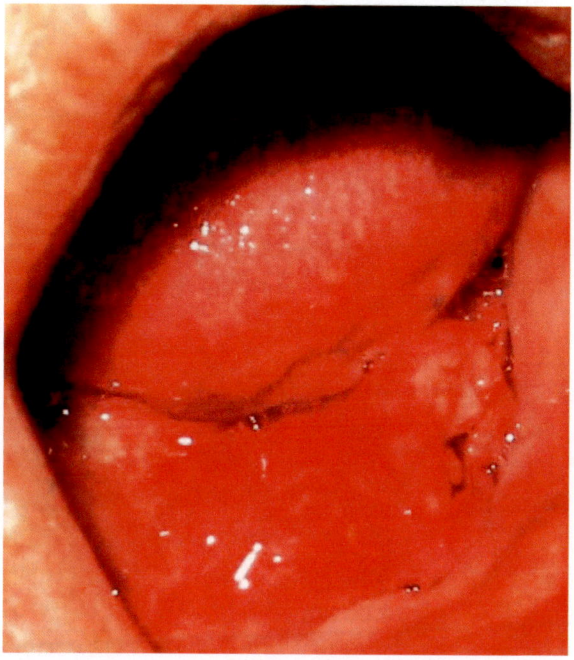

Figure 1. Floor of the mouth T2 squamous cell carcinoma.

Diagnosis

Oral cavity tumors are amenable to direct inspection, thus physical examination can provide early diagnosis. Evaluation for mouth neoplasms is based on history and physical examination, tissue sample for histological diagnosis and ancillary exams whenever indicated. A history of an ulcer lasting over 10 days, oral bleeding or mass, white or red mucosal plaques, difficulty in speech or swallowing (dysphagia), trismus, suggesting pterygoid and masticator space involvement; cranial nerve numbness such as inferior lip anesthesia, weight loss and enlarged cervical lymphnodes are clear signs of malignant disease. The history of risk factors exposure as commented above corroborates the clinical suspicion of mouth cancer. SCC may also develop from premalignant lesions such as leukoplakia or erythroplakia.

A thorough physical examination is mandatory to identify lesions that are predominantly painful and bleeding mucosal ulcerations, with or without verrucous or exophytic components. Figure 1 shows a small lateral floor of the mouth ulcerated lesion without mandibular involvement.

Oral cancers can involve bone, abutting the mandible, the hard palate or the retromolar trigone in a pushing margin involvement or, more aggressively, course with direct bone invasion [18]. The distance from the tumor to the mandible and the mobility of the lesion in relation to the mandible are critical elements in determining the management of perimandibular cancers.

Palpating neck nodes is part of routine examination for possible and often present metastatic disease in the nodal groups at risk. Neck nodes should be measured, characterized for cervical level, mobility and proximity to vital adjacent structures and deep planes, consistency and skin involvement.

At our Institution, flexible esophagoscopy with a 2% lugol dye solution is routinely used in patients undergoing treatment to detect second primary cancers [19,20] due to the high prevalence of synchronous and metachronous SCC in upper aerodigestive tract mucosa in this studied patient population [21].

To better assess the invasion of deep tissues by oral cancer, especially the bony structures; the use of imaging exams is preferred. Imaging studies, however, can not exquisitely identify the superficial mucosal extent of disease, which is best evaluated by visual inspection, palpation and incisional biopsy. Plain radiographs such as panorex or dental films can demonstrate gross bone involvement but do not show early cortical invasion.

Imaging exams may include Computed Tomography (CT) for detailed evaluation of disease extension, whether the tumor invades the bony structures of the oral cavity, and to properly assess invasion of vital structures in the neck by nodal metastases. CT advantages are good soft-tissue discrimination and vessel identification with excellent definition of bone soft-tissue interfaces. Cortical destruction and tumor in the alveolar canal and the bone marrow can be seen on CT. Figure 2 exemplifies mandibular erosion by oral SCC. Important disadvantages include radiation exposure and imaging artifacts caused by amalgams and low quality coronal view.

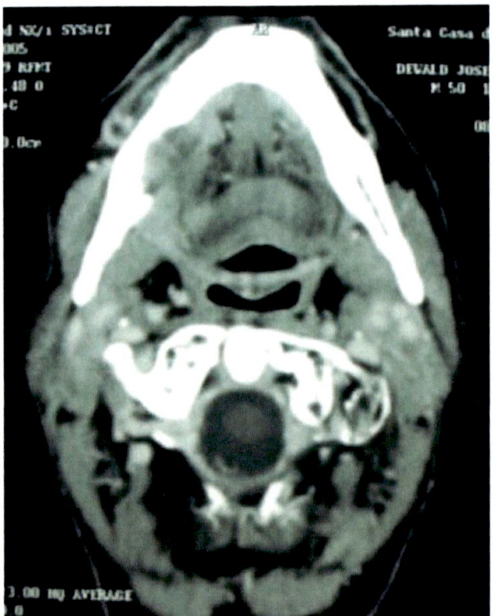

Figure 2. CT showing mandibular invasion by oral SCC.

Magnetic Resonance Imaging offers better soft tissue discrimination for tumor invasion, and enhanced assessment of central nervous system and skull base invasion. This is especially true when staging adenoid cystic carcinoma, a minor salivary gland tumor with early neural tropism and invasion [22].

Other less commonly utilized ancillary exams are PET-CT and Dentascan, which are seldom used in our practice because of the high cost. Even in the light of these exams, there is still no ideal method that identifies mandible invasion by SCC [23].

Tissue biopsy for histological confirmation is mandatory before planning treatment. Squamous cell carcinoma is histologically graded in well, moderately and poor differentiated, although these features do not alter disease survival.

After completion of data on disease extent, tumor staging according to TNM system is done to plan adequate treatment (Table 1).

Table 1. TNM staging for oral cavity cancer

Primary Tumor: T
TX Primary tumor cannot be assessed
T0 No evidence of primary tumor
Tis Carcinoma in situ
T1 Tumor 2 cm or less in greatest dimension
T2 Tumor more than 2 cm but not more than 4 cm in greatest dimension
T3 Tumor more than 4 cm in greatest dimension
T4 Tumor (lip) invades adjacent structures (through cortical bone, tongue, skin of neck)
Tumor (oral cavity) invades adjacent structures (through cortical bone, into deep [extrinsic] muscle of tongue, maxillary sinus, skin)
Regional Lymph Nodes: N
NX Regional lymph nodes cannot be assessed
N0 No regional lymph node metastasis
N1 Metastasis in a single ipsilateral lymph node, 3 cm or less in greatest dimension
N2a Metastasis in single ipsilateral lymph node more than 3 cm but not more than 6 cm in greatest dimension
N2b Metastasis in multiple ipsilateral lymph nodes, none more than 6 cm in greatest dimension
N2c Metastasis in bilateral or contralateral lymph nodes, none more than 6 cm in greatest dimension
N3 Metastasis in a lymph node more than 6 cm in greatest dimension
Distant Metastasis: M
MX Presence of distant metastasis cannot be assessed
M0 No distant metastasis
M1 Distant metastasis
Stage Grouping
Stage 0 Tis N0 M0
Stage I T1 N0 M0
Stage II T2 N0 M0
Stage III T3 N0 M0, T1 N1 M0, T2 N1 M0, T3 N1 M0
Stage IV T4 N0 MO, T4 N1 M0, Any T N2 M0, Any T N3 M0, Any T Any N M1

TREATMENT

Treatment options must take into consideration tumor and patient factors, such as primary tumor site, extent of disease, presence of positive neck nodes, bone invasion; and age, co-morbidities, performance status and patient's desire. The mainstay of oral cancer treatment is surgery (resection with wide surgical margins combined with proper neck dissection), with or without adjuvant radiotherapy. For advanced stages, adjuvant Radiotherapy is mandatory in order to reduce tumor recurrence.

External beam Radiotherapy should be used as single modality therapy when both survival and morbidity rates compare favorably with surgery treatment. Radiotherapy (RTX) is given as a daily application of 200 cGy (CentiGrays) over a 5 to 7 week period, for a total dose of 5,500 cGy to 6,500 cGy. RTX advantages include treating posterior tumors with difficult surgical exposure, equal efficacy for early T1 and T2 lesions and better outcome in terms of deglutition and speech.

Disadvantages are larger tumors (T3 and T4) respond poorly to RTX alone, should recurrences develop a second course of RTX can not be considered, high morbidity for salvage surgery in terms of infection and survival rates are extremely poor, side effects such as osteo and chondronecrosis, xerostomia and mucositis [24,25].

Interstitial irradiation or brachytherapy is commonly used combined with external RTX or surgery, mainly for cancers of the tongue and floor of the mouth. With brachytherapy larger doses of radiation can be delivered to specifically determined areas, with less morbidity to surrounding tissues and in less time. Disadvantages include the need of general anesthesia to proper position the brachytherapy catheters, risk of radiation to surrounding people, intra oral swelling, hemorrhage, severe mucositis and mandibular osteoradionecrosis.

Chemotherapy alone has no role in oral cavity cancer treatment: it is reserved for palliation only and for distant metastasis.

Surgical treatment options widely vary depending on tumor size, location in the mouth and involvement of adjacent structures, such as the mandible. Obtaining a surgical specimen for histopathological exam is of critical interest to analyze margins, histological tumor grade, vascular and perineural invasion and thus supply important information to prognostic outcome. Disadvantages are functional disabilities (speech, deglutition) and risk of postoperative complications in wide resections for advanced tumors.

Since the majority of surgical patients are middle age with a chronic history of tobacco use, preoperative management requires evaluation with blood tests, such as complete blood count, electrolytes, kidney and liver functions; chest X-rays and an electrocardiogram. Nutrition status should be emphasized, since a considerable amount of patients due to impairment to swallowing (trismus or odyphagia) and malnutrition secondary to alcoholism will be malnourished. Patients with a 10 percent or greater loss in total body weight should be put in enteral nutrition support via either nasogastric feeding tube or gastrostomy [26].

For head and neck cancer, neck dissection is performed either therapeutically or electively. In clinically positive neck nodes a therapeutic neck dissection is preferred, with a classical or modified radical neck dissection, resecting lymphnodes from level I to V. In patients with no clinically suspicious nodes (N0 neck), the procedure is indicated when there is a 15-20% risk of microscopic occult metastases. In oral cavity cancer management elective neck dissection plays an important role. The oral tongue and floor of the mouth are the two most common subsites or oral malignancies. Patients with lesions in these sites have high risk of nodal metastases. Even for T1 and T2 cancers, elective dissection is preferred. Other oral sites have minor risks of positive nodal disease and elective dissection is performed for advanced tumors [27,28]. The cervical nodes at greater risk of metastases are the lymphnodes in level I (submental and subdigastric nodes), II (jugulo-digastric) and III (mid jugular nodes), and selective neck dissection of these nodes is referred as supraomohyoid neck dissection (SOHND).

Oral Tongue Cancer

It is the most frequent site of oral cavity tumors after the lip, accounting for up to 50% of all cancers in the oral cavity. Most tumors affect the lateral border, between the middle and posterior thirds. Since the intrinsic tongue muscles offer no barrier to tumor spread, the adjacent structures (floor of the mouth, mandible, base of tongue, tonsillar pillar) are at risk for tumor involvement. Neck nodes are at risk for metastasis, and when the tumor reaches the mid line, bilateral neck metastasis can occur.

Although RTX can be used in T1 and some small T2 lesions, the majority of tongue cancers are treated surgically. For early T1 and T2 lesions, transoral resection with a partial glossectomy with 1.5cm margins of macroscopically normal tissue is the standard treatment. Intraoperative frozen sections of specimen margins is mandatory for optimizing surgical outcome. The tumor resection should be planned with a wedge like transversal incision and a horizontal suture line to close the surgical defect. Although this approach shortens the tongue in its anterior to posterior dimension, it offers a better functional result.

For larger and more advanced tumors (large and posterior T2, T3 and T4), a mandibulotomy approach is more reliable for oncologically sound resections. The paramedian mandibulotomy due to its low morbidity is the approach of choice. At our Institution, splitting the lip is not a routine, since with proper retraction, approach to larger lesions can be easily performed, even those with mandibular involvement. We reserve the lip splitting incisions for more posterior tumors, adjacent to the retromolar trigone and the tonsillar pillars.

In the N0 neck, neck dissection is indicated in T2 or larger lesions and even in thick T1 tumors. There is a 30% chance of occult nodal metastasis in tumors thicker than 5mm in depth [29], confirming its high potential for nodal disease. At Memorial Sloan-Kettering Cancer Center in New York, all T1 tumors thicker than 2mm receive adequate primary surgery plus elective SOHND, since it was demonstrated by Spiro et al. that there is a poorer survival in these patients [30,31]. Recent evidence suggests that there can be occult "skip" metastasis involving more inferior nodes (level IV), and recommendation is an "extended" SOHND, that is levels I to IV [32].

Lip Cancer

The majority of lip cancers is SCC and develops in patients chronically exposed to sun. The inferior lip is involved in 90% of cases due to incidence of sun rays. Only 7% arise in the upper lip, and 1% in the lip comissure. Inferior lesions are well differentiated T1 or T2 cancers that spread laterally rather than deeply. Upper lip and comissure tumors are more aggressive and tend to present with a deeper invasion pattern [33]. In lower lip tumors, nodal metastasis occur preferably to level I and peri-facial lymphnodes; when the lesion develops in the upper lip or comissure, nodes at risk are preauricular, periparotid and submental [34].

Lip cancer treatment is best performed by surgery. Since most lesions are T1 and T2, resection with adequate margins can almost always be performed with primary closure. RTX has the same local control, but immediate resection is a major advantage. For more advanced disease (T3 and T4) wide resection with bilateral SOHND (tumor abutting or crossing the mid line) and adjuvant RTX is necessary. Reconstruction varies on lip involvement: lesions smaller than 50% can be closed primarily, especially in the edentulous patient. In larger tumors, rotating flaps are the best choice. For lateral lip the Abbe-Estlander flap is the flap of choice; in mid line lesions, the Karapandzic advancement flap, based on the inferior labial artery, is often used.

Floor of the Mouth Cancer

The floor of the mouth accounts for 20% of all oral malignancies. Since it is a dependent site, pooling of carcinogens with a prolonged contact increases dramatically the risk of cancer. Lesions often involve the alveolar ridge, retromolar trigone or oral tongue, since this a limited small space within the oral cavity.

Treatment of T1 lesions can be effectively performed either by RTX or surgery. For small anterior tumors, the preferred treatment is transoral resection. For more advanced tumors, the mandible is usually involved and its management has a more important aspect in surgical resections. Shaha stated that in the FOM when tumors are close or adherent to the periosteum of the mandible a marginal mandibulectomy should be performed. Although he does not routinely perform a segmental mandibulectomy for more advanced lesions, preferring an oblique marginal mandibulectomy, good primary tumor control with optimum functional and cosmetic results [35]. In a study by McGregor et al., the route of mandibular invasion was analyzed. In the edentulous patients, the preferred tumor pathway is via the cortical deficiencies in the occlusal surface of bone. In the dentate nonirradiated mandible it occurs via tooth sockets, confirming that the presence of teeth is a natural barrier to cancer invasion [36]. In the irradiated mandible, invasion frequently occurs by two different routes: via the occlusal surface and directly through cortical bone, suggesting a decrease in the barrier to cancer spread effect of intact periosteum after RTX [37].

When there is gross tumor fixation in the occlusal surface of the mandible, with clinically or radiologicaly proven bone invasion, then the best approach is a segmental mandibulectomy, because when the occlusal cortical bone is invaded, no reliable barrier to vertical tumor spread via alveolar canal remains. With that in mind, there is a formal contraindication to marginal mandibulectomy when there is gross involvement of cortical bone, the inferior alveolar artery can not be preserved during surgery due to tumor involvement, the residual bone is thin and weak with a high risk of mandibular fracture, previous irradiation to the mandible and tumor abutting the bone on more than two surfaces.

Nodal metastases are present in up to 30 to 40% of FOM cancers, thus it is important to perform SOHND in all but small superficial T1 lesions [38]. In clinically positive neck metastases a more comprehensive dissection is preferred, either a modified radical or the classical radical neck dissection. Bilateral SOHND is indicated whenever the tumor is at or crosses the mid line.

Cancer of Buccal Mucosa

This specific oral tumor is associated with alcohol and tobacco consumption as well as with smokeless tobacco and betel nut chewing. Although rare in western societies, this site is frequently involved in India, where the habit of betel nut chewing is widely spread. Buccal mucosa cancers are commonly exophytic or verrucous in clinical presentation, rather than deeply infiltrative ulcerations. Advanced stage tumors in this site can involve the retromolar trigone, the alveolar ridge, hard palate and maxillary sinus.

Occult metastases occur in 10% of patients, although 50% can present with clinically palpable nodes. Frequent sites of lymphatic spread are submandibular nodes, and rarely periparotid and superior jugular lymphnodes [39].

Treatment for early tumors includes both RTX and surgery. RTX has a disadvantage because there is a risk of worsening preexisting trismus. Surgery is the treatment of choice in ulcerative lesions and tumors that involve bony structures. T1 and T2 cancers can be treated by per oral resection. T3 and T4 lesions often require a cheek flap and in more advanced cases maxillectomy or segmental mandibulectomy, depending on the invasiveness of these tumors. For larger tumors adjuvant RTX is mandatory.

Neck dissection in clinically negative patients is not recommended, since the rate of occult metastases is low (10%).

Cancer of Retromolar Trigone

The retromolar trigone is a portion of buccal mucosa that covers the ascending ramus of the mandible. Although it is very small in surface area, tumors in this site are not infrequent, accounting for 15% of all oral lesions. Cancers in this area are often difficult to diagnose due to its particular posterior situation within the oral cavity, besides the overlying mucosa is irregular and both dentition and the often verified trismus make inspection challenging. Tumors readily spread to adjacent structures such as the periosteum of the ascending ramus of the mandible, masticator space and pterygoid muscles, skull base and oropharynx. The inferior alveolar nerve is a route to central nervous system invasion.

Treatment comprehends surgery almost always including bone resection, contraindicating per oral resections. A segmental mandibulectomy of the ascending ramus is the surgical procedure of choice when there is gross tumor involvement in the mandible, although in selected cases a marginal mandibulectomy can be performed for early T1 cancers.

Occult metastases are found in 30-39% of patients. Elective neck dissection of levels I to III are indicated for T3 and T4 lesions. For clinically palpable nodes a modified radical neck dissection is indicated [40].

Cancer of the Alveolar Ridge

SCC of alveolar ridge accounts for 10% of oral cavity malignancies, frequently involving the lower portion, in the posterior dental arch of edentulous areas in the free margin of the gingiva. Advanced tumors commonly invade the floor of the mouth and buccal mucosa. Besides smoking and drinking, ill-fitting oral dentures seem to play a role in cancer development. Half the patients will have involvement of the mandible and lymphnode metastases will be present clinically in 30% and microscopically in 15% of patients [41]. Lymphatic metastases frequently involve the level II nodes.

Treatment is best performed with surgery, for bone invasion is not radiocurable. Small lesions of the superior alveolar ridge can be performed transoraly, and larger lesions will require a maxillectomy. For inferior tumors, the marginal mandibulectomy is adequate for early lesions and segmental mandibulectomy for advanced cancers. Elective SOHND is indicated for T3 and T4 lesions.

Cancer of the Hard Palate

Hard palate cancers are uncommon malignancies, accounting for less than 10% of oral cavity tumors. In areas of South East Asia the reverse smoking habit highly increases the risk of cancer in the palate [42]. The mucosal lining is firmly adherent to the periosteum, conferring a barrier to tumor spread and invasion.

Palatal cancers tend to be advanced lesions on diagnosis and neck metastases decrease the overall survival in five years from 70 to 30% [43]. Lesions are often from the well differentiated ulcerative type, with surrounding areas of leukoplakia. Occult metastases are rare, and clinically positive nodes are found in only 10 to 25% of patients [44]. Levels I and II are the most commonly involved.

Surgery is the first choice in treating palatal cancers, since invasive malignancies involve the mucoperiosteum of the underlying bone, reducing the success rate of exclusive RTX. Per oral resection with 1cm margins is satisfactory in early lesions with closure performed with posterior mucoperiosteum palatal flap based on the greater palatine artery. Advanced tumors with maxillary involvement require partial or total maxillectomy via a Weber-Ferguson or degloving approaches. Spiro et al. classified the maxillectomy in limited, when only one wall of the antrum was resected; subtotal when two or more were resected, including the palate;

and total when a complete resection is performed [45]. Rarely a radical maxillectomy with orbital exanteration is needed.

Due to low incidence of occult metastases, neck dissection is only performed in clinically suspicious nodes.

Adjuvant RTX is indicated with T3 and T4 cancers, positive or close margins and perineural invasion.

Reconstruction

For all oral cavity sites, surgical reconstruction is a challenge, often due to the extent of tissue resection. When reconstructive surgery is not properly planned defects will result in significant complications and decreased speech and deglutition abilities. Aesthetic mutilation is also of major concern and patients with disfigurement secondary to surgical resections may experience depression and loss of normal social activities.

Immediate reconstructive surgery at the time of tumor resection is always advised. It prevents scar retraction and fibrosis of the surgical defect, reducing the number of surgical procedures. Restoring function and form and minimize donor site deformity is the main goal for reconstructive surgeons.

The best option is free tissue transfer with microsurgical techniques, but pedicled myocutaneous flaps are used in some cases. For oromandibular defects the microvascular technique with either the composite fibular free flap or the iliac crest free flap has better functional results, and a comparison between techniques by Head et al. showed a clear advantage for microvascular option [46]. Urken et al. in his 11-year series of 210 patients with oromandibular reconstruction with microvascular bone free flaps, including immediate endosteal dental implants, had a success rate of 96%, with only 16 complications in vascular anastomosis [47].

Gullane [48] reported a series of 64 patients treated with bridging plates with excellent results and only 15.6% of complications defending its indication, but in a latter article he endorsed the routinely use of microvascular free flaps [49].

At out Institution bridging plates are used only for benign disease in which patients are not candidates for adjuvant treatment with RTX because the high index of complications in irradiated subjects [50].

Myocutaneous flap is a muscle segment that rotates to cover a surgical defect based in its own pedicle and blood supply, and an overlying skin paddle perfused by perforating vessels that arise from the main vascular pedicle. Advantages are simple harvesting technique, versatility, reliable pedicle and proximity to the head and neck area. Disadvantages include the limited arc of rotation with consequent inability to reach the farthermost portions of the scalp, risk of necrosis of the borders of the paddle and unaesthetic donor site defect.

The pectoralis major myocutaneous flap is the most frequently used pedicled flap in reconstructive head and neck surgery. Its pedicle is formed by branches of the thoracoacromial trunk that pierces the clavipectoral fascia. Advantages are its readily assessable pedicle, ease of harvesting, wide arc of rotation and the ease of primary closure of donor site. Disadvantages include its bulk for intraoral reconstruction and the thoracic wall scarring with nipple distortion. A new, safer and quicker harvesting technique is proposed the authors [51].

For intraoral reconstruction a more pliable flap is needed to replace the original lining, and the flap of choice is the infrahyoid myocutaneous flap described by Wang et al. [52]. Due to its thinness and malleability, its use for oral cavity reconstruction provides favorable cosmetic and functional results, and complications are easy to manage [53]. Other less used flaps are the lastissimus dorsi, temporalis and trapezius.

The routine use of pedicled flaps was studied by Vartanian et al. in a series of 437 patients, and the overall success was over 70%, although defects were not located solely in the oral cavity.

Current trend is to the broader use of microvascular free flaps, although pedicled flaps remain an important surgical tool in head and neck reconstruction due to its ease of harvest and low morbidity rates.

Rehabilitation

Following major oral cavity tumor resections, patients need to restore their ability to speak, chew and swallow as well as reestablish cosmesis. An important element after surgery is the combined efforts of a multidisciplinary team of head and neck surgeons, plastic reconstructive surgeons, speech therapists, nurses and dentists to achieve the best functional results in cancer therapy.

Mandibular reconstructive surgery has greatly improved after the microvascular free tissue transplants, allowing maximum quality in bone and mucosa reconstruction after radical surgery. Appropriate reconstructive procedures will enhance the postoperative abilities of speech and swallowing. Mastication is greatly dependent on oral competence and mandibular arch continuity, although segmental defects of the ascending ramus can be well tolerated by the patients.

A common complication after radiation therapy is xerostomia. Minor salivary glands are critically affected by RTX and a dry mouth will result. To avoid this inconvenience, the use of pilocarpine is indicated, which will facilitate food lubrication and swallowing.

Oral prosthodontist specialist is critical to achieve superior swallowing rehabilitation. Teeth play an important role in quality of mastication and deglutition, so a proper number and alignment is crucial to plan a proper denture. Oral obturators are ideal for coverage after hard palate and maxilla surgical resections, avoiding nasal regurgitation. Osseointegrated implants are important for obturator fixation. When there is adequate bone surface, titanium implants can be placed to better hold prosthesis in place.

Speech therapists play an important role in rehabilitation. Specialists practice exercises with the patients to improve speech and help the prosthodontist to manufacture the best obturator for each case. They can as well help the patient enhance the ability to swallow and chew recommending the best individualized food consistency to be served in meals.

Nutritionists are essential in patients with dietary negative balance. Proper nutrition therapy maintains a positive balance and sometimes it depends on nutritional supplements combined with everyday food. If oral intake is insufficient tube feeding via nasogastric tube or temporary gastrostomy is often required. Monitoring the patient's weight is crucial to reevaluate dietary intake needs.

Team effort is the key to success in rehabilitating oral cavity cancer patients after radical tumor resection.

PROGNOSIS

Patients treated for oral cavity cancer have different survivals depending on clinical stage. Low T stage, low N stage and absence of co-morbidities enhance overall survival. Early T1 and T2 lesions have 70-90% 5-year survival and the presence of nodal disease reduces survival in 50%. For advanced disease, especially large T4 with bilateral positive nodes survival ranges no farther than 20% [54,55]. For resectable advanced T3 and T4, even with N1 neck, with high dose adjuvant RTX survival increased to 50% in five years [56]. Better local control has increased deaths by distant metastases or second primary tumors.

As mentioned earlier in this chapter, currently there is no biological marker that can accurately predict survival. In coming years markers will be sensitive enough to predict cancer behavior and to better select treatment options with Chemorradiation or surgery and RTX.

REFERENCES

[1] Boyle J, Strong EW. Oral Cavity Cancer. In: Shah JP. *Cancer of the Head and Neck*. BC Decker. Hamilton, London. 2001. pg 100-126.

[2] www.inca.gov.br/

[3] www.nccn.org/professionals/physician_gls/PDF/head-and-neck.pdf

[4] Slaughter DP, Southwick HW, Smejkal J. "Field cancerization" in oral stratified squamous epithelium. *Cancer*. 1953; 5:963-8.

[5] International Agency for Research on Cancer. *Tobacco smoking: IARC Monograph on the evaluation of the carcinogenic risk of chemicals to humans*. Washington (DC): IARC; 1986.

[6] Maier H, Sennewald E, Heller GF, Weidauer H. Chronic alcohol consumption- the key risk factor for pharyngeal cancer. *Otalaryngol Head Neck Surg*. 1994; 110:168-73.

[7] Brugere J, Guenel P, Leclerc A, Rodriguez J. Differential effects of tobacco and alcohol in cancer of the larynx, pharynx and mouth. *Cancer*. 1986; 57:391-5.

[8] Velly AM, Franco EL, Schlecht N. Relationship between dental factors and risk of upper aerodigestive tract cancer. *Oral Oncol*. 1998; 34:284-91.

[9] McKaig RG, Baric RS, Olshan AF. Human papillomavirus and head and neck cancer: epidemiology and molecular biology. *Head Neck*. 1998 May;20(3):250-65.

[10] Kassim KH, Daley TD. Herpes simplex virus type proteins in human oral squamous cell carcinoma. *Oral Surg Oral Med Oral Pathil Oral Radiol Endod*. 1988; 65: 445-8.

[11] Liavaag PG, Cheung RK, Kerrebijin JD, Freeman JL, Irish JC, Dosch HM. The physiologic reservoir of Epstein-Barr virus does not map to upper aerodigestive tissues. *Laryngoscope*. 1998 Jan;108(1Pt 1):42-6.

[12] Parise Junior O, Carvalho LV, Miguel RE, Kowalski LP. Prognostic impact of p53, c-erbB-2 and epidermal growth factor receptor on head and neck carcinoma. *Sao Paulo Med J*. 2004 Nov 4;122(6):264-8.

[13] Xia W, Lau YK, Zhang HZ, Liu AR, Li L, Kiyokawa N, Clayman GL, Katz RL, Hung MC. Strong correlation between c-erbB-2 overexpression and overall survival of patients with oral squamous cell carcinoma. *Clin Cancer Res*. 1997; 3(1):3-9.

[14] Geisler SA, Olshan AF, Weissler MC, Cai J, Funkhouser WK, Smith J, Vick K. p16 and p53 Protein expression as prognostic indicators of survival and disease recurrence from head and neck cancer. *Clin Cancer Res*. 2002.8(11):3445-53.

[15] Akervall J, Bockmuhl U, Petersen I, Yang K, Carey TE, Kurnit DM. The gene ratios c-MYC:cyclin-dependent kinase (CDK)N2A and CCND1:CDKN2A correlate with poor prognosis in squamous cell carcinoma of the head and neck. *Clin Cancer Res*. 2003;9(5):1750-5.

[16] Denhart BC, Guidi AJ, Tognazzi K, Dvorak HF, Brown LF. Vascular permeability factor/vascular endothelial growth factor and its receptors in oral and laryngeal squamous cell carcinoma and dysplasia. *Lab Invest*. 1997;77(6):659-64.

[17] Smith BD, Smith GL, Carter D, Sasaki CT, Haffty BG. Prognostic significance of vascular endothelial growth factor protein levels in oral and oropharyngeal squamous cell carcinoma. *J Clin Oncol*. 2000;18(10):2046-52.

[18] Wong RJ, Keel SB, Glynn RJ, Varvares MA. Histological pattern of mandibular invasion by oral squamous cell carcinoma. *Laryngoscope*. 2000;110(1):65-72.

[19] Tincani AJ, Brandalise N, Altemani A, Scanavini RC, Valerio JB, Lage HT, Molina G, Martins AS. Diagnosis of superficial esophageal cancer and dysplasia using endoscopic screening with a 2% lugol dye solution in patients with head and neck cancer. *Head Neck*. 2000;22(2):170-4.

[20] Tincani AJ, Brandalise N, Andreollo NA, Lopes LR, Montes CG, Altemani A, Martins AS. Importance of upper digestive endoscopy using lugol dye solution for the diagnosis of superficial esophageal cancer and dysplasia in patients with head and neck neoplasms. *Arq Gastroenterol*. 2000;37(2):107-13. Portuguese.

[21] Martins AS. Multicentricity in pharyngoesophageal tumors: argument for total pharyngolaryngoesophagectomy and gastric transposition. *Head Neck*. 2000; 37(3):156-63.

[22] Fodice J, Kershaw C, El-Naggar A, Goepfert H. Adenoid cystic carcinoma of the head and neck: predictors of morbidity and mortality. *Arch Otolaryngol Head Neck Surg*. 1999;125(2):149-52.

[23] Acton CH, Layt C, Gwynne R, Cooke R, Seaton D. Investigative modalities of mandibular invasion by squamous cell carcinoma. *Laryngoscope*. 2000; 110(12):2050-5.

[24] Goodwin WJ Jr. Salvage surgery for patients with recurrent squamous cell carcinoma of the upper aerodigestive tract: when do the ends justify the means? *Laryngoscope*. 2000; 110(3 Pt 2 Suppl 93): 1-18.

[25] Schwartz GJ, Mehta RH, Wenig BL, Shaligram C, Portugal LG. Salvage treatment for recurrent squamous cell carcinoma of the oral cavity. *Head Neck.* 2000;22(1):34-41.

[26] Williams EF III, Meguid MM. Nutritional concepts and considerations in head and neck surgery. *Head Neck.* 1989;11: 393-9.

[27] Lydiatt DD, Robbins KT, Byers RM, Wolf PF. Treatment of stage I and II oral tongue cancer. *Head Neck.* 1993;15(4):308-12.

[28] Robbins KT. Indications for selective neck dissection: when, how, and why. *Oncology* (Williston Park). 2000;14(10):1455-64; discussion 1467-9.

[29] Fukano H, Matsuura H, Hasegawa Y, Nakamura S. Depth of invasion as a predictive factor for cervical lymph node metastasis in tongue carcinoma. *Head Neck.* 1997;19: 205-10.

[30] Spiro RH, Huvos AG, Wong GY, Spiro JD, Gnecco CA, Strong EW. Predictive value of tumor thickness in squamous carcinoma confined to the tongue and floor of the mouth. *Am J Surg.* 1986;152: 345-50.

[31] Spiro RH, Morgan GJ, Strong EW, Shah JP. Supraomohyoid neck dissection. *Am J Surg.* 1996;172(6): 650-3.

[32] Byers RM, Weber RS, Andrews T, McGill D, Kare R, Wolf P. Frequency and therapeutic implications of "skip metastases" in the neck from squamous carcinoma of the oral tongue. *Head Neck.* 1997;19(1):14-9.

[33] Zitsch RP. Carcinoma of the lip. *Otolaryngol Clin North Am.* 1993;26(2): 265-77.

[34] Jorgensen K, Elbrond O, Andersen AP. Carcinoma of the lip. A series of 869 cases. *Acta Radiol Ther Phys Biol.* 1973;12(3):177-90.

[35] Shaha AR. Marginal mandibulectomy for carcinoma of the floor of the mouth. *J Surg Oncol.* 1992;49(2):116-9.

[36] McGregor IA, MacDonald DG. Spread of squamous cell carcinoma to the nonirradiated edentulous mandible--a preliminary report. *Head Neck Surg.* 1987;9(3):157-61.

[37] McGregor AD, McDonald DG. Routes of entry of squamous cell carcinoma to the mandible. *Head Neck Surg.* 1988;10(5):294-301.

[38] Hudson DA, Stannard CE, Binnewald B, Price B. The role of suprahyoid block dissection in carcinoma of the floor of the mouth. *J Surg Oncol.* 1994;55(1):20-3.

[39] Bloom ND, Spiro RH. Carcinoma of the cheek mucosa. A retrospective analysis. *Am J Surg.* 1980;140(4):556-9.

[40] Byers RM, Anderson B, Schwarz EA, Fields RS, Meoz R. Treatment of squamous carcinoma of the retromolar trigone. *Am J Clin Oncol.* 1984;7(6):647-52.

[41] Byers RM, Newman R, Russell N, Yue A. Results of treatment for squamous carcinoma of the lower gum. *Cancer.* 1981 May 1;47(9):2236-8.

[42] Petruzzelli GJ, Myers EN. Malignant neoplasms of the hard palate and upper alveolar ridge. *Oncology.* 1994;8(4):43-8; discussion 50, 53.

[43] Evans JF, Shah JP. Epidermoid carcinoma of the palate. *Am J Surg.* 1981; 142:415-5.

[44] Ratzer ER, Schweitzer RJ, Frazell EL. Epidermoid carcinoma of the palate. *Am J Surg.* 1970;119(3):294-7

[45] Spiro RH, Strong EW, Shah JP. Maxillectomy and its classification. *Head Neck.* 1997;19(4):309-14.

[46] Head C, Alam D, Sercarz JA, Lee JT, Rawnsley JD, Berke GS, Blackwell KE. Microvascular flap reconstruction of the mandible: a comparison of bone grafts and bridging plates for restoration of mandibular continuity. *Otolaryngol Head Neck Surg*. 2003;129(1):48-54.

[47] Urken ML, Buchbinder D, Costantino PD, Sinha U, Okay D, Lawson W, Biller HF. Oromandibular reconstruction using microvascular composite flaps: report of 210 cases. *Arch Otolaryngol Head Neck Surg*. 1998;124(1):46-55.

[48] Gullane PJ. Primary mandibular reconstruction: analysis of 64 cases and evaluation of interface radiation dosimetry on bridging plates. *Laryngoscope*. 1991;101(6 Pt 2 Suppl 54):1-24.

[49] Davidson J, Boyd B, Gullane P, Rotstein L, Freeman J, Manktelow R, Rosen I. A comparison of the results following oromandibular reconstruction using a radial forearm flap with either radial bone or a reconstruction plate. *Plast Reconstr Surg*. 1991;88(2):201-8.

[50] Del Negro A, Tincani AJ, Araujo PPC, Martins AS. Alternatives in mandibular reconstruction. *Rev Bras Cir Cabeça Pescoço*; 35(4):241-3.

[51] Tincani AJ, Del Negro A, Araújo PPC, Salata F, Martins AS.

[52] Wang HS, Shen JW, Ma DB, Wang JD, Tian AL. The infrahyoid myocutaneous flap for reconstruction after resection of head and neck cancer. *Cancer*. 1986. 1;57(3):663-8.

[53] Tincani AJ, Del Negro A, Araujo PP, Akashi HK, Neves F da S, Martins AS. Head and neck reconstruction using infrahyoid myocutaneous flaps. *Sao Paulo Med J*. 2006 Sep 7;124(5):271-4.

[54] Franceschi D, Gupta R, Spiro RH, Shah JP. Improved survival in the treatment of squamous carcinoma of the oral tongue. *Am J Surg*. 1993 Oct;166(4):360-5.

[55] Kowalski LP, Bagietto R, Lara JR, Santos RL, Silva JF Jr, Magrin J. Prognostic significance of the distribution of neck node metastasis from oral carcinoma. *Head Neck*. 2000 May;22(3):207-14.

[56] Vikram B, Strong EW, Shah JP, Spiro R. Failure in the neck following multimodality treatment for advanced head and neck cancer. *Head Neck Surg*. 1984;6(3):724-9.

In: Progress in Oral Cancer Research
Editor: Frederik L. Nielsen, pp 91-106

ISBN 978-1-60021-865-1

Chapter IV

CHRONIC PERIODONTITIS AND THE RISK OF ORAL CANCER

***Mine Tezal*[1, 2] *and Maureen A. Sullivan*[1, 2]**
[1]State University of New York at Buffalo, Buffalo, NY, USA;
[2]Roswell Park Cancer Institute, Buffalo, NY, USA.

ABSTRACT

Morbidity and mortality from oral cancer are high and this has not improved in decades in spite of extensive research. A significant portion of research is concentrated on chemoprevention. However, advances in this field have not translated into a visible change in mortality and morbidity. In addition, existing chemoprevention strategies have two important obstacles: toxicity and reversal of the effects after cessation of treatment. Chronic infection and inflammation have been linked to carcinogenesis in a few organs. For oral cancer, substantial evidence has accumulated for the role of *human papillomavirus* (HPV). However, the development of an effective preventive vaccine strategy for oral cancer is still years away and the target population is largely unexplored. Therefore, safe and practical additional approaches are necessary to change the status quo of oral cancer. Periodontitis is a chronic oral infection caused by inflammatory reactions in response to gram negative anaerobic bacteria in the endogenous dental plaque. It leads to irreversible destruction of tissues around teeth clinically detectable as periodontal pockets and alveolar bone loss. Periodontal pockets have been suggested as reservoirs of HPV. Chronic proliferation and ulceration of the pocket epithelium may help HPV's initial infection and persistence. Our preliminary results from existing data at Roswell Park Cancer Institute suggest a robust independent association between the history of periodontitis and incident oral cancer. Our next step is to test the synergy between periodontitis and HPV for the risk of oral cancer. If this is true, it will translate to practical and safe prevention and treatment strategies. This chapter will review the evidence supporting the association between chronic periodontitis and oral cancer as well as HPV-periodontitis synergy.

INTRODUCTION

Oral cancer is a significant cause of morbidity and mortality and this has not changed for decades. It is estimated that 34,360 new cases of oral cancer and 7,550 deaths will occur in 2007 [1]. The incidence is open to debate because of the well-known field cancerization phenomenon in the head and neck region. Those with primary cancer of the oral cavity and pharynx are also at high risk for developing cancer of the esophagus, larynx, lung, and stomach. Oral cancer is notorious for its high rates of second primary cancers, recurrence, and distant metastases [2-4]. It often leaves the patients with disfiguration and loss of vital functions such as swallowing and breathing. Consequent psychological and social impairments are also very debilitating. The treatment is aggressive and often increases the morbidity without improving the survival significantly [5].

Even though oral cancer is largely preventable, the majority of funded research has been on treatment and diagnosis. However, advances in these fields have not translated into a visible change in grim oral cancer statistics. Primary prevention strategies against risk factors, mostly tobacco, alcohol and diet, are limited and have not been very effective. Most of the existing prevention strategies are secondary and tertiary. Preventive surgical resection, radiotherapy, photodynamic therapy and topical cytotoxic therapies had limited success [6, 7]. Chemoprevention, including retinoids, selenium, vitamin E, interferon- α (IFN-α), cyclo-oxygenase-2 (COX-2) and epidermal growth factor receptor (EGFR) tyrosine kinase inhibitors, have two important obstacles: toxicity and reversal of the effects after cessation of treatment [8-10]. Chronic infections with viruses, especially certain human papillomavirus strains (HPV 16 and 18) are another target for prevention. The vaccine targeting HPV types 6, 11, 16 and 18 became recently available for cervical cancer. However, the vaccine is prophylactic and is not effective for those who were previously exposed to the virus. It is expensive and requires 3 injections over a 6 month-period. Since the longest trial was 5 years, we don't know the length of immunity from the vaccine nor its long-term safety. Even though the vaccine is effective against infection, its effectiveness to prevent invasive cancer is not known [11-12]. Information concerning the role of viruses in oral cancer is fragmented and the development of an effective vaccine strategy may still be years away. The target population who would derive the most benefit from the vaccine is largely unexplored. Therefore, safe and practical additional approaches are necessary to change the status quo of oral cancer.

Although most studies assessing the infectious etiology of cancer are focused on viruses, the evidence on bacterial infections is also convincing [13-14]. Associations with *Helicobacter pylori* infection with gastric cancer and primary B-cell gastric lymphoma [15], *Chlamydia pneumonia* infection with lung cancer [16], *Salmonella typhi* infection with gallbladder cancer [17] and *Streptococcus bovis* infection with colon cancer [18] are a few examples. Recently, there are also a growing number of basic science studies identifying key molecular mechanisms [19-24].

Opposing effects of acute vs. chronic infection on cancer have been described. While chronic infection usually promotes cancer development, acute infection was shown to counteract cancer development. For example, a few studies showed that subjects who contracted *Salmonella typhi* but did not become carriers were not at higher risk for hepatobiliary carcinoma but only those who became chronic carriers were at high risk [25-27]. The process of acute infection is self-limiting. Pro-inflammatory cytokines give way to anti-inflammatory cytokines as healing progresses. In chronic infection, on the other hand, active tissue destruction and repair proceed simultaneously. Angiogenesis and fibrosis are the chief components of this process and chronic inflammatory cells and mediators persist in the environment [28, 29]. Therefore, chronicity of the infection/inflammation appears to be the key factor for carcinogenesis.

Chronic Periodontitis

Periodontitis is a chronic oral infection caused by inflammatory reactions in response to microorganisms in the endogenous dental plaque (Figure 1). The average prevalence of periodontitis in the general population is 30%; about 12% is a severe form [30-33].

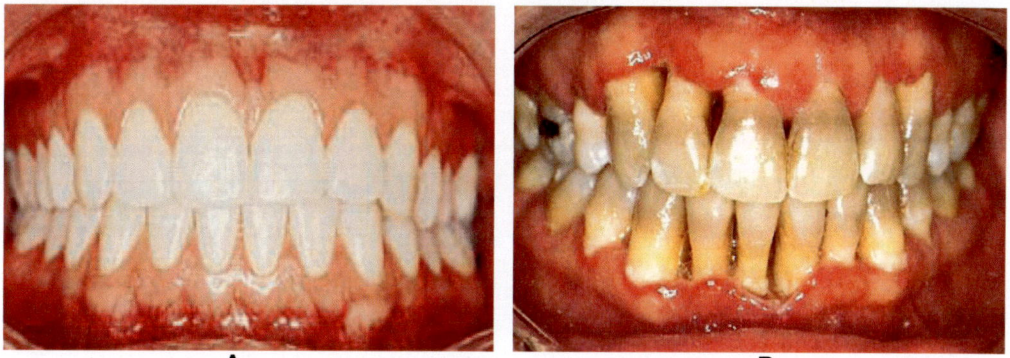

A. B.

Figure 1. Comparison of healthy periodontium (A) with periodontitis (B).

The dental plaque is a biofilm. It is critical to understand the characteristics of the biofilm to effectively control periodontitis as well as its systemic sequela. Biofilms are sessile community of various types of bacteria embedded in a polymeric matrix irreversibly attached to a surface. The majority of bacteria in the body exist in biofilms. A main characteristic of biofilms is quorum sensing which is communication and group behavior of bacteria residing in the biofilm. The bacteria in the biofilm differ profoundly from their free floating counterparts and are resistant to antimicrobials as well to host defense [34]. Mechanical removal of the biofilm, by brushing and flossing, is required. In the presence of periodontitis, however, biofilm in the periodontal pockets is inaccessible to personal oral hygiene practices and professional treatment is needed. It is important to note that biofilm properties of the dental plaque contribute to the persistence of periodontitis in the absence of treatment. Treatment of chronic periodontitis is safe and is based on mechanical removal of the biofilm. Chemotherapy alone is not effective [30].

Periodontitis results in a chronic release of inflammatory chemokines, cytokines, prostaglandins, growth factors and enzymes in saliva and to a lower degree in blood, all of which are also associated with carcinogenesis. The extent and severity of periodontitis are associated with the level of these inflammatory markers. The ensuing chronic inflammation is what leads to local pathologic anatomic changes, namely, periodontal pocket formation and alveolar bone loss [30]. As the disease progresses, epithelial attachment at the bottom of the periodontal pocket migrates apically along the root surface and the pocket depth increases. The pocket epithelium is characterized by continuous proliferation, formation of rete-ridges and ulcerations. In the connective tissue, there is increased angiogenesis, chronic inflammatory infiltrate, fibrosis and tissue loss (figure 2). Furthermore, periodontal pathogens and inflammatory mediators travel with saliva and blood from the affected tissues to distant sites and adversely affect systemic health. Multiple studies have shown that oral pathogens and cytokines are aspirated to lungs by saliva and are transported to arterial plaques by blood [31-38]. Most importantly, treatment of periodontal infections significantly prevents systemic adverse events [39-43]. We anticipate that the same mechanisms may play a part in the field cancerization of oral cancer.

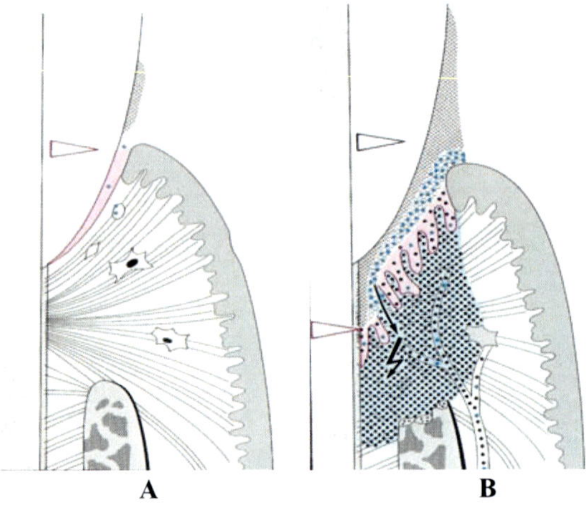

Figure 2. Tissue changes from periodontal health (A) to chronic periodontitis (B).

Poor oral hygiene (dental biofilm) is the cause of periodontitis but only small percentage of subjects with poor oral hygiene develops periodontitis [30]. A link between poor oral hygiene and the risk of oral cancer has also been suggested for a long time [44-54]. However, a definite association has not been established due to limited methodology of existing studies. We anticipate that among subjects with poor oral hygiene, those who develop periodontitis are at higher risk for oral cancer.

We are currently conducting an NIH funded study to test the hypothesis that chronic periodontitis is associated with increased risk of head and neck cancers using existing data at Roswell Park Cancer Institute (RPCI), Buffalo, NY. We have analyzed a subset of this population with a case-control study design. These preliminary analyses were restricted to subjects newly diagnosed with primary squamous cell carcinoma of tongue between June 15, 1999 and November 17, 2005. The control group consisted of subjects admitted during the same time period but not diagnosed with cancer. Children (age <21), edentulous, and those with prior history of cancer, cancer therapy and oral dysplasia were excluded. A total of 94 cases and 153 controls met the inclusion criteria. Histological diagnoses of cancer cases were available electronically from RPCI Tumor Registry. Cumulative history of periodontitis was measured by alveolar bone loss (ABL) from panoramic radiographs using an operator-interactive program on digitized radiographic images [55-58]. Accuracy and reliability of this technique have been established [59, 60]. ABL was measured in millimeter (mm) on mesial and distal sites of all teeth. One trained and calibrated examiner, blind to cancer status, performed all ABL measurements. Number of missing teeth, fillings, cavities and endodontic (root canal) treatments were also diagnosed from the radiographs. The independent effect of ABL on oral cancer was estimated from multiple logistic regression analysis by odds ratio (OR) and 95% confidence interval (CI). Each millimeter of alveolar bone loss was associated with 4.47 fold increase in the risk of tongue cancer (OR=4.47, 95% CI=2.80-7.15) after adjusting the effects of age at diagnosis, gender, race/ethnicity, smoking status, alcohol use and number of teeth. The remaining oral variables cavities, fillings, crowns and endodontic treatments were not significantly associated with the risk of tongue cancer (Table 1).

Table 1. Adjusted Odds Ratios for the Risk of Tongue Cancer (N=247)

	OR*	95% CI#	p
Mean ABL (per mm)	4.47	2.80 - 7.15	<0.001
At least 1 Site with ABL ≥4 mm (per site)	9.67	4.01 - 22.82	<0.001
Missing Teeth (per tooth)	1.02	0.98 - 1.05	0.357
Decayed Teeth (per tooth)	0.95	0.83 - 1.09	0.493
Filled Teeth (per tooth)	1.04	0.97 - 1.11	0.253
Crowns (per tooth)	0.91	0.83 - 1.01	0.080
Endodontic Treatments (per tooth)	0.89	0.74 - 1.06	0.197

*Odds ratios adjusted for age at diagnosis, gender, race, alcohol use, smoking status and number of teeth; # 95% Confidence intervals.

In summary, this study, analyzing existing patient records at a local comprehensive cancer center, confirmed our suspicions that the history of periodontitis may in fact be associated with oral cancer independent of smoking. However, the study had the classical shortcomings of secondary data analyses: Data on confounding variables was limited. In addition, the diagnosis of periodontitis was based on radiographs. Radiographic assessment of periodontal disease is not sensitive, does not reflect present disease status nor differentiate gingivitis from periodontitis. The encouraging results of this preliminary study provide the basis for further studies with quantitative clinical measures and comprehensive assessment of confounding.

Biological Mechanism

The question of how infections can influence cancer has interested scientists for over one and a half centuries, but only now are the general principles and the real complexity of this subject emerging. Chronic infections, such as periodontitis, can play a direct or indirect role in carcinogenesis:

1. Direct Toxic Effect of Microorganisms

Microorganisms and their products such as endotoxins (LPS), enzymes (proteases, collagenases, fibrinolysin and phospholipase A) and metabolic by-products (H_2S, NH_3 and fatty acids) are toxic to surrounding cells and may directly induce mutations in tumor suppressor genes and protooncogenes or alter signaling pathways that affect cell proliferation and/or survival of epithelial cells [27]. *Porphyromonas gingivalis* is a major periodontal pathogen that is capable of invading epithelial cells. In a recent study, *P.gingivalis* induced a transient increase in keratynocyte DNA fragmentation; however, after prolonged incubation, *P. gingivalis* blocked apoptosis in keratynocytes [61]. Another example of direct bacterial stimuli is the association between *Helicobacter pylori* and primary B-cell gastric lymphoma, where chronic infection causes persistent B-cell activation culminating in chromosomal rearrangements that ultimately cause cancer [15]. Numerous other studies support the evidence that commensal bacteria can directly affect various stages of cell cycle in carcinogenesis [62-64].

2. Indirect Effect through Inflammation

Chronic infection may stimulate carcinogenesis through an indirect mechanism involving activation of surrounding host cells (neutrophils, macrophages, monocytes, lymphocytes, fibroblasts and epithelial cells) to generate:

- Reactive oxygen species (hydrogen peroxide and oxy radicals), reactive nitrogen species (nitric oxides), reactive lipids and metabolites (malondialdehyhe, 4-hydroxy-2-nonenal) and matrix metalloproteases (MMPs) which can act as endogenous mutagens and can induce DNA damage in epithelial cells [28].
- Cytokines, chemokines, growth factors and other signals which provide an environment for cell survival, proliferation, migration, angiogenesis and inhibition of apoptosis [65]. This environment:
    - Help epithelial cells to accumulate mutations.
    - Drive these mutant epithelial cells to proliferate, migrate and give them a growth advantage

Recently, a key molecular mechanism connecting inflammation and cancer was identified. It was shown that a pro-inflammatory gene is involved in cancer development and that inactivation of this gene could dramatically (80%) reduce tumor development [22]. A subsequent study showed that cancer metastasis was halted with inhibition of a pro-inflammatory protein, nuclear factor-kappa B (NF-κB) or an inflammatory mediator, tumor necrosis factor alpha (TNF-α) [23]. Another study showed how prostaglandin E_2 (PGE_2) promotes colorectal adenoma growth [24]. Numerous other studies have confirmed the associations of various players in inflammation to carcinogenesis in several organs [66-68] including the oral cavity [69-72].

3. Biological Interactions of Periodontitis with Other Carcinogens

In addition to a plausible biological mechanism for an independent association, periodontitis may also biologically interact with other carcinogens such as tobacco, alcohol and certain viruses to increase the risk of oral cancer. For example, breaks in the mucosal barrier in the presence of periodontitis can lead to enhanced penetration of carcinogens [73]. An increased production of acetaldehyde (a known carcinogen) from ethanol was also shown in subjects with poor oral health [74, 75]. In addition, periodontal pockets may act as reservoirs for *human papillomavirus* (HPV), a suspected causal factor of oral cancer [76-78].

Periodontitis-HPV Synergy

HPV is a DNA virus with a specific tropism for squamous epithelia. More than 120 different HPV types have been isolated to date. Low-risk HPVs, such as HPV-6 and HPV-11, induce benign hyperproliferations of the epithelium such as papillomas or warts which rarely progress to cancer. High-risk oncogenic types such as HPV-16 and HPV-18 are associated with squamous cell carcinoma (SCC). HPV-16 and HPV-18 are capable of transforming epithelial cells. This transforming potential is largely a result of the function of two viral oncoproteins, E6 and E7, which functionally inactivate two human tumor suppressor proteins, p53 and pRb, respectively. Expression of high-risk HPV E6 and E7 results in cellular proliferation, loss of cell cycle regulation, impaired cellular differentiation, increased frequency of mutations, and chromosomal instability [79]. HPV-16 and HPV-18 are a central cause of cervical cancer and are also being investigated for head and neck cancers [80-85].

The average prevalence of HPV DNA in normal mucosa is 10% [80]. In a review of 60 studies, the prevalence of HPV DNA in head and neck SCCs was 25.9%. This was 23.5% in oral, 35.6% in oropharyngeal, and 24.0% in laryngeal SCCs. HPV-16 accounted for a larger majority of HPV+ oropharyngeal SCCs (86.7%) compared with HPV+ oral (68.2%) and HPV+ laryngeal (69.2%) SCCs. Conversely, HPV-18 was rare in HPV+ oropharyngeal SCCs (2.8%) compared with HPV+ oral (34.1%) and HPV+ laryngeal (17.0%) SCCs. Aside from HPV-16 and HPV-18, other oncogenic HPV DNAs were rarely detected in HNCs [82]. Probability of HPV DNA being detected in the oral mucosa increases with increasing degree of dysplasia. Overall, HPV DNA is 2 to 3 times more likely to be detected in precancerous lesions and 4.7 times more likely to be detected in HNCs than in normal mucosa [80].

HPV infection is a necessary but not sufficient cause of cervical cancer. Although majority of the population is infected with HPV at least once in their lives, most HPV infections are cleared rapidly by the immune system and do not result in pathology [86, 87]. Persistence of HPV infection is the strongest risk factor in the development of cancer. Thus, the identification of factors that influence the persistence of HPV infection is critical to facilitate efforts to prevent carcinogenesis. Certain bacterial co-infections in the cervix were shown to act synergistically with HPV infection. For example, several studies have shown that concurrent infection with *Chlamydia trachomatis* is associated with HPV persistence and increased the risk of cervical cancer [88, 89]. Studies suggest that viruses and bacteria, mostly studied in isolation, may in fact cooperate synergistically and should probably be considered as a pathogenic consortium in future investigations [90-96]. In addition, elevated levels of inflammatory cytokines IL-6, IL-1, and TNF-α were shown to modulate HPV E6/E7 gene expression and proliferation in human epithelial cells [97-102].

The strictly epitheliotropic nature of HPV, with a specific anatomic site preference, limits its range of infectivity. HPV infects exclusively the basal cells of the epithelium. Naturally occurring HPV infection begins when the virus gains access to permissive basal cells through wounds or abrasions [79]. In the presence of periodontitis, the periodontal pocket epithelium is usually ulcerated facilitating the access of the virus. In addition, replication of virus is associated with proliferation of the basal and parabasal cells. The junctional epithelium, located at the bottom of the periodontal pocket, has a very high mitotic rate and consists of basal and parabasal cell layers. It shares properties similar to the squamous-columnar junction of the cervix uteri, where the majority of HPV-associated cancers arise [103]. Integrin $\alpha_6\beta_4$ and syndecan-1, candidate receptors for HPV, are expressed during wound-healing and are found in the pocket and junctional epithelium in the presence of periodontitis [79, 91].

It is not clear where latent HPV resides in the head and neck region. This is an important factor in the effectiveness of therapeutic methods. Latent state would require the presence of infected cells which fail to differentiate [79]. Theoretically, the junctional epithelium fully fits these criteria. It has only basal and suprabasal cell layers and does not differentiate. HPV types 6, 11 and 16 DNA is detected in gingival tissue, gingival cervicular fluid and subgingival plaque from periodontitis sites [104-107]. These observations suggest that periodontal pockets may serve as a reservoir of HPV in the oral mucosa. This could explain the development of gingival papillomas and condylomas frequently found in patients with AIDS and in patients with organ transplants receiving cyclosporin treatment [107]. In these patients, local reactivation of latent HPV infection could occur in gingival tissues.

In summary, chronic periodontitis may facilitate HPVs initial infection and persistence by: 1- providing anatomical predisposition, 2- stimulation of chronic inflammation, 3- causing epithelial damage, and 4- being a source of bacterial co-infections. Evidence of periodontitis-HPV synergy is important to understand the natural history of HPV infection and oral cancer. It has practical implications for intervention since there is no treatment for HPV infection but there is a safe treatment for periodontitis. If this synergy is real, it will provide us a clinical high-risk profile for HPV status as well as for oral cancer.

Conclusion

In spite of long years of research, the research of specific microbial etiology has not translated into effective intervention and prevention strategies for oral cancer. In most cases, the infectious agents are ubiquitous, but only a small fraction of infected individuals develop cancer. Our approach is to clinically identify those who are at high-risk of developing oral cancer among infected individuals. We hypothesize that chronic periodontitis increases the risk of oral cancer independently as well as by helping HPVs initial infection and persistence. If this hypothesis is true, it will shed light to the etiology of oral cancer and the results will translate into immediate and safe prevention and treatment strategies. Subjects with periodontitis may be targeted as a "high-risk" population, and survival from oral cancer may be improved by early diagnosis and treatment. Preventing or treating periodontitis may result in a decreased incidence, morbidity and mortality of oral cancer.

REFERENCES

[1] Jemal A. Siegel R. Ward E. Murray T. Xu J. Thun MJ. Cancer statistics, 2007. *CA Cancer J Clin.* 2007;57(1):43-66.

[2] Schwartz LH, Ozsahin M, Zhang GN, et al. Synchronous and metachronous head and neck carcinomas. *Cancer* 1994;74:1933-8.

[3] Jones AS, Morar P, Phillips DE, et al. Second primary tumors in patients with head and neck squamous cell carcinoma. *Cancer* 1995;75:1343-53.

[4] Adami HO, Hunter D, Trichopoulos D. Oral and pharyngeal cancers. In: *Textbook of Cancer Epidemiology*. Oxford University Press, Inc. New York, NY. 2000. p. 115-136.

[5] Palme CE. Gullane PJ. Gilbert RW. Current treatment options in squamous cell carcinoma of the oral cavity. *Surgical Oncology Clinics of North America. 13(1):47-70, 2004 Jan.*

[6] Lippman SM, Sudbø J, Hong WK. Oral cancer prevention and the evolution of molecular-targeted drug development. *J Clin Oncol* 2005;23:346-356.

[7] Mignogna MD, Fedeleand S, Russo LL. The World Cancer Report and the burden of oral cancer. *European Journal of Cancer Prevention* 2004;13:139–142.

[8] Khuri FR, Lee JJ, Lippman SM et al. Randomized phase-II trial of low-dose isotretinoin for prevention of second primary tumors in stage I and II head and neck cancer patients. *J Natl Cancer Inst.* 2006;98:441-50.

[9] Kelloff GJ, Lippman SM, Dannenberg AJ. Progress in Chemoprevention Drug Development: The Promise of Molecular Biomarkers for Prevention of Intraepithelial Neoplasia and Cancer. A Plan to Move Forward. *Clin Cancer Res.* 2006;12(12):3661-3697.

[10] ChoeMS, Zhang X, Shin HJ, Shin DM, ChenZG. Interaction between epidermal growth factor receptor and cyclooxygenase 2-mediated pathways and its implications for the chemoprevention of head and neck cancer. *Mol Cancer Ther.* 2005;4:1448-1455.

[11] Muller M, Gissmann L. A long way: History of the prophylactic papillomavirus vaccine. *Dis Markers*. 2007;23(4):331-336

[12] Raffle AE. Challenges of implementing human papillomavirus (HPV) vaccination policy. *BMJ.* 2007;335(7616):375-377.

[13] Kuper H, Adami HO, Trichopoulos D: Infections as a major preventable cause of human cancer. *J Intern Med* 2000, 248:171-83.

[14] Lax AJ and Thomas W. How bacteria could cause cancer: one step at a time. Trends Microbiol. 2002, 10:293-9.

[15] Crowe SE:. Helicobacter infection, chronic inflammation, and the development of malignancy. *Curr Opin Gastroenterol.* 2005, 1:32-8.

[16] Littman AJ, White E, Jackson LA, Thornquist MD, Gaydos CA, Goodman GE, Vaughan TL: Chlamydia pneumoniae infection and risk of lung cancer. *Cancer Epidemiol Biomarkers Prev*. 2004;3:1624-1630.
[17] Vaishnavi C, Kochhar R, Singh G, Kumar S, Singh S, Singh K: Epidemiology of typhoid carriers among blood donors and patients with biliary, gastrointestinal and other related diseases. *Microbiol Immunol*. 2005; 49:107-112.
[18] Gold JS, Bayar S, Salem RR: Association of Streptococcus bovis bacteremia with colonic neoplasia and extracolonic malignancy. *Arch Surg*. 2004, 139: 760-765.
[19] Huycke MM, Gaskins HR: Commensal bacteria, redox stress, and colorectal cancer: mechanisms and models. *Exp Biol Med*. 2004, 229:586-97.
[20] Lax AJ and Thomas W. How bacteria could cause cancer: one step at a time. *Trends Microbiol*. 2002, 10:293-9.
[21] Jordan RCK, Macabeo-Ong M, Shiboski CH, Dekker N, Ginzinger DG, Wong DTW, Schmidt BL. Overexpression of matrix metalloproteinase-1 and -9 mRNA is associated with progression of oral dysplasia to cancer. *Clinical Cancer Research* 2004;10:6460-6465.
[22] Greten FR, Eckmann L, Greten TF, Park JM, Li ZW, Egan LJ, Kagnoff MF, Karin M. IKKβ links inflammation and tumorigenesis in a mouse model of colitis-Associated cancer. *Cell* 2004; 118 (3):285-296.
[23] Luo JL, Maeda S, Hsu LC, Yagita H, Karin M. Inhibition of NF-kappa B in cancer cells converts inflammation - induced tumor growth mediated by TNF alpha to TRAIL-mediated tumor regression. *Cancer Cell*. 2004;6(3):297-305.
[24] Wang D, Wang H, Shi Q, Katkuri S, Walhi W, Desvergne B, Das SK, Dey SK, DuBois RN. Prostaglandin E(2) promotes colorectal adenoma growth via transactivation of the nuclear peroxisome proliferator-activated receptor delta. [Journal Article] *Cancer Cell*. 2004;6(3):285-95.
[25] Caygill CP, Hill MJ, Braddick M, Sharp JC: Cancer mortality in chronic typhoid and paratyphoid carriers. *Lancet*. 1994, 343:83-4.
[26] Lazcano-Ponce EC, Miquel JF, Munoz N, Herrero R, Ferrecio C, Wistuba II, Alonso de Ruiz P, Aristi UG, Nervi F: Epidemiology and molecular pathology of gallbladder cancer. *CA Cancer J Clin*. 2001, 51: 349-364.
[27] Mager DL, Haffajee AD, Devlin PM, Norris CM, Posner MR, Goodson JM: The salivary microbiota as a diagnostic indicator of oral cancer: A descriptive, non-randomized study of cancer-free and oral squamous cell carcinoma subjects. *J Transl Med*. 2005, 3:27.
[28] Philip M, Rowley DA, Schreiber H. Inflammation as a tumor promoter in cancer induction. *Seminars in Cancer Biology*. 2004;14:433-439.
[29] Balkwill F and Mantovani A. Inflammation and cancer: back to Virchow? *Lancet*. 2001:357;539-545.
[30] Loesche WJ, Grossman NS. Periodontal disease as a specific, albeit chronic, infection: Diagnosis and treatment. *Clinical Microbiology Reviews*. 2001;14(4):727-752.
[31] Armitage GC. Periodontal diagnoses and classification of periodontal diseases. *Periodontology 2000*. 2004;34:9-21.

[32] Champagne CME, Buchanan W, Reddy MS, Preisser JS, Beck JD, Offenbacher S. Potential for gingival crevice fluid measures as predictors of risk for periodontal disease. *Periodontology 2000.* 2003;31:167-180.

[33] Burt B. Academy Report. Epidemiology of Periodontal Diseases. J Periodontol 2005;76:1406-1419.

[34] Socransky SS, Haffajee AD. Dental biofilms: Difficult therapeutic targets. *Periodontology 2000.* 2002;28:12-55.

[35] Scannapieco FA, Wang B, Shiau HJ. Oral bacteria and respiratory infection: Effects on respiratory pathogen adhesion and Epithelial Cell Proinflammatory Cytokine Production. *Annals of Periodontology.* 2001;6(1):78-86.

[36] Scannapieco FA, Ho AW, DiTolla M, Chen C Dentino AR. Exposure to the dental environment and respiratory illness in dental student populations. *J Can Dent Assoc.* 2004;70:198-202.

[37] Scannapieco FA. Pneumonia in Non-Ambulatory Patients: Role of oral bacteria and oral hygiene. *J Amer Dent Assoc.* 2006;137(10 supplement):21S-25S.

[38] Scannapieco FA, Bush RM, Paju S. Associations between periodontal disease and risk for nosocomial bacterial pneumonia and chronic obstructive pulmonary disease. A systematic review. *Annals Periodontol.* 2003;8:54-69.

[39] Scannapieco FA. Periodontal inflammation: From gingivitis to Systemic disease? *Compendium* 2004;25(7);16-25.

[40] Timothy C. Nichols, Thomas H. Fischer, Efthymios N. Deliargyris, Albert S. Baldwin Jr. Role of Nuclear Factor-Kappa B (NF-κB) in Inflammation, Periodontitis and Atherogenesis. *Annals of Periodontology.* 2001 6:1, 20-29.

[41] Anthony M. Iacopino. Periodontitis and Diabetes Interrelationships: Role of Inflammation. *Annals of Periodontology.* 2001 6:1, 125-137.

[42] López, Isabel Da Silva, Joaquín Ipinza, Jorge Gutiérrez. Periodontal Therapy Reduces the Rate of Preterm Low Birth Weight in Women With Pregnancy-Associated Gingivitis. *Journal of Periodontology.* 2005, 76;11: 2144-2153.

[43] Jeffcoat MK, Hauth JC, Geurs NC, Reddy MS, Cliver SP, Hodgkins PM, Goldenberg RL. Periodontal disease and preterm birth: Results of a pilot intervention study. *J Periodontol.* 2003;74:8:1214-1218.

[44] Graham S, Dayal H, Rohrer T. Dentition, diet, tobacco, and alcohol in the epidemiology of oral cancer. *J Natl Cancer Inst.* 1977;59(6):1611-1618.

[45] Zheng T, Boyle P, Hu H, Duan J, Jiang P, Ma D. Dentition, oral hygiene, and risk of oral cancer: A case-control study in Beijing, People's Republic of China. *Cancer Causes and Control.* 1990;1(3):235-241.

[46] Marshall JR, Graham S, Haughey BP, Shedd D, O'Shea R, Brasure J. Smoking, alcohol, dentition and diet in the epidemiology of oral cancer. *Oral Oncology, Eur J Cancer.* 1992;28B(1):9-15.

[47] Velly AM, Franco EL, Schlecht N, Pintos J, Kowalski LP, Oliveira BV and Curado MP. Relationship between dental factors and risk of upper aerodigestive tract cancer. *Oral Oncology.* 1998;34:284-291.

[48] Moreno-Lopez LA, Esparza-Gomez GC, Gonzalez-Navarro A, Cerero-Lapiedra R, Gonzalez-Hernandez MJ, Dominguez-Rojas V. Risk of oral cancer associated with

tobacco smoking, alcohol consumption and oral hygiene: A case-control study in Madrid, Spain. *Oral Oncology*. 2000;36:170-174.

[49] Homann N, Tillonen J, Rintamaki H, Salaspura M, Lindqvist C, Meurman JH. Poor dental status increases acetaldehyde production from ethanol in saliva: a possible link to increased oral cancer risk among heavy drinkers. *Oral Oncology*. 2001;37:153-158.

[50] Lissowska J, Pilarska A, Pilarski P, Samolczyk-Wanyura D, Piekarczyk J, Bardin-Mikollajczak A, Zatonski W, Herrero R, Munoz N, Franceschi S. Smoking, alcohol, diet, dentition and sexual practices in the epidemiology of oral cancer in Poland. *Eur J Cancer Prev*. 2003;12(1):25-33.

[51] Winn DM, Blot WJ, McLaughlin JK, Austin DF, Greenberg RS, Preston-Martin S. Mouthwash use and oral conditions in the risk of oral and pharyngeal cancer. *Cancer Research*. 1991;51:3044-3047.

[52] Talamini R, Vaccarella S, Barbone F, Tavani A, La Vecchia C, Herrero R. Oral hygiene, dentition, sexual habits and risk of oral cancer. *British Journal of Cancer*. 2000;83(9):1238-1242.

[53] Fernandez Garrote L, Herrero R, Ortiz Reyes RM, Vaccarella S, Lence Anta J, Ferbeye L. Risk factors for cancer of the oral cavity and oropharynx in Cuba. *British Journal of Cancer*. 2001;85(1):46-54.

[54] Balaram P, Sridhar H, Rajkumar T, Vaccarella S, Herrero R, Nandakumar A, Ravichandan K, Ramdas K, Sankaranarayanan R, Gajalakshmi V, Munoz N and Franceschi S. Oral cancer in southern India: the influence of smoking, drinking, paan-chewing and oral hygiene. *Int. J. Cancer*. 2002;98:440-445.

[55] Hausmann E, Allen K, Dunford R, Christersson L. A reliable computerized method to determine the level of the radiographic alveolar crest. *J Periodont Res.* 1989;24:368-369.

[56] Hausmann E, Allen K, Christersson L, Genco RJ. Effect of X-ray Beam Vertical Angulation on Radiographic Alveolar Crest Level Measurement. *J Periodontal Res.* 1989;24:8.

[57] Hausmann E, Allen K, Clerehugh V. What alveolar crest level on a bite-wing radiograph represents bone loss? *J Periodontol* .1991;62(9):570-2.

[58] Hausmann E, Allen K, Carpio L, Christersson LA, Clerehugh V. Computerized methodology for detection of alveolar crestal bone loss from serial intraoral radiographs. *J Periodontol.* 1992;63:657-662.

[59] Machtei EE, Christersson LA, Grossi SG, Dunford R, Zambon JJ, Genco RJ. Clinical criteria for the definition of "established periodontitis". *J Periodontol.* 1992;63:207-215.

[60] Grossi SG, Genco RJ, Machtei EE, Ho AW, Koch, Dunford RG, Zambon JJ and Hausmann E. Assessment of risk for periodontal disease (II), Risk indicators for alveolar bone loss. *J Periodontol.* 1995:66;23-29.

[61] Nakhjiri SF, Park Y, Yilmaz O, Chung WO, Watanabe K, El-Sabaeny A, Park K, Lamont RJ. Inhibition of epithelial cell apoptosis by Porphyromonas gingivalis. *FEMS Microbiology Letters*. 2001:200:145-149.

[62] Lara-Tejero M, Galan JE: A bacterial toxin that controls cell cycle progression as a deoxyribonuclease I-like protein. *Science.* 2000;290:354-357.

[63] Baik S.C, Youn HS, Chung MH, Lee WK, Cho MJ, Ko GH, Park CK, Kasai H, Rhee KH: Increased oxidative DNA damage in Helicobacter pylori infected human gastric mucosa. *Cancer Res.* 1996;56:1279-1282.

[64] Sasaki M. Yamaura C. Ohara-Nemoto Y. Tajika S. Kodama Y. Ohya T. Harada R. Kimura S. Streptococcus anginosus infection in oral cancer and its infection route. *Oral Diseases. 2005;11(3):151-6.*

[65] Karin M. Lawrence T. Nizet V. Innate immunity gone awry: linking microbial infections to chronic inflammation and cancer. *Cell.* 2006;124(4):823-35.

[66] Sparmann A. Bar-Sagi D. Ras-induced interleukin-8 expression plays a critical role in tumor growth and angiogenesis. *Cancer Cell.* 2004;6(5):447-58.

[67] Dauer DJ. Ferraro B. Song L. Yu B. Mora L. Buettner R. Enkemann S. Jove R. Haura EB. Stat3 regulates genes common to both wound healing and cancer. *Oncogene. 2005;24(21):3397-408.*

[68] Cassatella MA. Huber V. Calzetti F. Margotto D. Tamassia N. Peri G. Mantovani A. Rivoltini L. Tecchio C. Interferon-activated neutrophils store a TNF-related apoptosis-inducing ligand (TRAIL/Apo-2 ligand) intracellular pool that is readily mobilizable following exposure to proinflammatory mediators. *Journal of Leukocyte Biology. 2006;79(1):123-32.*

[69] St John MA, Li Y, Zhou X, Denny P, Ho CM, Montemagno C, Shi W, Qi F, Wu B, Sinha U, Jordan R, Wolinsky L, Park NH, Liu H, Abemayor E, Wong DT. Interleukin 6 and interleukin 8 as potential biomarkers for oral cavity and oropharyngeal squamous cell carcinoma. *Archives of Otolaryngology- Head & Neck Surgery.* 2004;130(8):929-35.

[70] Vucicevic Boras V. Cikes N. Lukac J. Virag M. Cekic-Arambasin A. Salivary and serum interleukin 6 and basic fibroblast growth factor levels in patients with oral squamous cell carcinoma. *Minerva Stomatologica.* 2005;54(10):569-73 .

[71] Rhodus NL. Cheng B. Myers S. Miller L. Ho V. Ondrey F. The feasibility of monitoring NF-kappaB associated cytokines: TNF-alpha, IL-1alpha, IL-6, and IL-8 in whole saliva for the malignant transformation of oral lichen planus. *Molecular Carcinogenesis.* 2005;44(2):77-82.

[72] Rhodus NL, Ho V, Miller CS, Myers S, Ondrey F. NF-kappa B dependent cytokine levels in saliva of patients with oral preneoplastic lesions and oral squamous cell carcinoma. *Cancer Detection & Prevention.* 2005;29(1):42-5.

[73] Pollanen MT, Salonen JI, Uitto VJ. Structure and function of the tooth–epithelial interface in health and disease. *Periodontology 2000.* 2003;31:12–31.

[74] Homann N, Tillonen J, Rintamaki H, Salaspura M, Lindqvist C, Meurman JH. Poor dental status 29. increases acetaldehyde production from ethanol in saliva: a possible link to increased oral cancer risk among heavy drinkers. *Oral Oncology.* 2001;37:153-158.

[75] Visapaa JP, Gotte K, Benesova M, Li J, Homann N, Conradt C, Inoue H, Tisch M, Horrmann K, Vakevainen S, Salaspuro M, Seitz HK. Increased cancer risk in heavy

drinkers with the alcohol dehydrogenase 1C*1 allele, possibly due to salivary acetaldehyde. *Gut. 2004;53(6):871-6.*

[76] Hormia M, Willberg J, Ruokonen H, Syrjanen S. Marginal periodontium as a potential reservoir of human papillomavirus in oral mucosa. *J Periodontol.* 2005;76(3):358-63.

[77] Saygun I, Kubar A, Ozdemir A, Slots J. Periodontitis lesions are a source of salivary cytomegalovirus and Epstein-Barr virus. *J Periodontal Res.* 2005;40(2):187-91.

[78] Pollanen MT, Salonen JI, Uitto VJ. Structure and function of the tooth–epithelial interface in health and disease. *Periodontology 2000.* 2003;31:12–31.

[79] Stubenrauch F, Laimins LA. Human papillomavirus life cycle: Active and latent phases. *Semin Cancer Biol.* 1999;9:379-386.

[80] Ragin CR, Modugno F, and Gollin SM. The Epidemiology and Risk Factors of Head and Neck Cancer: a Focus on Human Papillomavirus. *J Dent Res.* 2007;86(2):104-114.

[81] D'Souza G. Kreimer AR. Viscidi R. Pawlita M. Fakhry C. Koch WM. Westra WH. Gillison ML. Case-control study of human papillomavirus and oropharyngeal cancer. *N Engl J Med.* 2007;356(19):1944-1956.

[82] Miller CS, Johnstone B. Human papillomavirus as a riskfactor for oral squamous cell carcinoma: A meta-analysis,1982-1997. *Oral Surg Oral Med Oral Radiol Endod.* 2001;91:622-635.

[83] Puscas L. The role of human papilloma virus infection in the etiology of oropharyngeal carcinoma Curr Opin Otolaryngol HeadNeckSurg 13:212-216. 2005.

[84] Kreimer AR. Clifford GM. Boyle P. Franceschi S. Human papillomavirus types in head and neck squamous cell carcinomas worldwide: a systematic review. [Review]. *Cancer Epidemiology, Biomarkers & Prevention.* 14(2):467-75, 2005 Feb.

[85] Gillison ML, Koch WM, Capone RB, Spafford M, Westra WH, LiWu, Zahurak ML, Daniel RW, Viglione MI,.Symer DE, Shah KV, Sidransky D. Evidence for a causal association between human papilloma virus and a subset of head and neck cancers. J *Natl Cancer Inst.* 2000;92:709–20.

[86] Giuliano AR, Sedjo RL, Roe DJ. Clearance of oncogenic human papillomavirus (HPV) infection: effect of smoking (United States). *Cancer Cause Control.* 2002;13:839-846.

[87] Molano M, vanden Brule A, Plummer M. Determinants of clearance of human papillomavirus infections in Colombian women with normal cytology: a population-based, 5-year follow-up study. *Am J Epidemiol.* 2003;158:486-494.

[88] Madeleine MM, Anttila T, Schwartz SM, Saikku P, Leinonen M, Carter JJ, Wurscher M, Johnson LG, Galloway DA, Daling JR. Risk of cervical cancer associated with *Chlamydia trachomatis* antibodies by histology, HPV type and HPV cofactors. *Int J Cancer.* 2007;120(3):650-655.

[89] Samoff E, Koumans EH, Markowitz LE, Sternberg M, Sawyer MK, Swan D, Papp JR, Black CM, Unger ER. Association of *Chlamydia trachomatis* with persistence of high-risk types of human papillomavirus in a cohort of female adolescents. *Am J Epidemiol.* 2005;162(7):668-675.

[90] Saygun I, Kubar A, Ozdemir A, Slots J. Periodontitis lesions are a source of salivary cytomegalovirus and Epstein-Barr virus. *J Periodontal Res*. 2005;40(2):187-91.

[91] Hormia M, Willberg J, Ruokonen H, Syrjanen S. Marginal periodontium as a potential reservoir of human papillomavirus in oral mucosa. *J Periodontol.* 2005;76(3):358-63.

[92] Kumar PS, Griffen AL, Barton JA, Paster BJ, Moeschberger ML, Leys EJ. New bacterial species associated with chronic periodontitis. *J Dent Res*. 2003;82(5):338-344.

[93] Slots, Kamma JJ, Sugar C. The herpes virus-Porphyromonas gingivalis-periodontitis axis. *J Periodontal Res*. 2003;38(3):318-23.

[94] Slots J. Herpesviruses, the missing link between gingivitis and periodontitis? *Journal of the International Academy of Periodontology*. 2004;6(4):113-9.

[95] Kamma JJ, Slots J. Herpes viral-bacterial interactions in aggressive periodontitis. *Journal of Clinical Periodontology*. 2003;30(5):420-6.

[96] Sugano N, Ikeda K, Oshikaa M, Idesawa M, Tanaka H, Sato S, Ito K. Relationship between Porphyromonas gingivalis, Epstein-Barr virus infection and reactivation in periodontitis. *Journal of Oral Science*. 2004;46(4):203-6.

[97] Woodworth CD, Simpson S. Comparative lymphokine secretion by cultured normal human cervical keratinocytes, papillomavirus-immortalized, and carcinoma cell lines. *Am J Pathol*. 1993;142:1544-1555.

[98] Woodworth CD, Notario V, Di Paolo JA. Transforming growth factors beta 1 and 2 transcriptionally regulate human papillomavirus (HPV) type 16 early gene expression in HPV-immortalized human genital epithelial cells. *J Virol*. 1990;64:4767-4775.

[99] Woodworth CD, Lichti U, Simpson S, Evans CH, Di Paolo JA. Leukoregulin and gamma-interferon inhibit human papillomavirus type 16 gene transcription in human papillomavirus-immortalized human cervical cells. *Cancer Res*. 1992;52:456-463.

[100] Woodworth CD, Mc Mullin E, Iglesias M, Plowman GD. Interleukin 1 alpha and tumor necrosis factor alpha stimulate autocrine amphiregulin expression and proliferation of human papillomavirus-immortalized and carcinoma-derived cervical epithelial cells. *Proc Natl Acad Sci USA*. 1995;92:2840-2844.

[101] Iglesias M, Plowman GD, Woodworth CD. Interleukin-6 and interleukin-6 soluble receptor regulate proliferation of normal, human papillomavirus-immortalized, and carcinoma-derived cervical cells in vitro. *Am J Pathol*. 1995;146:944-952.

[102] Gaiotti D, Chung J, Iglesias M, Nees M, Baker PD, Evans CH. Tumor necrosis factor-alpha promotes human papillomavirus (HPV) E6/E7 RNA expression and cyclin-dependent kinase activity in HPV-immortalized keratinocytes by aras-dependent pathway. *Mol Carcinog*. 2000;27:97-109.

[103] Schroeder HE. The junctional epithelium: Origin, structure and significance. *Acta Med Dent Helv*. 1996;1:155-167.

[104] Madinier I, Doglio A, Cagnon L, Lefebvre JC, Monteil RA. Southern blot detection of human papillomaviruses (HPVs) DNA sequences in gingival tissues. *J Periodontol.* 1992;63:667-673.

[105] Parra B, Slots J. Detection of human viruses in periodontal pockets using polymerase chain reaction. *Oral Microbiol Immunol*. 1996;11:289-293.

[106] Saglam F, Onan U, Soydinc M, Yilmaz O, Kirac K, Sever MS. Human papillomavirus in a patient with severe gingival overgrowth associated with cyclosporine therapy. A case report. *J Periodontol.* 1996;67:528-531.

[107] Bustos DA, Grenon MS, Benitez M, de Boccardo G, PavanJV, Gendelman H. Human papillomavirus infection in cyclosporin-induced gingival overgrowth in renal allograft recipients. *J Periodontol.* 2001;72:741-744.

In: Progress in Oral Cancer Research
Editor: Frederik L. Nielsen, pp 107-124
ISBN 978-1-60021-865-1

Chapter V

LOWER LIP RECONSTRUCTION FOLLOWING RESECTION OF MALIGNANT TUMORS

Kenji Yano[*] and Ken Matsuda
Department of Plastic and Reconstructive Surgery, Osaka University Graduate School of Medicine, Osaka, Japan.

INTRODUCTION

The aim of this article was to review and describe techniques for reconstruction of the lower lip defects after resection of malignant tumors with emphasis on the cosmetic and functional outcome. The lower lip reconstruction must be considered individually because the methods employed are not always applicable to every defect conditions. Lip defects may be classified as partial (involving only skin or mucosa) or full thickness, which involve both skin and muscle (with or without mucosal involvement). The size of the defect is often the most important consideration because it is usually a strong indicator for the optimal method of reconstruction. Therefore, a defect of approximately 30% of the lower lip can be reconstructed with primary closure because of the great elasticity of the lips. If a horizontal defect is greater than 30% of the lip, the use of adjacent tissue is mandatory to reconstruct the deficiency. If there is total lower lip defect following tumor resection, other adjacent or distant flaps may be needed for lip reconstruction. The reconstructive procedures can be classified as follows:

1. Cutaneous defects
2. Defects of 30% or less of the lower lip
3. Defects of 30% to 50% of the lower lip
4. Defects of 50% to 75% of the lower lip
5. Transverse narrow defects in the lower lip
6. Total lower lip reconstruction

[*] Correspondence concerning this article should be addressed to: Kenji Yano, M.D., Ph.D. From the Department of Plastic and Reconstructive Surgery, Osaka University, e-mail: knjyano@psurg.med.osaka-u.ac.jp.

Anatomy

The lips not only separate the oral cavity from the outside but also play an important role in oral continence, eating, communication, oral access, and maintenance of the oral milieu. The lip sensation, muscular strength, and integrity of the lip curtain are essential to maintain these functions. The lower lip posture is controlled by an intricate complex of muscular slips including depressors, retractors, and evertors of the lower lip and the buccal angle. As antagonistic to the depressor labii inferioris, depressor anguli oris, and mentalis muscles, the orbicularis oris is the main muscle in the lip responsible for the complex sphincteric action. The main function of the lips, oral competence, is controlled by this orbicularis oris muscle. Its fibers decussate in the midline and at the commissures, and anatomically it consists of a pars peripheralis and a pars marginalis. The pars marginalis, which is uniquely developed in the human lips, consists of a single (or sometimes double) band of narrow-diameter muscle fibers lodged within the tissues of the red-lip margin. The larger pars peripheralis resembles a fan with its stem at the commissure (modiolus), which is open in peripheral segments, and the lowest fibers reach and attach to the mentolabial sulcus. The motor nerves arise from the buccal and marginal mandibular rami of the facial nerve. The sensation of the lower lip is provided by the mental nerve, a branch of the mandibular division of the trigeminal nerve. The mental nerve emerges from the mental foramen with the mental branch of the inferior alveolar artery. The blood supply is the superior and inferior labial arteries from the external maxillary artery, with venous drainage into the anterior facial vein. The mental branch of the inferior alveolar artery helps supply the chin and anastomoses with the submental and inferior labial vessels.

Cutaneous Defects

For relatively shallow cutaneous defects that do not involve the lip vermilion, local skin flaps or full-thickness skin grafts may be used. The donor sites for full-thickness skin grafts should be chosen considering the skin texture and color matching, and closed primarily. As donor sites, the preauricular, retroauricular, and supraclavicular regions are often used. Regarding mustache, skin grafting around the mouth is more suitable for female than male patients. For male patients, wedge excision or local skin flaps may be more preferable even for partial-thickness defects with small horizontal extent.

Defects of 30% or Less of the Lower Lip

For full-thickness defects of up to 30% of the lower lip, V-shaped or W-shaped wedge excision with primary closure provides good results (Figure 1). This is because of the tremendous flexibility and expandability of the vermillion tissue, and most cases with lower lip defects (by trauma or benign tumor excision) encountered are appropriately repaired by this procedure. Care must be taken with the primary closure to approximate the white roll and the vermillion border precisely. Each of the three layers (skin, orbicularis oris muscle, and oral mucosa) should be repaired meticulously not only for good aesthetic result but also for preserving the postoperative sphincteric muscle function around the oral region.

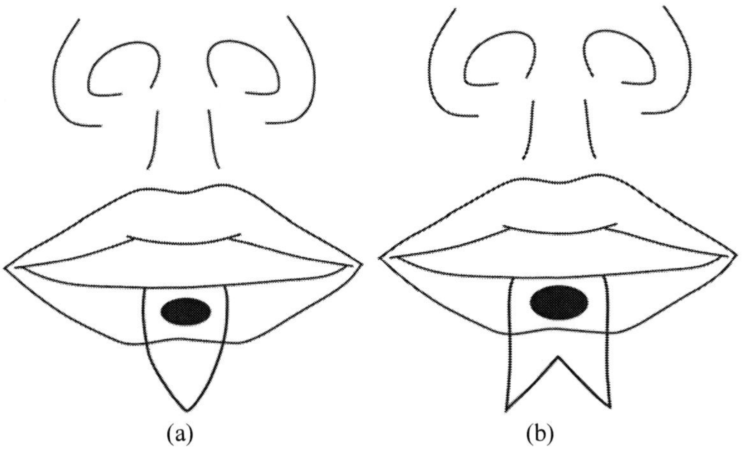

Figure 1. Designs for wedge excision and primary closure. (a) V-shaped design. (b) W-shaped design.

DEFECTS OF 30% TO 50% OF THE LOWER LIP

Defects more than 30% of the lower lip are often sequelae of excision of large benign tumor or relatively small malignant tumor with proper surgical margin. Since the defect can not be closed primarily, it should be reconstructed with neighboring tissue.

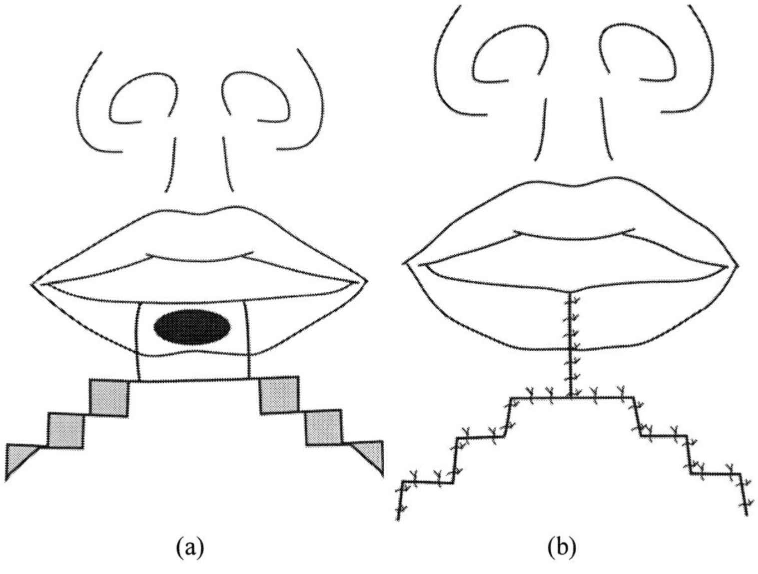

Figure 2. A stepladder flap. (a) Small skin is removed to correct the flap advancement. (b) Postoperative view.

A Stepladder-Flap and Schuchardt Procedure

This method was introduced by Johanson et al. [1]. for reconstruction of up to two-thirds of the lower lip (Figure 2). It may be applied for both central and lateral defects of the lower lip. According to the defect size, two to four steps are used for the closure. Since the muscle continuity and the sensation are well preserved, stepladder reconstruction achieves good function more quickly than the lip switch flap, but the tight lip and the noticeable scar in the mental region are drawbacks of this method. For the central part defect, Schuchardt procedure [2] is another option. This procedure includes rotation and advancement of the cheek and lip (Figure 3). The skin incision is extended around the labial mental fold to the submental region, and some skin is excised to correct the advancement. The scar around the mental region may be more inconspicuous than in the stepladder method, but the tight lip is a disadvantage of this method as well.

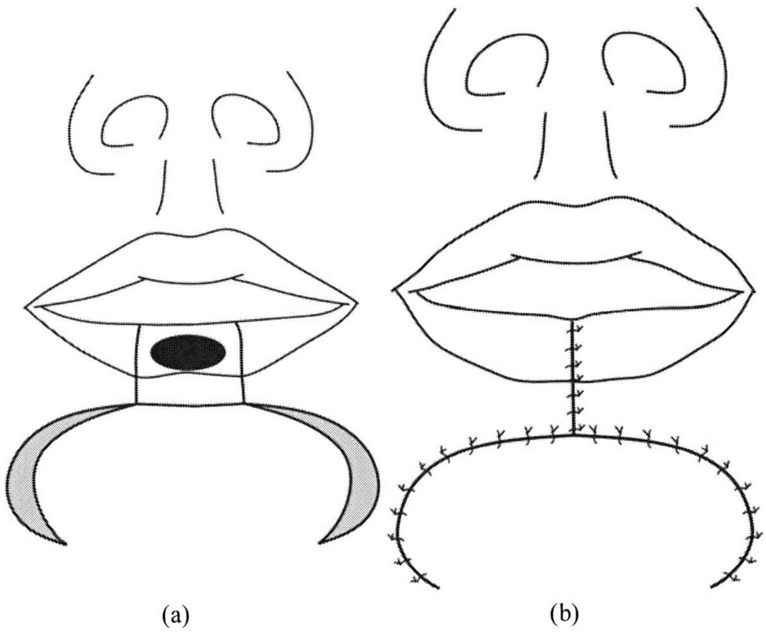

Figure 3. Schuchardt procedure. (a) Some skin is removed for the flap rotation and advancement. (b) Postoperative view.

Estlander Flap [3]

Estlander flap is a transposition flap from the upper lip and used mainly for the lateral part defects of the lower lip with or without enrollment of the commissure (Figure 4). The continuity of the orbicularis oris muscle and the sphincteric function are well preserved. However, the disadvantage of this flap is rounding of the reconstructed commissure which spoils the postoperative aesthetic result and requires secondary revision to reconstruct the obliterated commissure in most cases.

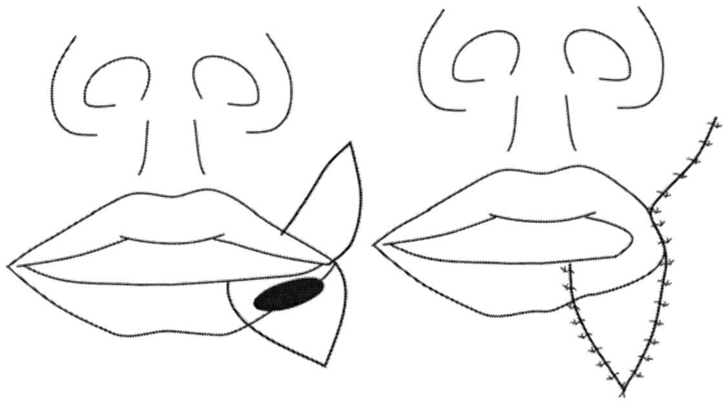

(a) (b)

Figure 4. Estlander flap. (a) Tumor resection and flap design. (b) Postoperative view.

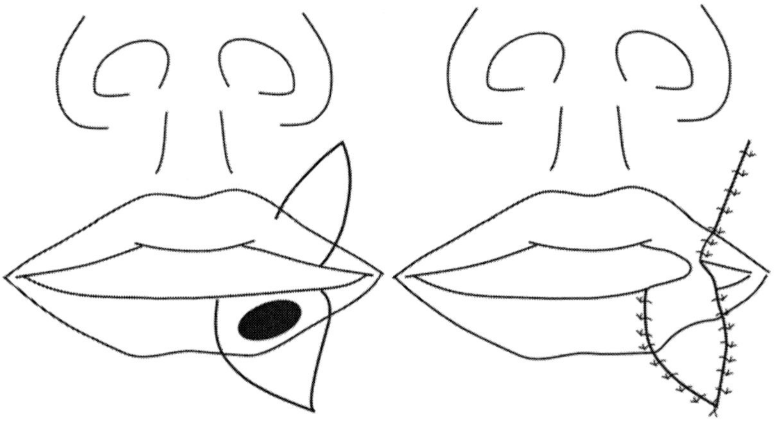

(a) (b)

Figure 5. Abbe flap. (a) Tumor resection and flap design. (b) Postoperative view.

Abbe Flap [4]

This is an opposing lip switch flap usually used for the upper lip defects, but in some cases this flap may be used to reconstruct the lower lip defect (Figure 5). The flap is elevated on its vascular pedicle, the superior labial artery. The donor site may be the lateral part of the upper lip to minimize the aesthetic morbidity of the upper lip. The transferred flap is divided on postoperative days 10 to 14. The transferred orbicularis oris muscle in the flap is once denervated by this procedure and acts only as a linkage of the broken orbicularis muscle chain in the early postoperative state, but it is reinnervated by nerve ingrowth from the adjacent orbicularis oris muscle in the late postoperative state [5]. The commissure is preserved in this method, and secondary revision for the commissure is unnecessary. However, since the upper lip has more complex anatomy and aesthetic priority than the lower lip, this procedure is mainly indicated for the upper lip defects and it should be limited for the lower lip defects.

DEFECTS OF 50% TO 75% OF THE LOWER LIP

Defects of 50% to 75% of the lower lip mainly result from excision of middle or large malignant tumors. For reconstruction of the defects, large flaps containing both the remaining lip and cheek tissue are necessary. Vermillion tissue defects are reconstructed by mucosal flap or tongue flap. Gillies fan flap [6] and its modifications or Karapandzic flap [7] is often used. Both of these flaps cause rounding of the commissure that compromises the postoperative aesthetic outcome.

Gilles Fan Flap and its Modifications

These procedures represent extended version of Estlander flap [3]. The flap is elevated in the nasolabial region, rotated, and transferred to the defect in V-Y advancement fashion (Figure 6). The original commissure is moved to the reconstructed lower lip, as it causes tight lip and rounding of the commissure. McGregor [8] modified the classic fan flap method to set the pivot of the rotation at the commissure (Figure 7). The flap is elevated on the superior labial artery, and as the flap rotates the muscle fiber direction changes and new vermillion is created by the mucosal flap or tongue flap which prevents tight lip. Since the facial nerve to the orbicularis oris is dissected, the muscle is denervated after the flap elevation although reinnervation occurs postoperatively. Nakajima [9] reported a modified fan-shaped flap method that maintains the facial vessels and nerve supplying the flap (Figure 8). Since preserving the superior labial artery as the vascular pedicle to the flap results in rounding of the commissure, the fan-shaped flap based on the facial vessels has an advantage of creating a sharp commissure by dividing the labial artery at the margin of the flap.

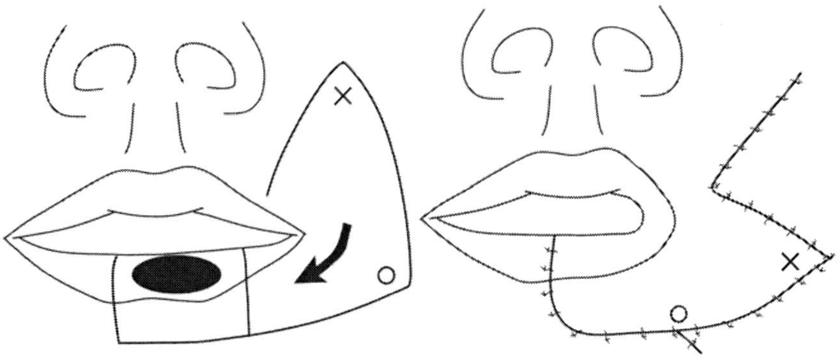

(a) (b)

Figure 6. Gillies fan flap. (a) Tumor resection and flap design. (b) Postoperative view.

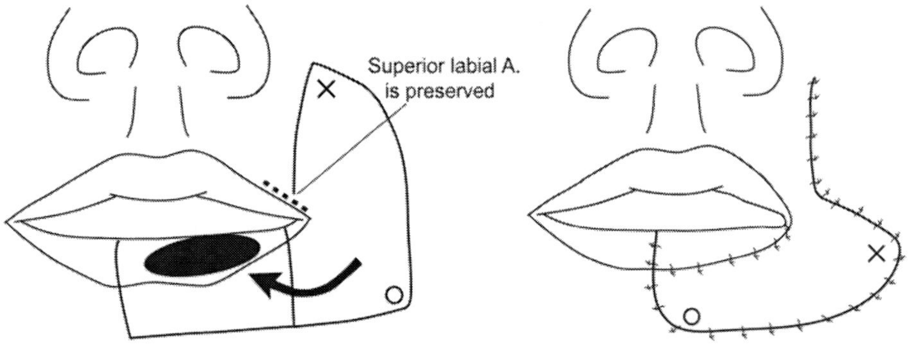

(a) (b)

Figure 7. Fan flap modified by McGregor. The flap is more rotated than Gillies fan flap, and the direction of the orbicularis oris muscle is changed. (a) Tumor resection and flap design. The pivot point of the flap lies at the commissure. (b) New vermillion is reconstructed with mucosal flap or tongue flap.

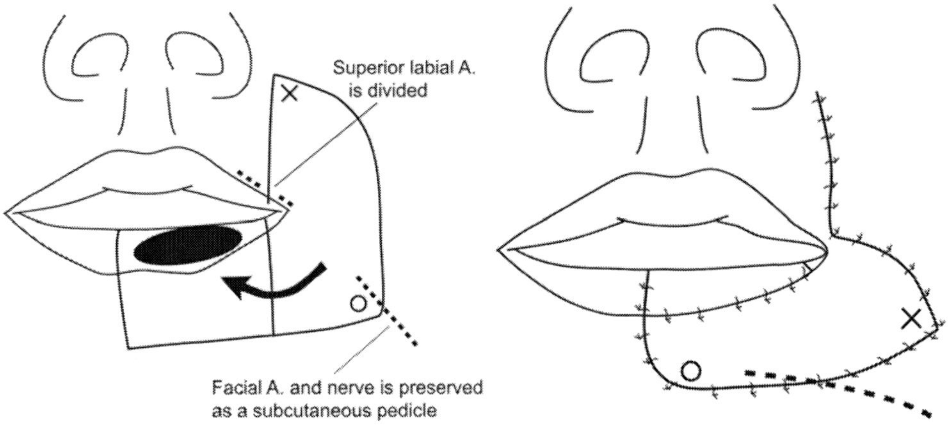

(a) (b)

Figure 8. Fan flap modified by Nakajima. (a) Tumor resection and flap design. The flap is supplied by the facial vessels and nerve, and the superior labial artery is divided to create a sharp commissure. (b) New vermillion is reconstructed with mucosal flap or tongue flap.

Karapandzic Flap [7]

Similar to Gilles fan flap [6], this is a flap with full-thickness pedicle, modified with emphasis on preservation of the underlying structure including the depressor muscles, facial vessels and nerves to the flap (Figure 9). The flaps may be used bilaterally and advanced medially to create proper orbicularis oris muscle continuity. Reconstruction with this method provides good muscle continuity and functioning sphincter, but tight lip, microstomia, and round commissure of the reconstructed lip are disadvantages of this method and secondary revision is often required.

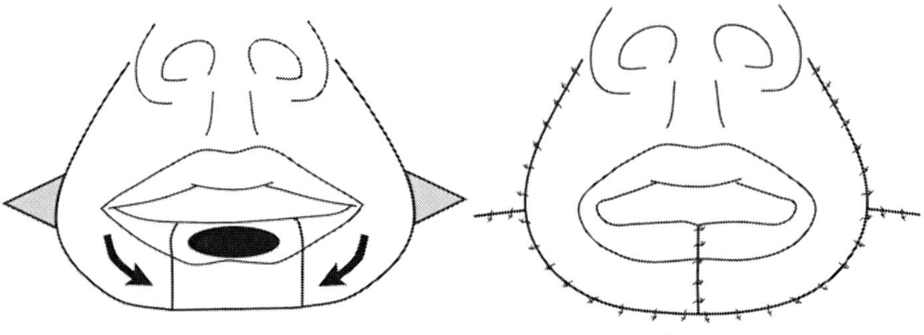

(a) (b)

Figure 9. Karapandzic flap. (a) Tumor resection and flap design. Bilateral flaps are advanced medially without injuring the facial vessels and nerves supplying the flap.

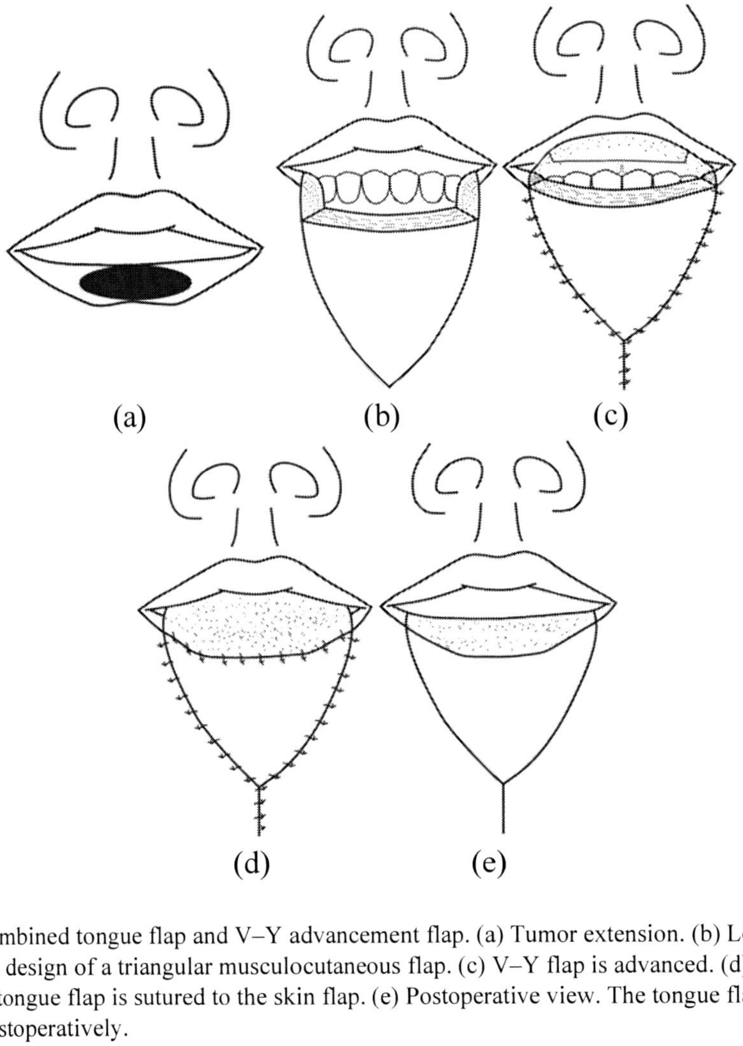

(a) (b) (c)

(d) (e)

Figure 10. Combined tongue flap and V–Y advancement flap. (a) Tumor extension. (b) Loss of substance and design of a triangular musculocutaneous flap. (c) V–Y flap is advanced. (d) Distal undersurface tongue flap is sutured to the skin flap. (e) Postoperative view. The tongue flap is divided two weeks postoperatively.

TRANSVERSE NARROW DEFECTS IN THE LOWER LIP

Various reconstructive approaches for defects of the lower lip have been described, but few studies addressed the wide transverse narrow defects. Herein, we introduce the procedures for transverse narrow defects of the lower lip.

Combined Tongue Flap and V-Y Advancement Flap for Lower Lip Defects [10] (Figure 10(a)-(e))

The full-thickness lesion is resected according to the radical criteria for malignant tumors of vermilion or vermilion border, which require an approximately 1.0-cm free margin. The excision is carried out in a rectangular shape and includes only a thin layer of the orbicularis oris pars marginalis muscle. The mental 'V'-shaped advancement flap is designed in the form of a triangle with its apex inferiorly, at the edge of the mandible. Only the skin and subcutaneous tissue are incised, thus preserving the orbicularis oris, depressor labii inferioris, and mentalis muscles. For upward advancement of the flap, it is necessary to dissect the orbicularis oris muscle plane at least 1 or 2 cm lateral to the flap and to dissect subcutaneously the apex of the flap. The flap is advanced upward to the lip defect as an orbicularis oris musculocutaneous flap while preserving the oral sphincter. The skin and subcutaneous tissue are sutured in two layers in a 'Y' fashion, joining the remaining vermilion border and the upper end of the flap. Next, mucosal coverage is provided by the tongue flap. A rectangular tongue flap is designed on the inferior surface to fit the vermilion defect. The tongue flap is elevated and inset to the vermilion defect. The tongue flap is cut off after two weeks, and the oral side of the vermilion is sutured. The donor site of the tongue is closed primarily.

Double V-Y Advancement Flap in the Lower Lip Reconstruction [12,13] (Figure 11(a)-(f))

A V-shaped flap is incised in the mentum up to the lower maxillary margin below the defect. The dermis is resected completely down to the muscular threshold, thus freeing the flap margins laterally. A similar incision is carried out in the vestibular mucosa up to the fornix. Two advancement flaps are thus obtained and then sutured above the defect. Because no muscular dissection is carried out during this reconstructive procedure, motor innervation from the facial nerve is preserved on both sides. From the vascular standpoint, both flaps receive blood by means of several small perforators that terminate in a fine reticular pattern characterizing the labial artery territories. The cutaneous donor site is sutured, whereas the vestibular side is left free to heal. A buccinator muscle mucosal flap is then elevated for reconstruction of the lower lip vermilion [13]. Once again, when the flap is raised, it must be ensured that the flap contains a branch of the facial artery. The mucosa immediately above the branch should also be included, along with the buccinator muscle fibers. The flap is then transposed to the lower vermilion defect. The two cutaneous and mucous flaps are sutured together distally while ensuring continuity with the stump margins.

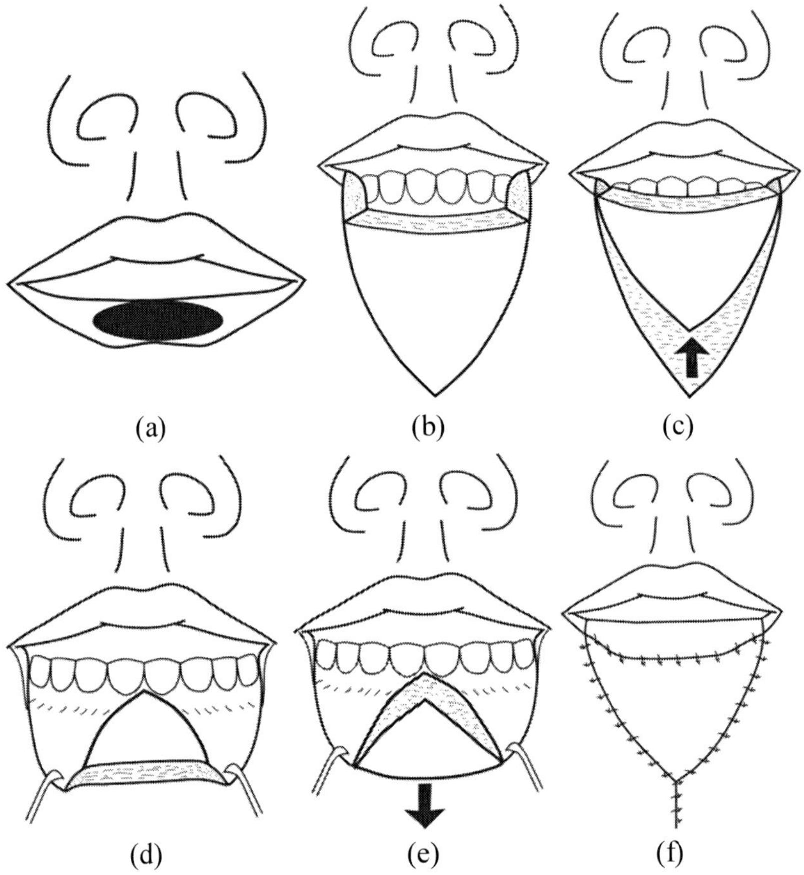

Figure 11. Double V-Y advancement flap. (a) Tumor extension. (b) Tumor resection and design of the cutaneous V-Y flap. (c) Dissection and advancement of the cutaneous V-Y flap to the defect. (d) Design of the mucous V-Y advancement flap. (e) Advancement of the mucous V-Y flap. (f) Postoperative view.

Mental Neurovascular V-Y Advancement Island Flap [11] (Figure 12)

Before making the flap design, which may be unilateral or bilateral depending upon the nature of the defect, the position of the mental foramen is marked on the skin. The mental neurovascular V-Y advancement island flap is designed in the form of a triangle with its apex inferiorly and incorporating the mental nerve. The base of the triangle abuts onto the inferior border of the excision, and the apex lies below the edge of the mandible. Following ablation of the tumor, only the skin is incised down to the subdermal tissues on the planned borders of the unilateral or bilateral V-Y flaps. Elevation of the flap from the bone is carried out from a medial to lateral direction after deepening the medial incision down to the periosteum. Careful attention is paid to preserve the integrity of the mental neurovascular bundle. The mandibular attachments of the depressor muscles are separated from the bone during elevation of the apex of the flap. Then, the dissection is carried out superiorly at the lateral border, preserving the orbicularis oris and depressor anguli oris muscles intact. Thus, a V-Y island flap is created and ready to be advanced superomedially, based on the integrity of the neurovascular bundle and above-mentioned two muscles. A new oral sphincter is created with these muscles. In wide transverse narrow defects, the pars peripheralis of the orbicularis oris muscle remains intact, and upon advancing the flap upward, these muscle fibers oppose the marginal orbicularis oris fibers of the remaining lower lip.

The mucosal coverage is provided by local mucosal flaps. The width of this flap may extend up to 3 cm, thus potentially creating a 3 × 6-cm mucosal flap. Muscle is included in the proximal 2 cm of the flap, and the donor site is closed primarily. Different mucosal flap techniques including the tongue flap can also be used to reconstruct the mucosal surface. The muscle and skin are sutured separately as two layers in Y fashion after advancement of the triangular flap.

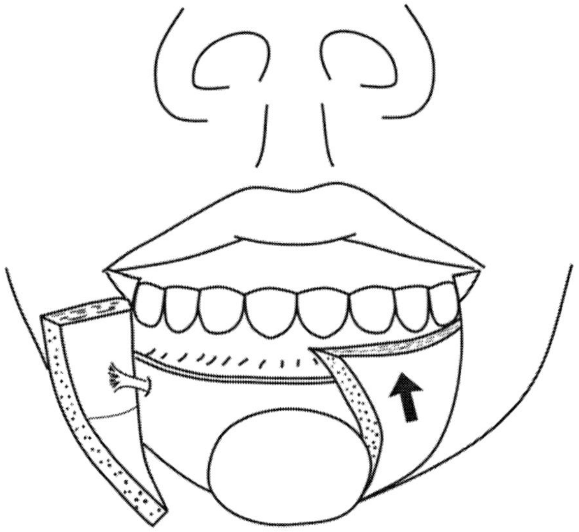

Figure 12. Mental neurovascular V-Y advancement island flap.

Total Lower Lip Reconstruction

Total lower lip defects after malignant skin tumor resection continue to be a challenge for reconstructive surgeons. The reconstructive goals in treating total lower lip defects are to restore the external skin and mucosal lining and maintenance of oral competence and sphincter function. Many techniques can be used in primary reconstruction of total lower lip defects, and most of them are functional. If a total lower lip defect is reconstructed with a static, dysfunctional technique, then the patient is prone to some problems such as drooling and gingival show.

There are two kinds of techniques for reconstruction of total lower lip defects. Local flap techniques can be used for total lower lip reconstruction. It is important to distinguish lower lip from chin or mental reconstruction. The lower lip is approximately 7.0 cm wide and 2.0

cm high. The local flap techniques described herein is adequate for total lip reconstruction, but the reconstructed lip is frequently too tight. They sometimes lead to a small mouth (microstomia), which makes it difficult to wear dentures especially for elderly patients. Larger defects that involve removal of the chin may require additional or alternate methods for reconstruction. Free flap techniques allow a functional reconstruction of extensive lower lip defects in one stage [14].

Webster Method [15] (Figure 13(a)-(b))

Essentially the entire lower lip is excised. Bilateral cheek-lip flaps are advanced medially. The skin and subcutaneous tissue are excised only for removal of tissue excesses. Minimal incisions are performed laterally through the muscle. Buccal mucosa flaps are folded forward to provide new red border. Z-plasty is performed on all vertical suture lines to prevent vertical contraction such as lip notching.

Wechselberger et al. presented a minor modification in the dissection of the orbicularis oris muscle in an attempt to improve the motor innervation and to provide adequate oral competence and labial functioning in expression and speaking. The motor function and innervation of the lips after reconstruction are documented by clinical findings as well as electrophysiological methods [16].

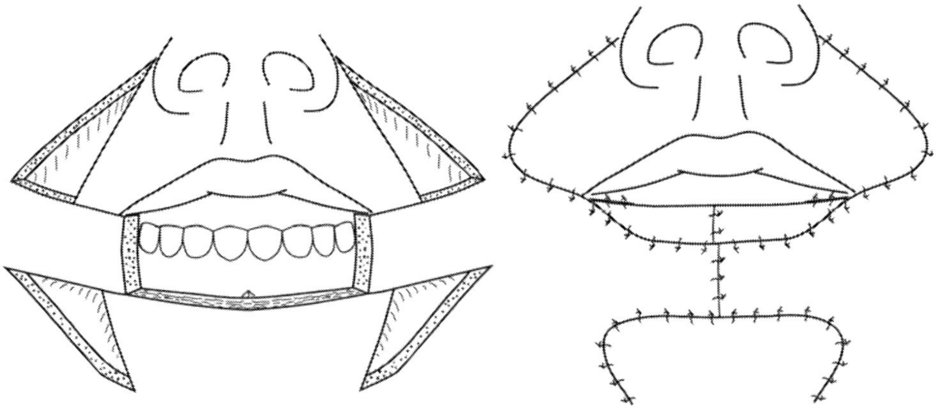

(a) (b)

Figure 13. Webster method. (a) Extent of resection and excision of half-crescents of skin and fat. (b) Postoperative view.

Nasolabial Flap (Figure 14(a)-(b))

A banner-shaped flap is designed within the nasolabial fold immediately superior and lateral to the nasolabial crease. Because hair follicles seldom extend lateral to the nasolabial crease in men, this design avoids the transfer of hair-bearing skin to the lower lip. The length of the flap is sufficient to bridge the entire lip in its transverse dimension. The width of the flap at its widest point measures approximately 2.5 cm. However, in the elderly patients with lax facial skin, the width can be extended to 3.5 cm as needed.

Proper flap design necessitates an understanding of the effect of tissue rotation at the pivot point. To minimize the incidence of creation of dog-ears at the oral commissure, the flap should be based immediately superior and lateral to the defect, and discrepancies between the medial and lateral flap length should be kept to a minimum. Placing the flap base superior and lateral to the commissure effectively suspends the reconstructed lip and prevents any downward traction.

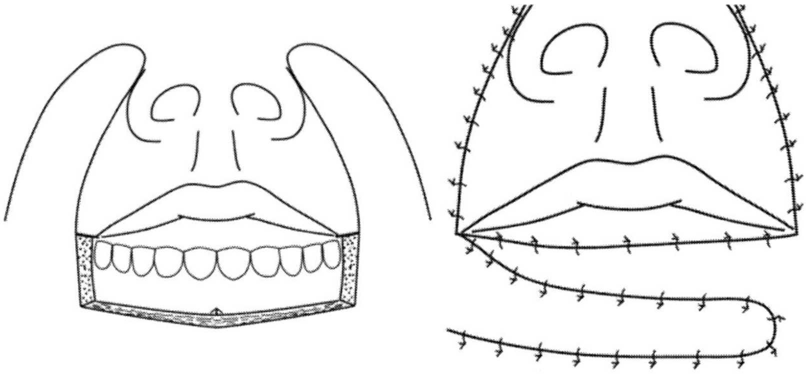

(a) (b)

Figure 14. Bilateral subcutaneous nasolabial flaps. (a) Preoperative design. (b) Postoperative view.

The flap is elevated in the subcutaneous plane, immediately superficial to the facial musculature. The distal flap is tapered to provide simple closure without distortion of the lower eyelid. After transposition into the defect, the distal flap is often trimmed and discarded. The donor site is closed primarily, with modest lateral cheek undermining as required.

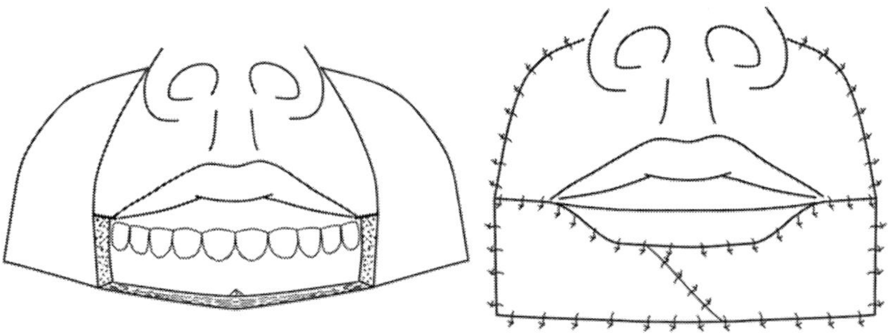

(a) (b)

Figure 15. Gate flap. (a) Preoperative design. (b) Postoperative view.

The flap(s) are easily transposed into the lip defect. If the commissure remains intact, the flap pedicle can be divided as early as 9 days after the procedure. In defects that are vertically short, a single flap may suffice to adequately restore the lower lip height. When vertical deficit is large, bilateral flaps may be interposed to reconstruct the entire vertical dimension of the lip. One flap serves as skin coverage, and the other serves as lining. Occasionally, the use of supplementary buccal mucosal flaps may provide additional lining. The transposed nasolabial flap nicely simulates the resected vermilion in shape. In addition, medical tattooing can later be used to simulate the vermilion color, if desired [17]. Fujimori presented a minor modification using transposed nasolabial island flaps; the so called "gate flap" [18]. (Figure 15(a)-(b))

Cervicofacial Flap

The lower lip defects are reconstructed with cervicofacial flaps raised with supraomohyoid neck dissections and anterior based dorsal tongue flaps. The cervicofacial flap is used to replace the skin of the lower lip, and the tongue flap is used to replace the mucosal surface and the vermilion. The tongue flap is separated from its pedicle after three weeks [19].

Yu's Technique (Figure 16(a)-(b))

A horizontal incision is made laterally from the corner of the mouth. The length of the incision is slightly longer than the defect if the flap is unilateral, or slightly longer than the half of the defect if the flap is bilateral. This incision continues up to the nasolabial fold and should be slightly curved. Meanwhile, we continue the horizontal incision in an inferior direction for about 1.5 cm. From the end of the curved upper part, an incision is drawn perpendicular to the horizontal line, which is almost half the distance between them. The horizontal line on its medial half is composed of full-thickness tissue of the oral mucosa. The lateral half includes skin and subcutaneous tissue, superficial to the underlying musculature. This reconstruction provides skin and muscle in the medial part and skin only in the lateral part. a new labial vermilion is created by means of a flap from the oral mucosa in the form of a parallelogram coming from the commissure [20,21].

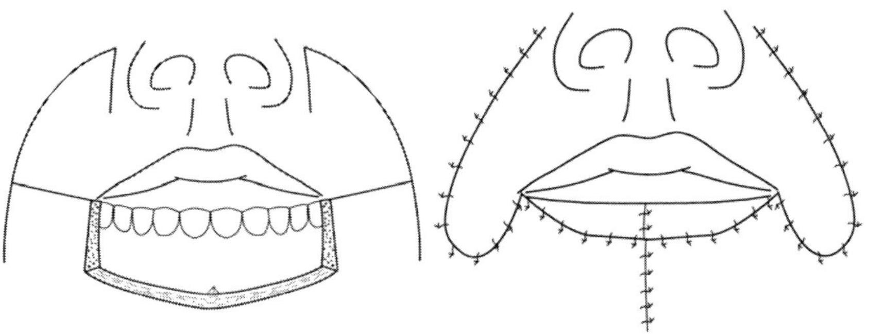

(a) (b)

Figure 16. Yu's technique. (a) Preoperative design. (b) Postoperative view.

Forearm Flap

Sakai et al. [22] and Sadove et al. [23] reported on the use of a composite radial forearm-palmaris longus free flap for total lower lip reconstruction. Ozdemir et al. recommended the sensate radial forearm-palmaris longus free flap for total lower lip reconstruction [24]. The most preferred free flap for reconstruction of total lower lip defects is the composite radial forearm and palmaris longus tendon flap [25]. The described refinement of the composite radial palmaris longus free flap technique allows reconstruction of the lower lip with a functioning oral sphincter, and this technique can be recommended for patients who need large lower lip resection. It provides functional recovery of the reconstructed lower lip synchronizing with the remaining upper lip.

A composite radial forearm flap including the palmaris longus tendon is designed. The skin flap for reconstruction of the intra-oral lining and the skin defect is folded over the palmaris longus tendon. Both ends of the vascularized tendon are laid through the bilateral modiolus and anchored with adequate tension to the intact orbicularis muscle of the upper lip.

A Forearm Flap Combined with a free Gracilis Muscle Transfer

The composite radial forearm-palmaris longus free flap, which provides static suspension and coverage of the defect, can be performed simultaneously. By the use of a firm support, sagging of the lower lip can be prevented but the results are not acceptable functionally. The lower lip contains the orbicularis oris musclethat plays an important role in oral sphincter function, which is essential for speech, facial expression, and eating. A prefabricated and reinnervated gracilis free flap was used to simultaneously reconstruct the labial muscular sling and cover both skin and lining mucosa [26]. Ueda et al. devised a novel method; namely, synchronized reconstruction with a forearm flap combined with transfer of the free gracilis muscle [27]. The pedicle vessels of the gracilis muscle are anastomosed to the radial artery and vein at the top of the flap. Its motor nerve is anastomosed to the buccal branch in the cheek, and both cut ends of the muscle flap are sutured to the cut end of the orbicularis oris muscle. This resulted in an excellent sphincter function.

There were some attempts of dynamic reconstruction using various flaps combined with the masseter muscle [28,29], depressor anguli oris muscle [16], rectus abdominis musculocutaneous free flap transfer [30], and temporal muscle transfer [31].

Anterolateral Thigh-Fascia Lata Flap [32]

The anterolateral thigh flap is a fasciocutaneous flap based on the musculocutaneous and septocutaneous perforators of the descending branch of the lateral circumflex femoral artery and its venae comitantes. The flap is harvested with 5-cm fascial extensions at the superior and inferior margins. The flap is folded over the fascia lata to restore the intra-oral lining and cover the external skin defect. The fascia lata extensions are divided longitudinally into two fascial strips at both margins of the flap. Two strips are tunneled through the orbicularis oris muscle in the upper lip and sutured to each other and to the orbicularis oris muscle. The remaining two strips are anchored to the zygomatic bone periosteum by permanent sutures. An anterolateral thigh flap is used for cheek and lip defects. Then, a sheet of fascia lata graft is used to reconstruct the oral sphincter. The tendon graft is passed into the subcutaneous layers of the reconstructed lip, woven into the remaining orbicularis oris muscle of the lip, and anchored to the upper lip near the philtral columns to complete the oral ring with adequate tension.

CONCLUSION

Regarding the cosmetic appearance, the new lip should eliminate the original one as much as possible with: good thickness and projection, minimal deformities produced by rearrangement of the facial muscles, sufficient height to cover the teeth, and acceptable scars following the reconstructive procedure, possibly hidden in the anatomic folds. Finally, the repair should be carried out at the time of the excision and in one stage.

We can summarize the reconstructive procedures as follows:

Cutaneous Defects

For shallow cutaneous defects that do not involve the lip vermilion and the orbicularis oris muscle, full-thickness skin grafts may be used. Care must be taken with the skin grafts to ensure that the repair does not appear "patched" and unnatural. Choose donor sites for full-thickness grafts that are inconspicuous and easily closed primarily.

Defects of 30% or Less of the Lower Lip

Defects of up to one third of the lower lip can usually be closed primarily, because of the tremendous distensibility of the three elements of the lip (skin, orbicularis oris muscle, and buccal mucosa).

Defects of 30% to 50% of the Lower Lip

Defects of 30% to 50% of the lower lip can be closed with a stepladder or lip switch flap. In most circumstances, stepladder reconstruction achieves good function more quickly than the lip switch flap and has a better aesthetic outcome.

Defects of 50% to 75% of the Lower Lip

Defects of 50% to 75% of the lower lip can be closed with Gillies fan flap or Karapandzic flap. The latter flap generally provides a better functional result. Both of these flaps cause rounding of the corner of the mouth that compromises the aesthetic outcome.

Transverse Narrow Defects in the Lower Lip

V-Y advancement flap with tongue flap or mucosal flap is safe and can be used to reconstruct transverse narrow defects in the lower lip with good functional and aesthetic outcomes.

Total Lower Lip Reconstruction

Total lower lip defects after large malignant tumor excision continue to be a challenge for reconstructive surgeons. The reconstructive goals are to restore the oral lining, the external cheek, oral competence, and function. The local flap techniques can be used for total lower lip reconstruction, but the reconstructed lip is frequently very tight. The free flap technique allows a functional reconstruction of extensive lower lip defects in one stage.

REFERENCES

[1] Johanson B, Aspelund E, Breine U, et al. Surgical treatment of non-traumatic lower lip lesions with special reference to the step technique. A follow-up on 149 patients. *Scand J Plast Reconstr Surg.* 1974; 8: 232-240.

[2] Schuchardt K. Operationen im Gesicht und im kieferbereich Operationen an den Lippen. In Bier A, Braun H, Kummel H (eds): Chirurgische Operationslehre. Leipzig, JA Barth. 1954. (in German)

[3] Estlander JA. Eine Methode aus der einen Lippe Substanzverluste der anderen zu eresetzen. *Arch Klin Chir.* 1872; 14: 622. (in German)

[4] Abbe R. A new plastic operation for the relief of deformity due to double harelip. *Plast Reconstr Surg.* 1968; 42: 481-483.

[5] Smith JW. The anatomical and physiologic acclimatization of tissue transplanted by the lip switch technique. *Plast Reconstr Surg.* 1960; 26: 40-56.

[6] Gillies H, Millard DR: The Principle and Art of Plastic Surgery. Little Brown & Co., Boston (1957).

[7] Karapandzic M. Reconstruction of lip defects by local arterial flaps. *Br J Plast Surg.* 1974; 27: 93-97.

[8] McGregor IA. Reconstruction of the lower lip. *Br J Plast Surg.* 1983; 36: 40-47.

[9] Nakajima T, Yoshimura Y, Kami T. Reconstruction of the lower lip with a fan-shaped flap based on the facial artery. *Br J Plast Surg.* 1984; 37: 52-54.

[10] Yano K, Hosokawa K, Kubo T. Combined tongue flap and V-Y advancement flap for lower lip defects. *Br J Plast Surg.* 2005; 58: 258-262.

[11] Bayramicli M, Numanoglu A, Tezel E. The mental V-Y island advancement flap in functional lower lip reconstruction. *Plast Reconstr Surg.* 1997; 100: 1682-1690.

[12] Bocchi A, Baccarani A, Bianco G, et al. Double V-Y advancement flap in the management of lower lip reconstruction. *Ann Plast Surg.* 2003; 51: 205-209.

[13] Ono I, Yamashita T, Kamiya T, et al. Lower lip and vermilion reconstruction with buccal musculomucosal flap combined with V-Y plasty after malignant tumor excision. *Plast Reconstr Surg.* 2006; 117: 133e-139e.

[14] Jeng SF, Kuo YR, Wei FC, et al. Reconstruction of concomitant lip and cheek through-and-through defects with combined free flap and an advancement flap from the remaining lip. *Plast Reconstr Surg.* 2004; 113: 491-498.

[15] Webster RC, Coffey RJ, Kelleher RE. Total and partial reconstruction of the lower lip with innervated musclebearing flaps. *Plast Reconstr Surg.* 1960; 25: 360-371.

[16] Kushima H, Iwasawa M, Kiyono M, et al. Functional reconstruction of total lower lip defects with a radial forearm free flap combined with a depressor anguli oris muscle transfer. *Ann Plast Surg.* 1997; 39: 182-185.

[17] Rudkin GH, Carlsen BT, Miller TA. Nasolabial flap reconstruction of large defects of the lower lip. *Plast Reconstr Surg.* 2003; 111: 810-817.

[18] Fujimori R. "Gate flap" for the total reconstruction of the lower lip. *Br J Plast Surg.* 1980; 33: 340-345.

[19] Akbas H, Karacaoglan N. Reconstruction of large lower lip defects: a new method. *Otolaryngol Head Neck Surg.* 2001; 124: 456-458.

[20] Lopez AC, Ruiz PC, Campo FJ, et al. Reconstruction of lower lip defects after tumor excision: an aesthetic and functional evaluation. *Otolaryngol Head Neck Surg.* 2000; 123: 317-323.

[21] Yu JM. A new method for the reconstruction of the lower lip after tumor excision. *Eur J Plast Surg.* 1989; 12: 155-159.

[22] Sakai S, Soeda S, Endo T, et al. A compound radial artery forearm flap for the reconstruction of lip and chin defect. *Br J Plast Surg.* 1989; 42: 337-338.

[23] Sadove RC, Luce EA, McGrath PC. Reconstruction of the lower lip and chin with the composite radial forearm-palmaris longus free flap. *Plast Reconstr Surg.* 1991; 88: 209-214.

[24] Ozdemir R, Ortak T, Kocer U, et al. Total lower lip reconstruction using sensate composite radial forearm flap. *J Craniofac Surg.* 2003; 14: 393-405.

[25] Jeng SF, Kuo YR, Wei FC, et al. Total lower lip reconstruction with a composite radial forearm-palmaris longus tendon flap: a clinical series. *Plast Reconstr Surg.* 2004; 113: 19-23.

[26] Lengele BG, Testelin S, Bayet B, et al. Total lower lip functional reconstruction with a prefabricated gracilis muscle free flap. *Int J Oral Maxillofac Surg.* 2004; 33: 396-401.

[27] Ueda K, Oba S, Ohtani K, et al. Functional lower lip reconstruction with a forearm flap combined with a free gracilis muscle transfer. *J Plast Reconstr Aesthet Surg.* 2006; 59: 867-870.

[28] Shinohara H, Iwasawa M, Kitazawa T, et al. Functional lip reconstruction with a radial forearm free flap combined with a masseter muscle transfer after wide total excision of the chin. *Ann Plast Surg.* 2000; 45: 71-73.

[29] Demir Y, Latifoglu O, Yavuzer R, et al. Oral commissure reconstruction with split masseter muscle transposition and cheek skin flap. *J Craniomaxillofac Surg.* 2001; 29: 351-354.

[30] Kiyokawa K, Hayakawa K, Yanaga H, et al. Primary reconstruction after resection of a buccal mucosal malignant tumor with dynamic reconstruction of the angulus oris. *J Jpn Plast Reconstr Surg.* 1998; 18: 9-14.

[31] Yamauchi M, Yotsuyanagi T, Yokoi K, et al. One-stage reconstruction of a large defect of the lower lip and oral commissure. *Br J Plast Surg.* 2005; 58: 614-618.

[32] Yildirim S, Gideroglu K, Aydogdu E, et al. Composite anterolateral thigh-fascia lata flap: a good alternative to radial forearm-palmaris longus flap for total lower lip reconstruction. *Plast Reconstr Surg.* 2006; 117: 2033-2041.

In: Progress in Oral Cancer Research
Editor: Frederik L. Nielsen, pp 125-142

ISBN 978-1-60021-865-1

Chapter VI

Epidemiological Research: An Essential, Integral Component of Patient Care

E.M. O'Sullivan
Oral & Maxillofacial Surgery Dept., Cork University Dental Hospital, Cork, Ireland.

Abstract

Epidemiology is often seen as a rather remote entity, far removed from the real world of patient care. While it is frequently identified with narrow epidemiological aims such as the publication of large tomes of incidence and mortality rates, epidemiology has a critical role to play in the fight against cancer. It is difficult, if not impossible, to properly organise and implement a response to a specific disease without detailed information on its aetiology, epidemiology, natural history, therapeutic options and patient outcome. This is particularly true in the fight against oral cancer. Analysis of relevant patient details may lead to the identification of aetiological factors, regional variation in incidence and mortality rates, and assist in the development of preventive strategies and improved services.

However, epidemiological analysis can only be as good as the quality of the data collected. The validity of the incidence data depends on full case ascertainment with microscopic confirmation, accurate ICD classification including sub-code or 4th digit, as well as exact dates of diagnosis and death. Meaningful comparative survival analysis requires treatment related details, and accurate staging data. This is dependent on three issues: (i) the accuracy, completeness and availability of the original medical notes, (ii) intensity of the diagnostic work-up and (iii), the regional cancer registration protocols. While international research has continuously highlighted the importance of appropriate staging of tumours to facilitate stratification of definitive treatment and evaluation of results, the availability of tumour-related variables such as staging and sub-site location is generally disappointing.

A high resolution study of Oral and Pharyngeal Cancer in Southern Ireland revealed sub-optimal recording of vital details. This phenomenon is by no means unique to

Ireland, or even, to head and neck cancer. Indeed, international reports indicate that survival comparisons are frequently limited by the quality of the staging information available and the accuracy with which it is recorded. Clearly, the current level of missing data undermines the power of epidemiological research and the evaluation of patient care. We must all accept responsibility for ensuring that accurate and complete data on disease stage, management and outcomes are recorded as information collection and audit are crucial to improving services.

Introduction

While the practice of medicine has been constantly evolving since the days of Hippocrates (430 BC), the last 150 years have been termed the golden age of medicine as it has been a period of unprecedented growth and development. At the beginning of the 19th century, the field of medicine had relatively little to offer in the face of the virtual plague of infectious diseases that were a major source of premature mortality. The traditional therapeutic practices of bleeding and purging gradually gave way to the practice of close clinical observation, the establishment of a definitive diagnosis and the estimation of a probable prognosis (Le Fanu, 2000). Between 1880 and 1947, the field of microbiology was formally established, initially in the face of stiff opposition and ridicule, and specific microbes were identified as the cause of many of the common infectious diseases. The introduction of immunization processes ended centuries of fear associated with diseases such as smallpox, tuberculosis, typhoid, cholera, polio, and plague (Atchley, 1988). However, low average life expectancies, malnutrition, poor sanitation and minimal formal medical services contributed to a predominant focus on perceived priorities such as obstetrics, infectious disease control, and pain management for much of that time period.

The 20th century, and particularly the period around World War II, witnessed a quantum leap in the practice of medical science with the introduction of antibiotics, intravenous fluids, blood banks, increased sophistication and safety in anaesthesia, and the harnessing of irradiation for diagnostic and therapeutic purposes. Other major advances came about with the formalisation of state involvement in medical welfare, for example the establishment of the National Health Service in the UK in 1945, the introduction of steroids, the discovery of DNA by Crick and Watson, and of course, major advances such as open heart surgery, and organ transplantation. Increasing success at a variety of macro levels – socio-economic, medical science, state services and education – contributed to an order of magnitude increase in the quality of life, a dramatic decrease in perinatal and perioperative mortality, and an increase in the average life expectancy, particularly among developed societies. Indeed, the average life expectancy at birth in developed countries is currently 71.0 years for males and 78.1 years for females, representing a substantial improvement (13%-15%) on figures quoted for 1950 when a male infant was expected to live only 62.9 years, and the average female survived 68.1 years (U.N, 2005). Although rates in developing countries still lag behind those of the more affluent regions, a 50% improvement has been achieved in recent decades bringing the male life expectancy rate to 63.4 years (females, 66.8) compared with 40.6 years in 1950 (females, 42.3 years).

The pronounced shift in global disease burden, and subsequent reduction in mortality from infectious or communicable diseases, has resulted in the situation where cancer has now come to the fore as a major public health challenge. Since the risk of cancer increases substantially with age (Parkin et al., 1992), the risk doubling in each successive decade of life, enhanced longevity has resulted in the current situation where cancer is second only to cardiovascular disease as the major cause of death in most developed regions. In 2000, approx. 10 million new cancer diagnoses and 6 million cancer deaths occurred worldwide, representing 13% of all deaths (Horton, 2005), with almost 2.8 million new cases and 1.9 million deaths annually throughout Europe (Sancho-Garnier et al., 2004). Furthermore, current estimates suggest that by the year 2020, the number of new cases will grow to between 15 and 20 million, with as many as 12 million deaths (Sener, 2005; Sikora, 1999). Indeed, Phillip Sharp (2007) recently predicted that, given the highly age-specific nature of cancer incidence and the aging profile of the population, cancer is likely to displace heart disease as the most common cause of death. Clearly, the major challenge facing medical science in the 21st century is to optimize the development and delivery of oncologic interventions to patients in the face of this increased disease burden, across political and socio-economic divides.

Epidemiology

In today's post-genomic scientific environment, with constantly advancing technologies and the promise of highly targeted personalized therapies, it is easy to look to the tremendous advances in biomedical research for the optimal response to the life-threatening and relatively ubiquitous challenge of human cancer. Epidemiology, on the other hand, is often seen as a rather remote entity, far removed from the real world of patient care. While it is frequently identified with narrow epidemiological aims, such as the publication of large tomes of incidence and mortality rates, epidemiology has a critical role to play in the fight against cancer. Indeed, it is difficult, if not impossible, to properly organise and implement a response to a specific disease without detailed information on its aetiology, epidemiology, natural history, therapeutic options and patient outcome.

Basic Principles

Epidemiology deals with the frequency and occurrence of specific diseases within defined populations. Epidemiological studies are generally classified under three headings namely, descriptive, analytical and experimental. Descriptive epidemiology examines the frequency of a particular disease within a specific group of individuals or 'population' defined by the classic epidemiological triad of 'person, place and time'. Analytical epidemiology explores potential aetiological factors and seeks to ascertain causation in a non-interventional manner while experimental epidemiology tests the impact of a specific intervention on disease outcome. However, it is worth noting that all epidemiological studies will, by their very nature, contain a descriptive component. The most frequently used descriptive measures are:

The crude incidence rate	This is the number of new cases of a specific disease recorded during a given time interval, divided by the total population at risk. In cancer epidemiology, incidence rates are generally calculated on the basis of a denominator of 100,000 people, over a time interval of one year. The crude rate does not taken the overall age structure of that specific community into consideration.
Age-specific incidence rate	For any given age category, this is 100,000 times the number of cases identified within the age category, divided by the associated Population Number.
Age-adjusted incidence rate	This measure involves the artificial application of the age-specific rates to a theoretical, standard world population structure rather than using the demographic characteristics of the original study area. This standardisation technique facilitates inter-registry comparisons of annual cancer incidence rates (Boyle & Parkin, 1991).
Prevalence	This is the number of cases living with a specific disease, regardless of the time since diagnosis or whether the condition is considered cured.
Crude survival rate	The crude (observed) survival rate measures the proportion of the study population alive after a specific time period-generally measured in 1, 3, 5 and 10 year intervals. All deaths are counted, regardless of the cause.
Adjusted survival rate	This is defined as the proportion of the initial study population that escape death due to the specific cause (cancer) if all other causes of death were not operating. When reliable cause of death data is available, an adjustment can be made for those that die from other causes - only those who died of the specific disease are counted i.e. disease specific deaths.
Relative survival rate	This survival measure is used when reliable information on cause of death is unavailable and is calculated by adjusting for all other causes of death. It therefore represents the ratio of a person's chance of surviving with a specific disease relative to that of an 'average person' of the same sex and age who does not have this particular disease

Origins of Cancer Registration

While historical records indicate a certain awareness of the need to establish reliable cancer statistics dating back to the early 18th century when the forward-thinking but unsuccessful London Cancer Census (1728) was attempted, attempts at establishing reliable and comparative mortality or morbidity statistics were abortive and little factual knowledge was obtained until the beginning of the 20th century (Wagner, 1985). The first efficient efforts to obtain reliable population-based estimates of cancer incidence and prevalence are attributed to the Mecklenburg and Hamburg registries in the late 1930s (Crowley, 1995).

From the outset, both these registries placed a major emphasis on comprehensive standardised data collection procedures and integrated central administration, adopting a systematic and aggressive approach to data collection and patient follow-up. The task of the registry was outlined as the collection of data serving as a basis for (a) follow-up of individual patients, (b) reliable morbidity statistics with a view to an accurate estimation of therapeutic results, and (c) an accurate evaluation of variations in incidence of malignant neoplasms, secular as well as geographical, occupational etc. (Clemmesen, 1965).

The success of the Hamburg registry led to a steady expansion in cancer registration in the USA, Canada and throughout Europe over the next decade. Undoubtedly, the establishment of the Danish Cancer Registry in 1942 is one of the major landmarks in the history of cancer registration. It was the first cancer registry set up covering a national population, it remains the oldest functioning national cancer registry, and is considered by many to be the 'gold standard' for cancer registration. Furthermore, the Director of the Danish Cancer Registry, Dr J. Clemmesen, was among the first to highlight the benefit of establishing an international network of cancer registries. He convened a conference in Copenhagen in 1946, at which a group of twelve internationally renowned cancer experts urged the World Health Organization (WHO) to adopt cancer registration as a key global health care instrument (Crowley, 1995; Clemmesen, 1974). They suggested that:

(i) Great benefit would follow from the collection of data about cancer patients from as many different countries as possible.
(ii) Such data should be recorded on an agreed plan so as to be comparable.
(iii) Each nation should have a central registry to arrange for the recording and collection of such data.
(iv) There should be an international body whose duty it should be to correlate the data and statistics obtained in each country.

These proposals ultimately lead to the establishment of the International Agency for Research on Cancer (IARC), as the specialised cancer research centre for the WHO in 1965 and to the launch of its sister organization, the International Association of Cancer Registries (IACR) in 1966. Today, these two organizations continue to promote the ongoing development of population-based cancer registries, and the collection and analysis of reliable and accurate cancer morbidity data from a wide range of populations. Every five years, the two groups jointly produce "Cancer Incidence in Five Continents" (CI5), a reference publication which has done much to increase the availability of standardised cancer statistics from registries around the world. The stated objective of the project is "to provide comparable data on the incidence of cancer in different geographical locations, and distinct sub-populations (especially ethnic) within these locations, as a source of reference for studies requiring information on international variations in cancer risk" (Parkin et al., 2002).

Current Level of World Coverage

The most recent volume of Cancer in Five Continents (CI5, Volume VIII) contains data from 186 registries, and 214 diverse populations in 57 countries for the period 1993-1997. Thus, approximately 9.3% of the world's population is currently covered by cancer registration (Table 1). This represents a steady progression in cancer registration worldwide since the first volume, covering just 32 cancer registries, was published in 1966 (Parkin et al., 2002).

The rate of registration coverage varies substantially by location, the variation roughly reflecting regional economic development. The highest rates of registration are seen in Oceania (over 70% coverage), while very low rates are evident for the continents of Asia (4.2%) and Africa (0.8%) as illustrated in Figure 1.

Table 1: Population & Cancer Incidence Coverage in CI5, VIII (Parkin et al., 2002)

Number of Registries	186
Total Population Covered	581 million
Estimated World Population	6.25 billion
Worldwide Coverage (%)	9.3%

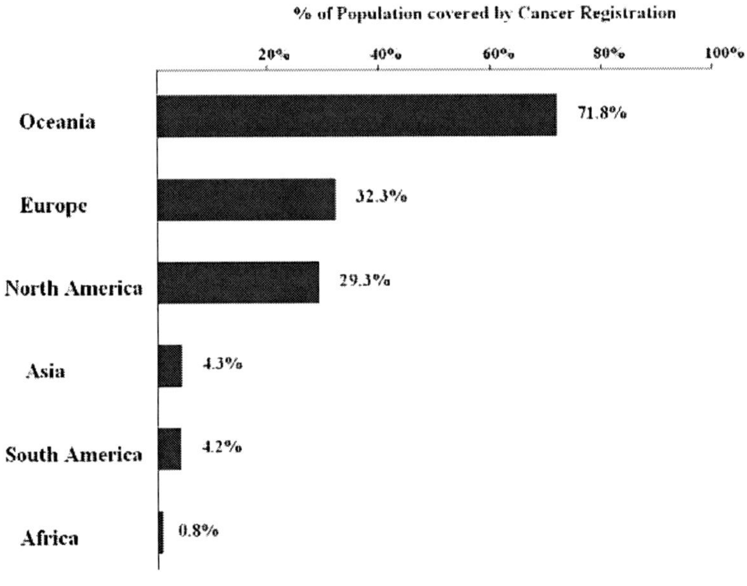

Figure 1: Worldwide Cancer Registration Cover.

The extent of this variation is further illustrated in Figure 2. Here, the sharp contrast between the proportion of the world's population resident in each region compared with the contribution made by that area to world-wide cancer registration is evident. Thus, it is seen that while Africa, South America and Asia collectively account for over 80% of the world's population, these regions contribute just over 25% of all cancer registrations. Conversely, the world's two most affluent regions, North America and Europe, contribute almost two-thirds of world-wide cancer registrations although they account for just less than one-fifth of the world's population.

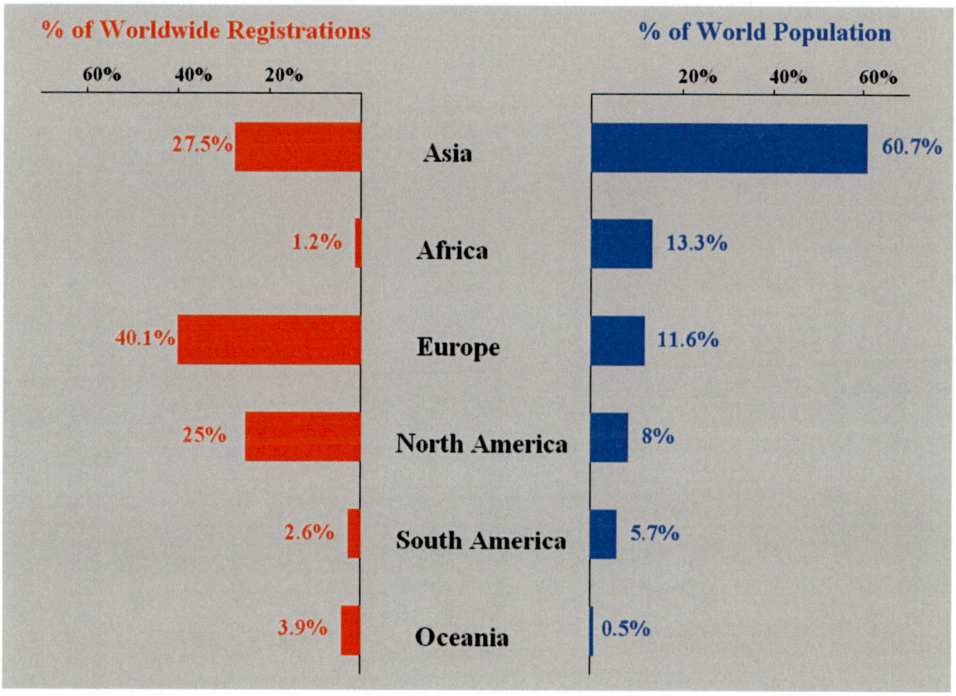

Figure 2: World Population & Cancer Registration Cover.

International Variation in Incidence Rates

When conducting an epidemiological examination of any cancer, one is immediately presented with huge variations in the disease across different geographical locations and ethnic groups. Parkin et al., (2002) reported marked international variations in risk for all cancers, stating that "for some cancer sites, these are very large (well over one hundred-fold for oesophageal cancer, for example)". Indeed, detailed analysis of the international site specific incidence rates for oral cancer revealed highly significant geographical based trends with up to a 20-fold variation between countries in annual incidence rates for individual oral and pharyngeal sites (O'Sullivan, in press). Figure 3 illustrates the variability in international age-standardised incidence rates for all oral and pharyngeal sites combined (ICD-10, C01-C14).

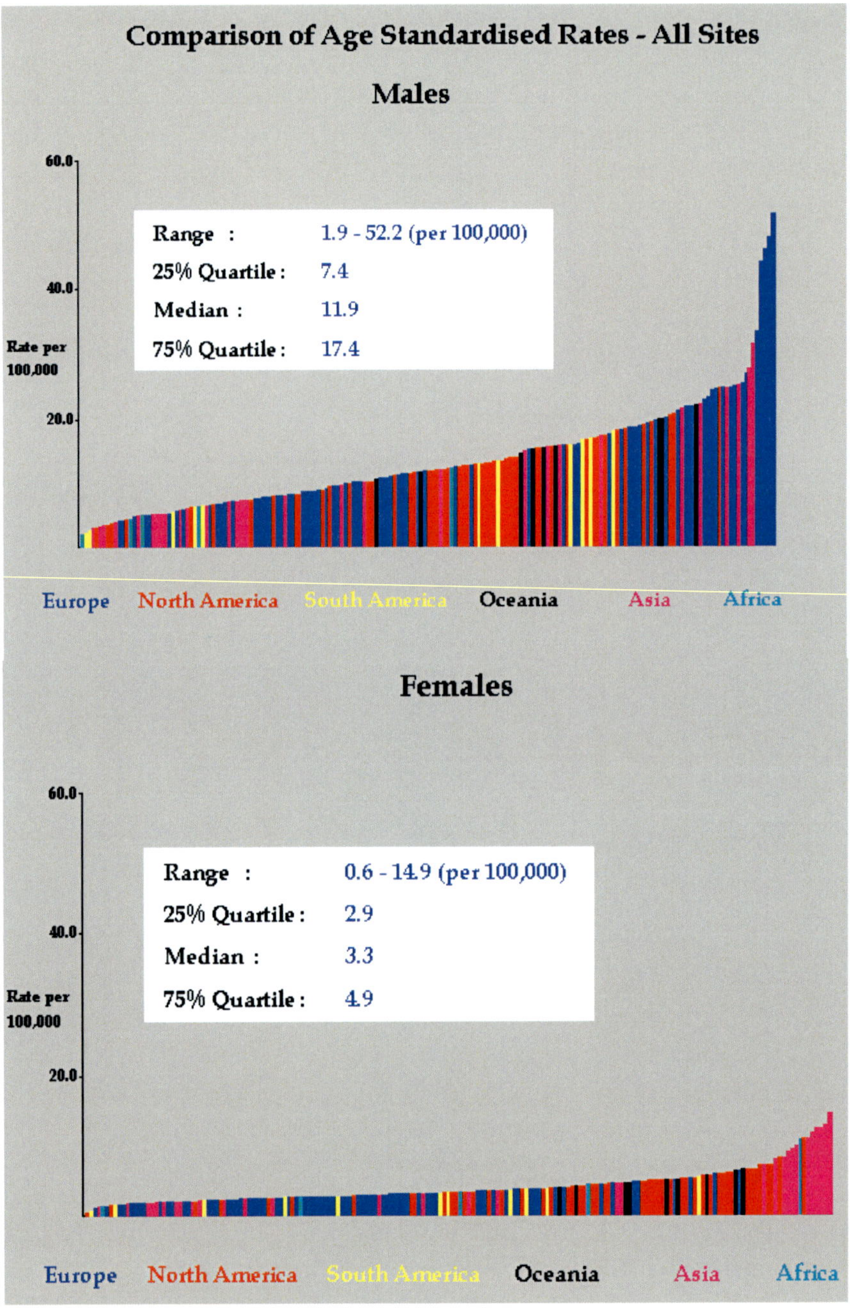

Figure 3: Comparison of ASRs for All OPC Sites (ICD-10, C00-C14) by Sex: CI5, VII.

A global insight into the pattern of the disease can be obtained by an examination of the 183 coloured bars in this comb graph, each representing the age-standardised rate (ASR) for a particular registry as listed in CI5-VII. By using the same scale for both sexes, the difference in the susceptibility to the disease between males and females is immediately evident. Thus it can be seen that the ASRs for males range from 1.9 to 52.2 per 100,000 (median 11.9), while the corresponding rates for females are considerably lower – ranging from 0.6 to 14.9 per

100,000 (median 3.3). Indeed, approximately 75% of the registries have male ASRs exceeding 7.4 per 100,000 (IQR 7.4 to 17.4); however, less than a quarter of all registries reported female rates in excess of 5.0 per 100,000 (IQR 2.9 to 4.9).

This comb graph (Figure 3) also clearly demonstrates the high European rates of oral and pharyngeal cancer in males; indeed, the five highest such rates in this series were all recorded by registries in Northern France; epidemiological research indicates that the geographical variations in mortality of head and neck cancer in France are closely linked to those for alcohol mortality (Menegoz, 2002). On the other hand, female rates follow quite a different pattern and show greater uniformity (as well as being considerably lower) with European rates being generally well below the median while the higher rates are recorded almost entirely by Asian registries.

The next comb graph (Figure 4), highlights some interesting differences in the pattern of age standardised incidence rates for specific oral and pharyngeal sites for males, namely lip, oropharynx, nasopharynx and hypopharynx (O'Sullivan, In press, reproduced by the kind permission of editor). The wide spectrum of international experience is quite evident, namely:

(i) The highest rates of lip cancer in males are recorded in South Australia and in areas of North America, as is in keeping with the known aetiological links between lip cancer and UV exposure.

(ii) Nasopharyngeal cancer (NPC) on the other hand is a rare event in most regions as displayed by the IQR 0.4-1.0, with high male rates recorded only in Asia (Hong Kong, 24.3) and in areas with a strong immigrant Asian population such as San Francisco, and Los Angeles. Unlike most OPC sites, the aetiology of NPC has not been linked to alcohol and tobacco consumption, but rather to the Epstein-Barr virus and the consumption of unusual dietary items (such as salted fish, principally in southern China and Tunisia). Indeed, the geographic and ethnic distribution of NPC illustrated here also suggests that the disease is associated with specific genetic and environmental factors as postulated by Grulich et al., (1995) and Muir & Weiland, (1995).

(iii) In contrast, the comb graphs for male oropharyngeal and hypopharyngeal cancer highlight the significance of the European experience, as few other registries record a rate in excess of 5.0 per 100,000. In fact, the five highest recorded rates are all from French registries and the majority of the top fifteen incidence rates are reported by European registries. These trends have been linked with very high levels of alcohol and tobacco consumption in those regions, and particularly to the combined usage of these substances, highlighting the immense impact of behavioural issues such as alcohol abuse in male oropharyngeal and hypopharyngeal cancer (Menegoz, 2002). High male rates were also reported in areas of Central and Eastern Europe, and Latin America (Francheschi et al., 2000).

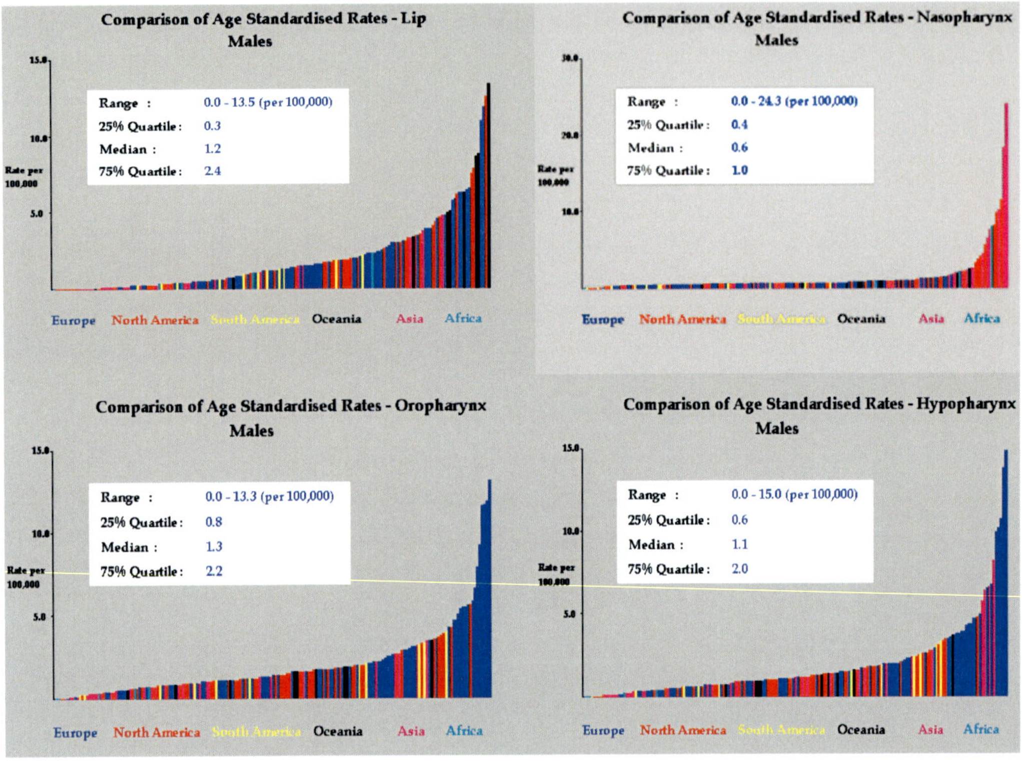

Figure 4: Comparison of ASRs for Lip, Oropharyngeal & Nasopharyngeal and Hypopharyngeal Cancer in Males (O'Sullivan, in press).

Epidemiological research of this nature, particularly when combined with behavioural data and information on temporal trends, may provide vital clues that assist in the identification of further aetiological factors. Indeed, examination of incidence trends in oral cancer over the past few decades reveals several significant changes, including the dramatic reduction in the M: F ratio from 6:1 to < 2:1, and site specific changes such as the decline in lip and salivary gland cancer in most countries and the increase in tongue and intra-oral lesions (Neville & Day, 2002; La Vecchia et al., 2004; Levi et al., 2003). Analysis of regional and temporal variation in the incidence of oral and pharyngeal cancer confirms the significant aetiological role of tobacco and alcohol. Furthermore, such analysis may provide the answers to currently unresolved issues such as the observed increased incidence in females and younger males and among those lacking the traditionally established risk factors (Partridge, 2000; Johnson, 1999); ultimately, this should enable us to develop and implement effective preventive strategies and to evaluate the effectiveness of existing preventive interventions.

Mortality Rates

Incidence rates alone, however, do not provide the full story. Accurate mortality rates are also critically important as they allow researchers to:

- Estimate disease prevalence i.e. the number of subjects requiring clinical surveillance or active therapeutic intervention, an essential step in determining healthcare investment and research priorities.
- Prevalence estimates also facilitate assessment of the relative burden of cancer with respect to morbidity, mortality, as well as the socio-economic impact of the disease.
- Comparative survival analysis may highlight treatment related prognostic factors associated either with the particular treatment modality, a specific regimen or an individual treatment centre/physician. Similarly, analysis of national and international variation in survival rates may underscore the potentialities for future improvement.
- Finally, accurate survival data allow researchers to monitor the global impact of diagnostic or therapeutic advances, to plan and assess clinical trials and to undertake studies on the equity of the health service.

Factors Influencing the Quality of Epidemiological Data

While epidemiological research clearly has a pivotal role to play in any long term strategy to cure, palliate, or prevent the disease, the quality of research is highly dependent upon the quality of the data collected, which is in turn determined largely by the accuracy and completeness of the medical case files. In 2003, James S. Marks, the Director of the US National Centre of Chronic Disease Prevention and Health Promotion declared:

> *"Having complete, timely, high-quality cancer data from throughout the United States is essential to identifying, understanding, and controlling our nation's cancer burden" (Marks, 2003).*

Moreover, as Brewster (1995) pointed out, it is not enough to generate high quality data: they must be seen to be of high quality if they are to be interpreted with confidence. The validity of the incidence data depends principally on the following factors: (i) full case ascertainment, (ii) the rate of microscopic confirmation, (iii) the availability of exact dates of diagnosis and death, and, (iv) precise ICD classification. Unfortunately, research indicates that several of these basic requirements are currently not being met.

Completeness of registration, that is, the proportion of all incident cancers in the target population which are included in the registry database, should ideally be as close to 100% as possible to ensure that analysis of inter-registry variation reflects true differences in cancer risk, rather than artefacts of the registration process. Despite the rapid advances in information technology and a growing appreciation of the importance of cancer registration, full case ascertainment remains problematic. This has been attributed to international disparity in cancer registration coverage, inter-registry variation in reporting requirements, as well as variations in state and registry ethos regarding issues such as patient confidentiality, voluntary versus compulsory reporting, and the availability and extent of state support. In fact, the conflict between an individual's right to privacy and the national need for full disclosure in medical issues is becoming increasingly contentious; it is sobering to note that the introduction of legislation requiring informed consent from patients in Hamburg and Nordrhein-Westfalen in the mid-1980s resulted in a drop of approx. 30% in cancer registration in these areas (Dudeck, 2001).

Indeed, even in highly developed and well resourced countries such as the United States, the cancer registry system is far from comprehensive, existing as multiple overlapping, hierarchical systems, with diverse purposes, variable speeds of reporting and different governing bodies (Pearson et al., 2002; NPCR, 1999). Furthermore, many registries are not population-based identifying only a specific site (e.g. GIT), specific age group (childhood cancer registries) or a 'convenient-to-gather' but non-representative portion of cases – a case in point being the American College of Surgeons NCDB, the largest cancer registry in the US (Partridge, 1998).

While cancer registries may adopt different approaches to the issue of Quality Assurance, certain derivable indicators are routinely employed to monitor data for evidence of regional or site specific variation in quality and completeness. These include:

- The historic data method which compares the observed number of cases with those expected in a similar population, reviewing the stability of temporal trends in incidence rates, age-specific incidence curves and the rates of childhood cancer (Parkin & Plummer, 2002).
- An analysis of the proportion of cases with histological confirmation, a high proportion being indicative of good quality data. High rates of verification (>95%) are routinely recorded in the US (SEER) and in many Northern European registries. However, considerably lower rates (<90%) were recently recorded for many European registries including Poland, Slovakia, most English registries, South Portugal and in Italy (Ragusa) by Capocaccia et al. (2003) in the EUROCARE-III study. It is also interesting to note that while the majority of male OPC cases (94.7%) were histological confirmed, the rate of morphological verification was significantly lower rate in females (88.5%) in the most recent edition of Cancer in Five Continents (Parkin & Plummer, 2002).
- The proportion of cases registered solely on the basis of death certification (DCOs) is routinely examined as these cases represent the residuum of cases – those for which no other cancer related information was available. As the diagnostic information on death certificates is well known to suffer from a lack of precision, a high percentage of DCOs is considered a negative correlate of validity. High DCO rates (>10%) were recorded for oral and pharyngeal cancer by seven registries in CI5 VIII namely, Argentinia (Bahia), Ecuador, Italy, Japan, Korea, Philippines, and Zaragoza, Spain.
- Finally, the mortality/incidence ratio (M/I) is considered an important indicator of completeness and quality, as it is an example of the independent case ascertainment method (Parkin et al., 1994). The rates are analysed using mortality data generated by an *independent* data source (national or municipal body). The M/I should be less that one, unless the incidence is declining dramatically, and should be consistent with prevailing survival rates.

ICD classification - Oral and pharyngeal cancer registration continues to be characterised by significant site misclassification, particularly a lack of ICD fourth digit sub-site coding despite the well known prognostic significance of this information. For example, the prognosis is considerably less favourable for tumours situated in base of tongue, floor of mouth, glosso-epiglottic vallecula, pyriform sinus and supraglottic larynx than for lesions in other sub-sites within their respective ICD categories (Sant et al., 2003). While the high level of standardization attained by participating registries, and the extensive checking procedures employed by EUROCARE-3 virtually eliminated extensive misclassification for most cancers, information on anatomical sub-coding was largely unavailable for head and neck cancers. Indeed, Berrino (2003) declared that "few cancer registries have [even] recognised the importance of properly classifying the site of origin of the tumour within head and neck organs".

A chart audit undertaken as part of a high resolution study on Irish oral and pharyngeal cancer (n, 370) by the author in 2006, also highlighted this issue as over two-thirds of the lesions (67%) were coded as NOS (Not otherwise specified). Indeed, although most of the lip and salivary gland lesions were allocated a sub-site classification, the majority of tongue, floor of mouth and nasopharyngeal lesions were simply coded as NOS. Repeated use of the NOS soubriquet also featured in the recent report of the Irish National Cancer Registry (NCRI, 2007) as 100% of tongue base lesions, 100% of nasopharyngeal, 84% of tonsil and 57% of floor of mouth cancers were thus recorded. The current lack of accurate information of specific tumour location clearly compromises the value of detailed analysis of incidence trends and significantly undermines national and international efforts to produce much needed, accurate survival estimates for head and neck cancer. Ideally, such survival estimates would be adjusted for case-mix taking all possible factors into consideration, particularly the stage of disease at diagnosis and the degree of therapeutic intervention. However, adjustment for these issues is complex and is highly dependent upon (i) the availability and quality of the medical records (ii) the intensity of the diagnostic work-up and (iii) regional cancer registration protocols.

(i) Medical Records

The accuracy, completeness and availability of the original medical notes has a critical role to play in determining the availability of staging data. While international research has continuously highlighted the importance of appropriate staging of tumours to facilitate stratification of definitive treatment and evaluation of results, the availability of staging information remains generally disappointing as highlighted by the following international oral cancer studies:

- Ireland – staging information unavailable for 91% of cases, tumour size unavailable for 75% cases (O'Sullivan, 2006).
- Irish National Cancer Registry (NCRI, 2007) – TNM staging unavailable for 57.7% of females with oral cancer and 50.2% of males; while T-stage was reported missing for just 27%, this still compares most unfavourably with rates routinely reported NCI SEER staging rates (94%).

- Brazil – tumour size missing for 48%, nodal status unavailable for 49% (Cervasio et al., 2001)
- Western Australia Cancer Registry – stage unavailable for 63% of lip cancers and 50% of oesophageal cancers (Threlfall et al., 2005)

However, this phenomenon is by no means unique to Ireland, or even, to head and neck cancer. Indeed, international reports indicate that survival comparisons are frequently limited by the quality of the staging information available and the accuracy with which it is recorded (Visser & van Leeuwen, 2005). Indeed, staging information was available for only 19% of the 151,244 cases of colorectal cancer recorded in EUROCARE-3, while the SEER registry achieved 100% staging (Gatta et al., 2003). Similarly, staging data was largely unavailable for stomach cancer as the majority (76.2%) of the EUROCARE-3 registries had staging data for less than 50% of their cases (Capocaccia, 2003).

(ii) The Intensity of the Diagnostic Work-up:

The clinical stage recorded at diagnosis depends on the extent of investigation, which varies considerably between centres and countries; the continuing development of more sensitive techniques for the detection of regional and distant metastases can therefore confound comparisons of stage-specific survival over time or between countries. The diagnostic basis for the recorded clinical stage must therefore be taken into consideration as it allows researchers to control of the 'stage migration phenomenon' in their analysis. This phenomenon explains the improved survival rates observed for patients who undergo extensive staging procedures (MRI/ CT/ PET etc) as those with subtle advanced disease are upstaged, leading to improved survival rates for all stages. Conversely, a less vigorous staging process tends to lower the survival rates across all stages. The availability and usage of these facilities worldwide varies widely and the current variability in the intensity of the staging protocols is thought to account for much of the unexplained variation in survival for many cancers, including colorectal (Gatta et al., 2000).

(iii) The Regional Cancer Registration Protocols

Finally, it must be acknowledged that the availability of accurate staging data is also dependent upon specific regional cancer registration protocols as not all cancer registries have systematically recorded clinical stage at diagnosis over long periods; furthermore, the diagnostic basis for the recorded clinical stage is not routinely available.

Recommendations for the Future

Clearly, the current level of missing data undermines the power of epidemiological research and the evaluation of patient care. Changes are required on several fronts namely, the cancer registries, treatment centres and, of course, the clinicians.

- Firstly, cancer registries must expand their datasets to include sub-site classification (4th digit ICD), accurate stage at diagnosis, information on diagnostic basis for staging, as well as treatment related information
- Secondly, cancer registries need to become an integral part of the clinical community, providing feedback to clinicians, health administrators and politicians, guiding policy change and helping to direct resources to create high quality care. Rapid feedback on treatment outcomes will increase interest in epidemiological research and promote a positive approach to data collection. However, registries also need to be willing to highlight areas where data collection is poor and to demand completeness
- Thirdly, while as clinicians we all know that clinical best practice demands comprehensive accurate medical records, the cancer centres and hospital management need to actively promote the benefits of comprehensive medical records and of capturing accurate staging information – both for accreditation purposes and to facilitate the estimation of the number of cases potentially available for prospective trials and retrospective studies.

    - They need to introduce policies and procedures to facilitate compliance. Even relatively simple changes such as the introduction of clearly defined roles in relation to the completion of staging forms and physician reminder systems to ensure staging forms are completed at or near the time of diagnosis have been shown to be effective.
    - The introduction of proforma forms for all hospital admissions and oncology clinics would standardise data collection, reduce missing details, and could also be used to audit existing standards. This type of reporting has been introduced successfully in many pathology labs, often alongside the traditional essay type report. Increasing focus on standardization has led to the introduction of uniform data sets and audit services in several regions, including the DAHNO (National Data for H& N Oncology) audit service in the UK (Bradley & MacKenzie, 2005). Completion of these data sets is an essential step towards evidence based treatment modification which may offer significant benefits to these patients.

- Fourthly, hospitals need to provide increased medical records resources in areas such as computerisation, staffing, training and even by simply providing adequate storage facilities. Hospitals are coming under increasing pressure from accreditation schemes to ensure that all aspects of clinical care including medical records are of the highest quality. This has led to the introduction of compulsory staging in some centres. Indeed, while the introduction of compulsory TNM staging as a condition of employment at the Ottawa Regional Cancer met with considerable resistance initially, compliance improved within a short period of time and physicians began using the data for research purposes and for program planning (Evans, 2000).

Conclusion

In any given environment, the establishment of an accurate epidemiological disease profile is fundamental to the overall planning and specification of the appropriate response of medical systems to (i) optimise patient outcome, and (ii) successfully implement preventive strategies. Accurate cancer staging is vital both at an individual level and a population level while analysis of relevant patient details may lead to the identification of aetiological factors, regional variation in incidence and mortality rates, and assist in the development of preventive strategies and improved services.

Epidemiological research and analysis must therefore be viewed as an implicit component of patient care and not simply as an optional extra. This is particularly true in the field of oral and pharyngeal cancer as the wide distribution of sub-sites and varied presenting stages suggest that multi-centre data collection and meta-analysis may hold the key to future progress. However, as already intimated, epidemiological analysis can only be as good as the quality of the data collected. Clearly, the current level of missing data undermines the power of epidemiological research and the evaluation of patient care. We must all accept responsibility for ensuring that accurate and complete data on disease stage, management and outcomes are recorded as information collection and audit are crucial to improving services.

References

Atchley, R. (1988). Social forces and aging. Ed.5. *Wadsworth Pub Co. Belmont Calif. P.23.*

Berrino, F. (2003). The EUROCARE Study: strengths, limitations and perspectives of population-based, comparative survival studies. Editorial DOI: 2003 European Society for Medical Oncology. *Annals of Oncology; 14* (Supplement 5): v9–v13.

Boyle, P; Parkin, DM. (1991). Statistical methods for registries. In: Jensen, OM; Parkin, DM; MacLennan, R. et al Eds. Cancer registration – principles and methods. *IARC Scientific Publication No. 95. Lyon: IARC.*

Bradley, PJ; Mackenzie, K. (2005). Head and neck cancer in the United Kingdom: the current documents. *Clinical Otolaryngol; 30*, 451–457.

Brewster, J. (1995). Improving the quality of cancer registration data. *R Soc Med; May; 88(5)*:268-71

Capocaccia, R; Gatta, G; Roazzi, P. et al. (2003). The EUROCARE-3 database: methodology of data collection, standardisation, quality control and statistical analysis. *Annals of Oncology 14* (Supplement 5): v14–v27.

Cervasio, SOL; Dutra, RA; Tartaglia, S. et al. (2001). Oral squamous cell carcinoma: a retrospective study of 740 cases in a Brazilian population. *Braz Dent J; 12(1)*:57-61.

Clemmesen, J. (1965). Statistical studies in the aetiology of malignant neoplasms. Acta Pathol Microbiol Scand; 1 (Suppl. 174). In: Crowley, MJ. (1995). *Cancer – The Irish Experience*. Ed 1.

Clemmesen, J. (1974). Statistical studies in the aetiology of malignant neoplasms. *Acta Pathol Microbiol Scand; 4* (Suppl. 247).

Crowley, MJ. (1995). *Cancer – The Irish Experience.* Ed 1.

Dudeck, J. (2001). Informed consent for cancer registration. *Lancet Oncol; 2*: 8-9.

Evans, B. (2000). Lessons Learned in Implementing the Capture of Stage Information in a Regional Cancer Centre, Ottawa Regional Cancer Centre. In: National Initiative to Improve Cancer Survival Information – Workshop Report. *Chronic Diseases in Canada; Vol. 19: No.2.*

Francheschi, S; Bidoli, E; Herrero, R. et al (2000). Comparison of cancers of the oral cavity and pharynx worldwide: etiological clues. *Oral Oncol, Eur J Canc; 36*:106-115.

Gatta, G; Capocaccia, R; Sant, M. et al. (2000). Understanding variations in survival for colorectal cancer in Europe: a Eurocare high resolution study. *Gut 2000; 47:533–8.*

Gatta, G; Ciccolallo, L; R. Capocaccia R. et al. (2003). Differences in colorectal cancer survival between European and US populations: the importance of sub-site and morphology. *European Journal of Cancer; 39:2214–22.*

Johnson, NW. (1999). Oral cancer. *FDI World Dental Press Ltd.*

NCI - SIG, (1999). Cancer Surveillance Research Implementation Plan. Prepared by the Surveillance Implementation Group, National Cancer Institute, National Institutes of Health. Full Text Available online at www.cancercontrol.cancer.gov/sig/appb.htm

NCRI. (2007). National Cancer Registry of Ireland. *Data on Cancer Incidence in Ireland 1994-2004*. Unpublished data obtained from Ms. S. Deasy, NCRI on request.

Grulich, AE; McCredie, M; Coates, M. (1995). Cancer incidence in Asian migrants in New South Wales, Australia. *Br J Canc*; *Feb: 71(2): 400-8.*

Horton, R. (2005). The neglected epidemic of chronic disease. *Lancet. Online Publication, 5 October 2005, 67454-5.*

La Vecchia, C; Lucchini, F; Negri, E; Levi, F. (2004). Trends in oral cancer mortality in Europe. *Oral Oncol; 40:4:433-9.*

Le Fanu, J. (2000). *The rise and fall of modern medicine*. Carroll & Graf Publishers.

Levi, F; Lucchni, F; Negri, E; La Vecchia, C. (2003). The end of the tobacco related lung epidemic in Europe. *J Natl Cancer Inst; 95:631-2.*

Marks, JS. (2003). Cancer Registries: The Foundation for Cancer Prevention and Control. *NCR 2003 Fact Sheet.*

Menegoz, F; Lessec'H, JM; Rame, JP et al. (2002). Lip, oral cavity and pharynx cancers in France: incidence, mortality and trends (period 1975-95). *Bull Canc; Apr:89:4:419-29.*

Muir, C; Weiland, L. (1995). Upper aerodigestive tract cancers. *Cancer; 75: 147-53.*

Neville, BW; Day, TA. (2002). Oral cancer and precancerous lesions. *CA Cancer J Clin; 52*: *195-215.*

NPCR (1999). National Program of Cancer Registries: Cancer Surveillance System (NPCR-CSS) Rationale and Approach. Atlanta, GA, National Program of Cancer Registries.

O'Sullivan, EM. (In press). International Variation in the Incidence of Oral and Pharyngeal Cancer. *Community Dental Health.*

O'Sullivan, EM. (2006). Availability & Accuracy of Staging Information in Oral & Pharyngeal Cancer in Southern Ireland Presented at: 14th Annual Research Conference CUH/UCC, Ireland. 21-06-2006.

Parkin, DM; Plummer, M. (2002). Comparability and quality of data. Ch. 5 In: Parkin, DM; Whelan, SL; Ferlay, J. et al. Eds. (2002). *Cancer Incidence in Five Continents, Vol. VIII. (IARC Scientific publication No. 155). Lyon, IARC.*

Parkin, DM; Whelan, SL; Ferlay, J. et al. Eds. (2002). *Cancer Incidence in Five Continents, Vol. VIII. (IARC Scientific publication No. 155). Lyon, IARC.*

Parkin, DM; Muir, CS; Whelan, SL. et al. Eds. (1992). *Cancer Incidence in Five Continents, Vol. VI. (IARC Scientific publication No. 120). Lyon, IARC.*

Partridge, EE. (1998). The National Cancer Database: Ten years of growth and commitment. *CA Cancer J Clin; 48:131-133.*

Partridge, M. (2000). Oral cancer: 1. The genetic basis of the disease. *Dental Update; 27:242-8.*

Pearson, ML; Ganz, PA; McGuigan, K. et al. (2002). The case identification challenge in measuring quality of cancer care. *J Clin Oncol; 20:4353-60.*

Sancho-Garnier, H; Levi, F; Pisani, P; Lynge, E. (2004). Europe's Cancer Burden. In: *Evidence-Based Cancer Prevention Strategies for NGOs. UICC; p.17-35.*

Sant, M; Aareleid, T; Berrino, F. et al. (2003). EUROCARE-3: survival of cancer patients diagnosed 1990–94—results and commentary. *Annals of Oncology; 14 (Suppl. 5): v61–v118.*

SEER NCI (2004). November 2004, SEER 9 Registries Data.

Sener, SF. (2005). Disease without borders. *CA Canc J Clin; 55:7-9.*

Sharp, PA. (2007). The Science of Cancer Beyond 2006. Lecture given at the investiture of Dr. John Niederhuber as Director of the National Cancer Institute. *Published online in The Oncologist; 12:136–141 www.TheOncologist.com.*

Sikora, K. (1999). Developing a global stategy for cancer. Millenium review 2000. *Eur J Cancer; 35: 14: 1870-7.*

Threlfall, T; Wittorff, J; Padabphet, B. et al. (2005). Collection of population-based cancer staging information in Western Australia – a feasibility study. Population Health Metrics 2005, 3:9. Full text available online at: http://www.pophealthmetrics.com/content/3/1/9

U.N. (2005). Earth Trends Demographics. http://earthtrends.wri.org/searchable_db/index

Visser, O; van Leeuwen FE. (2005). Stage-specific survival of epithelial cancer in North-Holland/Flevoland, The Netherlands. *Eur J Canc; 41:2351-2330.*

Wagner, G. (1985). Cancer registration: historical aspects. In: Parkin, DM; Wagner, G; Muir, CS. Eds. The Role of the Registry in Cancer Control. *IARC Publication No. 66. Lyon: International Agency for Research on Cancer. 3-12.*

In: Progress in Oral Cancer Research
Editor: Frederik L. Nielsen, pp 143-156
ISBN 978-1-60021-865-1

Chapter VII

GENOTOXIC POTENTIAL OF COMPOUNDS USED IN DENTAL PRACTICE: A CONTROVERSAL ISSUE

Daniel Araki Ribeiro[1,*] and Daisy Maria Favero Salvadori[2]
[1]Department of Health Sciences, Federal University of Sao Paulo, UNIFESP, SP, Brazil;
[2]Department of Pathology, Botucatu Medical School, Sao Paulo State University, UNESP, SP, Brazil.

ABSTRACT

Toxicology and risk assessments rely upon various testing systems to estimate risks of adverse effects from chemical exposures. In this regard, genotoxicity tests have become a fundamental tool for regulatory decisions, since the data have typically been important in regulatory schemes and decisions involving the identification of potentially DNA-damaging agents and in supporting concerns for carcinogenicity. Recently, a number of dental materials have entered the market. Such compounds have the potential to be in contact with oral tissues over extended periods of time. However, studies on the genotoxicity of dental agents are limited and contradictory. The purpose of this paper is to provide an overview on the genotoxic potential of compounds currently used in dentistry, such as fluoride, chlorhexidine, endodontic compounds, dental bleaching agents, and glass ionomer cements based on our recent research. Some of these compounds appear capable of exerting noxious activity on the genetic material. The action mechanisms are discussed. Therefore, this is an area that warrants investigation since the risk assessment of these substances with respect to genotoxicity certainly will improve oral health as far as will prevent oral carcinogenesis.

Keywords: genotoxicity; fluoride; chlorhexidine; endodontic compounds; dental bleaching agents; glass ionomer cements

INTRODUCTION

Toxicology and risk assessments rely upon various testing systems to estimate risks of adverse effects from chemical exposures. Risk managers use those estimations to help protect people from potential harm (Lamb and Brown, 2000). Regulatory agencies such as the United States Environmental Protection Agency (EPA) and the Food and Drug Administration (FDA) interpret the available toxicity data in risk assessments for regulatory decision-making.

In recent decades, genotoxicity tests have become a fundamental tool for regulatory decisions, since the data have typically been important in regulatory schemes and decisions involving the identification of potentially DNA-damaging agents and in supporting concerns for carcinogenicity (USEPA, 1986). Therefore, the use of genotoxicity testing is essential for evaluation of potential human toxicity so that hazards can be prevented. Moreover, these data contribute to significant understanding of the mode of toxic action. A variety of assays can measure genotoxicity, such as the bacterial reverse gene mutation assay (Salmonella reversion assay or Ames test), the mouse lymphoma gene mutation assay, the micronucleus test, the chromosome aberration test, and the single cell gel (comet) assay.

Recently, a number of dental materials have entered the market. Such compounds have the potential to be in contact with oral tissues over extended periods of time. Herein, genotoxicity data of dental agents are of special importance, particularly due to conflicting results so far and because many of them have not yet been investigated. As a result, the purpose of the present article is to provide an overview on the genotoxic potential of some most important compounds currently used in dental practice based on our recent research.

FLUORIDE

Fluoride intake in low concentrations during tooth development results in formation of dental enamel, which is more resistant to caries (Bartlett et al., 2005). According to the Centers for Diseases Control, fluoridation by drinking water to prevent dental caries was considered to be one of the ten most important public health achievements of the 20th century (Everett et al., 2002). It was established that a concentration of 0.7 ppm fluoride in drinking water reduces caries by 40-49% in primary teeth and 50-59% in permanent teeth, with no clinical appearance of adverse effects (WHO, 1984).

Nevertheless, some human populations are exposed to high doses of fluoride, mainly in developing countries. In this context, some studies focusing on possible genotoxic effect of excess fluoride are contradictory and inconclusive. According to some authors, lack of toxicogenetic effects was verified in Salmonella under high doses of sodium fluoride (Martin et al., 1979). Furthermore, fluoride did not induce DNA damage in mammalian cells (Matsuda, 1980; Li et al., 1989; 1995; Sato et al., 1989; Slamenova et al., 1992; Kleinsasser

* Correspondence concerning this article should be addressed to: Dr. Daniel A Ribeiro, DDS, PhD, Departamento de Ciências da Saúde, Universidade Federal de São Paulo – UNIFESP, Av. Ana Costa, 95 Vila Mathias, Santos – SP, Zip code: 11060-001. Phone +13 32222040; Fax: + 13 32222048; e-mail:daribeiro@unifesp.br.

et al., 2001; Ribeiro et al., 2004a; 2006a). On the other hand, some authors have reported the mutagenic potential of fluoride in *Drosophila melanogaster*, plants and mice (Mohamed and Chandler, 1977). Chromosome aberrations were also increased by fluoride at doses of 25-100 μg/mL in CHO cells, in cultured human lymphocytes and fibroblasts at doses of 20-40 μg/mL and by using the short-term experimental test system *in vivo* (Albanesi, 1987; Aarderma et al., 1989; Velazquez-Guadarrama et al., 2005). Sodium fluoride was able to induce morphological and neoplastic transformation of Syrian hamster embryo cells (Jones et al., 1988). Yet investigators have mentioned both synergistic and antagonist effects with known mutagens (Voegel, 1973). Taking into account the few *in vivo* genotoxicity data available, we have designed a study aiming to evaluate a possible genotoxic potential of sodium fluoride in Wistar rats. The single cell gel (comet) assay was performed in peripheral blood leukocytes, oral mucosa and brain cells of animals treated with two different doses of sodium fluoride in drinking water (7 and 100 ppm) for six weeks. No measurable genotoxicity was found by sodium fluoride in all the cellular types evaluated (Ribeiro et al., 2004b).

Fluoride is rapidly and extensively absorbed from the gastrointestinal tract after ingestion. Owing to the action of clearance mechanisms, fluoride may be transported to the liver, kidney and urinary bladder until it is ultimately excreted. In this regard, Buzalaf *et al.* (2006) have recently investigated the genotoxic effects of sodium fluoride in liver, kidney and urinary bladder of Wistar rats treated with 5, 15 and 100 ppm of sodium fluoride in drinking water for six weeks. The results showed no detectable genotoxicity as depicted by the single cell gel (comet) assay. Conversely, other authors have reported DNA damage in oral mucosa cells and hepatocytes of rats exposed to NaF at 150 mg/L when compared to control group (He et al., 2006).

Considering the hallmark of apoptosis, DNA fragmentation, some authors have verified that fluoride produced large DNA fragments, possibly due to activation of caspases and p53 with consequent up-regulation of MDM2 and p21 genes (Anuradha et al., 2000; Morgan et al., 2002; Wang et al., 2004; Otsuki et al., 2005; Satoh et al., 2005). Since these genes play an important role in the apoptotic pathways, the dysregulation of apoptosis in cells induced by fluoride could be one of the mechanisms involved in the transformation from benign to malignant phenotype. In addition, studies have shown that fluoride is able to inhibit both protein and DNA synthesis in cultured mammalian cells and promotes oxidative stress and/or lipid peroxidation *in vitro* and *in vivo* (Guan et al., 2000; Anuradha et al., 2001; Ghlsh et al., 2002; Kubota et al., 2005; He et al., 2006). Particularly, the inhibition of DNA synthesis may be a secondary effect of the inhibition of protein synthesis, or a result of the direct inhibition of DNA polymerase or other DNA-synthesis-associated enzymes. These hypotheses are relevant since there is no strong mechanism by which the genotoxic effects can be induced by direct interaction of fluoride with DNA.

CHLORHEXIDINE

Chlorhexidine is a symmetrical cationic molecule containing two 4-chlorophenyl rings and two biguanide groups connected by a central hexamethylene chain. In 1970, chlorhexidine was first reported as an effective antimicrobial agent by Loe and Schiott

(1970). To date, no other agent besides fluoride has received more attention in dentistry. Its actions include anti-dental plaque formation, gingivitis control and root-canal disinfection. However, data about the genotoxic potential of chlorhexidine are very limited and controversial. Increased DNA damage in peripheral leukocytes and buccal cells was detected by the single cell gel (comet) assay in individuals that rinsed their mouths with chlorhexidine at 0.12% concentration (Eren et al., 2001). Gene mutations were also induced by the breakdown products of chlorhexidine in microorganisms (Prasad, 1970). Furthermore, the mouse lymphoma assay detected a positive response after chrlohexidine exposure *in vitro* (Withrow et al., 1989; Mitchell et al., 1997). Nevertheless, negative results were detected in the SOS chromotest and UMU test (Sakagami et al., 1988; Klimm et al., 1989). An earlier study using SHE cells treated with chlorhexidine at concentrations up to 10 μM also showed no increase of sister-chromatid exchanges (Miyachi and Tsutsui, 2005).

On the basis of inappropriate evidence about the genotoxic potential of chrorhexidine, we designed an experimental study in order to evaluate whether this antiseptic compound can cause DNA damage in rat oral mucosa and peripheral blood cells *in vivo* (Ribeiro et al., 2004c). Statistically significant increase of DNA damage was detected either in peripheral leukocytes or in oral mucosa cells of the animals exposed to chlorhexidine at 0.12% concentration (Ribeiro et al., 2004c). However, it is not still clear how chlorhexidine is absorbed from the oral mucosa and gastrointestinal tract and then promotes these biological actions. In an attempt to elucidate this issue, the micronucleus test was applied in this setting. The results showed no increase of micronucleated cells in reticulocytes, indicating that chlorhexidine did not induce chromosome breakage or loss in erythrocytes. Recently, we assayed the genotoxic potential of chlorhexidine at concentrations ranging from 0.01 to 1 % on CHO cells. It was clearly observed that chlorhexidine at all concentrations tested did not cause an increase of DNA injury (Ribeiro et al., 2005a). In addition, we have observed that chlorhexidine was able to induce genomic damage in multiple organs such as kidney in vivo (Grassi et al., 2007). However, it is important to emphasize that *in vitro* test systems do not consider the complex homeostatic situation that occurs *in vivo*.

Some authors have provided evidence on the mode of action of chlorhexidine. The interaction between chlorhexidine and metals is assumed (Warner et al., 1993). According Negrello-Newton *et al.* (2004), the possibility of an interaction between chlorhexidine and iron must be considered. Iron mobilization has long been known to induce oxidative stress, leading to lipid peroxidation, oxidative DNA damage, and possibly plays a role in iron-induced carcinogenesis. Further studies are necessary in order to demonstrate the hazard that this compound may induce DNA damage.

Endodontic Compounds

The main purposes of endodontic therapy are to eliminate microorganisms in root canals and fillings in order to restore dental function. To best of our knowledge, only a few studies on putative genotoxicity of endodontic agents have been conducted and those report with divergent findings. Huang *et al.* (2001) have reported that zinc oxide eugenol-based sealers do not induce DNA damage in oral carcinoma cells *in vitro*. However, they have detected a dose-dependent increase of genotoxicity when cells were exposed to resin-based sealers. These data are largely of the same magnitude as those reviewed by Geurtsen *et al.* (1997). Later, Tai *et al.* (2002) found that N2-, AH26-, and AH-Plus-based root canal sealers exhibited genotoxicity by causing DNA single-strand breaks. However, Huang *et al.* (2002a,b) have demmonstrated that resin-based sealers such as AH26 and AH-Plus sealers exhibited cytotoxicity and a dose-dependent increase of DNA damage *in vitro* assessed by single cell gel (comet) assay. More recently, this research group has evidenced that toxicity of these root canal sealers is regulated by cell death (Huang et al., 2004).

In human dental pulp fibroblasts exposed to phenolic compounds, potent antimicrobial agents, no DNA breakage was detected (Chang et al., 2000; do Céu Silva et al., 2003). Conversely, these same substances were able to induce unscheduled DNA synthesis in a concentration-dependent manner on SHE cells (Hamaguchi and Tsutsui, 2000). Recently, we investigated whether formocresol, paramonochlorophenol or calcium hydroxide could induce DNA damage in mouse lymphoma cells and primary human fibroblasts by the single cell gel (comet) assay *in vitro*. These materials are widely used in endodontic practice to eradicate bacteria and consequently to produce root canal disinfection. Our data demonstrated that the single treatment with formocresol, paramonochlorofenol and calcium hydroxide at concentrations of 20, 40 and 80 μg/mL did not induce strand breaks in DNA (Ribeiro et al., 2004d). Similar results were observed in CHO cells after exposure to formocresol, paramonochlorophenol and calcium hydroxide adjusted to 100 μg/mL (Ribeiro et al., 2005a). In fact, it has been reported that chlorophenol failed to promote unscheduled DNA synthesis in the presence or absence of exogenous metabolic activation (Hagiwara et al., 2006), although cresol induced unscheduled DNA synthesis in the presence of exogenous metabolic activation (Hamaguchi and Tsutsui, 2000). By contrast, statistically significant differences in the frequencies of sister-chromatid exchanges were observed in SHE cells treated with chlorophenol or formaldehyde (Miyachi and Tsutsui, 2005) and chromossomal aberrations were induced by formocresol, with chlorophenol being a significant chromosomal aberration inducer in the presence of exogenous metabolic activation only (Hagiwara et al., 2006). Besides cresol, formocresol is also composed of formaldehyde that is a known genotoxic substance (Casanova et al., 1994). The primary genotoxic effect seems to be the formation of DNA-protein crosslinks (Merck and Speit, 1999). This finding emphasizes our negative results, since the standard alkaline single cell gel (comet) assay protocol used is not well-suited for detecting DNA-crosslinks lesions.

Under the assumption that endogenous and exogenous agents are able to generate genetic damage continuously, it would be useful to know whether, and to what extent, these antimicrobial endodontic compounds possess synergistic and/or antagonist effects with known genotoxins. Thus, we have performed assays to investigate the ability of formocresol, paramonochlorophenol and calcium hydroxide to modulate the genotoxic effects induced by the oxidatively damaging agent hydrogen peroxide and the alkylating agent methyl methanesulfonate *in vitro*. The addition of methyl methanesulfonate in increasing concentrations to cells incubated with formocresol, paramonochlorophenol or calcium hydroxide did not contribute to genetic damage (Ribeiro et al., 2006f). No changes were also observed with respect to hydrogen peroxide for all endodontic compounds evaluated (Ribeiro et al., 2006f).

Gutta-percha has been used in endodontics for more than 100 years and is today the most frequently used core material for permanent obturation of root canals (Wenberg & Ostravik, 1989). In cases of endodontic failure, however, it is necessary the endodontic re-treatment that fundamentally consists of the removal of gutta-percha cones from inside root canals. There are several methods for gutta-percha removal: thermal, mechanical and chemical solvent. Chloroform is one of chemical agents widely used for gutta-percha softening or dissolving. However, side health effects from exposure to chloroform have been reported in literature (Wourns et al., 1990). Among them, studies have addressed that the chloroform is possibly carcinogenic to humans (Hunter et al., 1991). Because of the concerns about the chloroform, clinicians and researchers have developed a renewed interest in finding alternative solvents (Kaplovitz, 1991). Eucalyptol, a widely used substance for flavoring and fragrance, has been used herein as a solvent without apparent harmful effects (Uemura et al., 1997). Taking into consideration that DNA damage and cellular death play important role during carcinogenesis, studies on genotoxic or cytotoxic effects of chloroform and other gutta-percha solvents as for example eucalyptol are needed for the comprehensive risk assessment of these compounds. The results pointed out that both gutta-percha solvents were cytotoxic at concentrations of 2.5, 5 and 10 μl/mL ($p<0.05$). On the other hand, both solvents did not induce DNA breakage at 1.25μl/mL concentration (Ribeiro et al., 2006h).

In the 1990s, mineral trioxide aggregate was developed as a root-end-filling material. A number of biocompatibility studies has been conducted either *in vitro* or *in vivo* showing that mineral trioxide aggregate has good sealing ability and tissue healing properties. Nevertheless, genotoxicity data are needed to complete risk assessment of mineral trioxide aggregate. Herein, we have investigated whether regular and white mineral trioxide aggregate can induce DNA damage in vitro by means of mouse lymphoma and CHO cells. The results showed that the materials tested did not induce DNA strand breaks at concentrations ranging from 1-1000 μg/mL as depicted by the single cell gel (comet) assay (Ribeiro et al., 2005b;2006b,c). These findings confirmed and extended the data already published showing a good biocompatibility of mineral trioxide aggregate.

Nowadays, studies have compared mineral trioxide aggregate with Portland cement. The findings suggest that they seem almost identical macroscopically, microscopically and by x-ray diffraction analysis, and contain the same chemical elements. This information indicates that Portland cement has the potential to be used as a less expensive root-end-filling material in dental practice. We have observed the absence of genotoxicity in rodent neoplastic cells exposed to regular and white Portland cements at concentrations ranging from 1-1000 μg/mL To verify the genotoxicity in ordinary human cells, we exposed lymphocytes to these compounds *in vitro* (Ribeiro et al., 2006c). Mineral trioxide aggregate at concentrations up to 1000μg/mL did not induce genotoxic effect (Braz et al., 2006; Silva et al., 2006). Furthermore, no DNA damage was found for ordinary and white Portland cements (Braz et al., 2006). In summary, these data are consistent with the notion that mineral trioxide aggregate and Portland cements had no genotoxic effect.

Dental Bleaching Agents

Dental bleaching is a simple and conservative procedure for esthetic restoration of vital or non-vital discolored teeth. There are many bleaching agents commercially available with various constituents, such as hydrogen peroxide and carbamide peroxide. Carbamide peroxide decomposes to produce hydrogen peroxide, which may be considered the active ingredient of choice for bleaching because of its low molecular weight and its ability to denature proteins. Nevertheless, a number of studies has demonstrated the risk of tissue damage from contact of these agents with the oral mucosa (Floyd, 1997). In light of these considerations, few efforts have been made to establish the putative genotoxicity of these agents. Zouain-Ferreira *et al.* (2002) have evaluated the genotoxic effects of four commercial dental bleaching agents: Insta-Brite, Karisma, Opalescence and Whiteness using bacterial mutation assay as end-point. The bleaching agents were capable of inducing DNA damage. The authors concluded that dental bleaching compounds can generate biological effects like those from ionizing radiations. To verify the genotoxicity of these agents on eukaryotic cells, experiments were designed by our group. The results showed that all dental bleaching tested (Clarigel Gold; Whitespeed; Nite White Excel 2; Magic Bleaching; Whiteness HP and Lase Peroxide) induced DNA damage as detected by the single cell gel (comet) assay either to CHO cells or to L5178Y mouse lymphoma cells (Ribeiro et al., 2005d; 2006d). A clear dose-response relationship was observed, with the strongest effect obtained at the highest dose of hydrogen peroxide (Whiteness HP and Lase Peroxide, at 35% concentration). In fact, the hydrogen peroxide molecule easily permeates the cell membrane and is transformed into hydroxyl radicals by a non-enzymatic process in the presence of metal ions ($Fe2+$ or $Cu2+$) occurring in the cytoplasm, known as the Haber-Weiss or Fenton reaction. Hydroxyl radicals, a potent derived free radical species, can induce single-strand breaks, double-strand breaks, alkali-labile sites and various species of oxidized purines and pyrimidines. Other reactive oxygen species derived from hydrogen peroxide can also interact with DNA and induce a broad spectrum of DNA lesions.

Glass Ionomer Cements

Since glass ionomer cements were first introduced in the early 70s by Wilson and Kent (1972), they have been used extensively in dentistry as restorative materials and adhesives for composite restorations. Their usage also includes prosthetic and orthodontic devices. Some studies have demonstrated that glass ionomer cements are able to induce DNA damage in various test systems such as the bacterial UMU-test, eukaryotic DNA synthesis inhibition test, *in vivo* alkaline filter elution technique as well as sister chromatid exchange test in human lymphocytes (Heil et al., 1996; Stea et al., 1998; Muller et al., 2003). However, negative results were also observed under *in vitro* experiments (Schweikl et al., 1994; 1998). Such discrepancies have been attracting attention to new studies on genotoxicity of these cements. Data obtained in our laboratory using CHO cells or L5178Y mouse lymphoma cells demonstrated that the powder from Ketac Molar displayed genotoxicity only at the maximum concentration tested (100 μg/mL) (Ribeiro et al., 2006e; Ribeiro et al., 2006g). Similarly, liquid from Vitrebond at 0.1% dilution caused an increase of DNA damage. These data are in accordance with those described by Kleinsasser *et al.* (2004; 2006) who found only a small genotoxicity induced by 2-hydroxyethyl methacrylate (HEMA), a component of liquid Vitrebond. No significant DNA damage was noted at concentrations possibly relevant to *in vivo* situations (10^{-4} M) (Spahl et al., 1998) Nevertheless, studies reported that HEMA induced apoptotic death, probably affecting the intrinsic apoptotic pathway (Paranjpe et al., 2005). In conclusion, these results support the rationale that some glass ionomer cements induced DNA migration detected by single cell gel (comet) assay as a sign for limited genotoxic effects in higher concentrations. With the highest levels of DNA migration being combined with elevated cytotoxic effects, a low *in vivo* noxious activity could be observed. Further studies must be conducted with isolated substances of these glass ionomer cements in order to clarify the action mechanism.

Conclusion

In this review, we have highlighted recent advances on the genotoxic potential of some compounds widely used in dental practice. Although their possible action mechanisms have been purposed, much remains to be examined. Therefore, this is an area that warrants investigation since the risk assessment of these substances with respect to genotoxicity will be added to those used for regulatory purposes in improving oral health and preventing oral carcinogenesis.

Acknowledgements

This study was supported by Fundação de Amparo à Pesquisa do Estado de São Paulo (FAPESP, Grant number: 05/52567-8).

References

Aardema MJ, Gibson DP, LeBoeuf RA (1989). Sodium fluoride-induced chromosome aberrations in different stages of the cell cycle, a proposed mechanism. *Mutation Research 223*,191-203.

Albanese R (1987). Sodium fluoride and chromosome damage (in vitro human lymphocyte and in vivo micronucleus assays). *Mutagenesis 2*,497-499.

Anuradha CD, Kanno S, Hirano S (2000). Fluoride induces apoptosis by caspase-3 activation in human leukemia HL-60 cells. *Archives of Toxicology 74*,226-230.

Anuradha CD, Kanno S, Hirano S (2001). Oxidative damage to mitochondria is a preliminary step to caspase-3 activation in fluoride-induced apoptosis in HL-60 cells. *Free Radical Biology and Medicine 31*,367-373.

Bartlett JD, Dwyer SE, Beniash E, Skobe Z, Payne-Ferreira TL (2005). Fluorosis, a new model and new insights. *Journal of Dental Research 84*,832-836.

Braz MG, Camargo EA, Salvadori DM, Marques ME, Ribeiro DA (2006). Evaluation of genetic damage in human peripheral lymphocytes exposed to mineral trioxide aggregate and Portland cements. *Journal of Oral Rehabilitation 33*,234-239.

Buzalaf MA, Salvadori DM, Marques ME, Caroselli EE, Leite AL, Camargo EA, Ribeiro DA (2006). *Bulletin of Environmental Contamination and Toxicology 77*, 700-706..

Casanova M, Morgan KT, Steinhagem WH, Everitt JI, Popp JA, Heck Hd'A. DNA-protein cross-links and cell replication at specific sites in the nose of F344 rats exposed subchronically to formaldehyde (1994). *Fundamental Apply Toxicology 23*,525-536.

Chang YC, Tai KW, Huang FM, Huang MF (2000). Cytotoxic and nongenotoxic effects of phenolic compounds in human pulp cell cultures. *Journal of Endodontics 26*,440-443.

do Ceu Silva M, Gaspar J, Silva ID, Leao D, Rueff J (2003). Induction of chromosomal aberrations by phenolic compounds, possible role of reactive oxygen species. *Mutation Research 540*,29-42.

Eren K,Ozmeric N, Sardas S (2001). Monitoring of buccal epithelial cells by alkaline comet assay (single cell gel electrophoresis technique) in cytogenetic evaluation of chlorhexidine. *Clinical Oral Investigation 6*,150-154.

Everett ET, McHenry MA, Reynolds N, Eggertsson H, Sullivan J, Kantmann C, Martinez-Mier EA, Warrick JM (2002). Dental fluorosis, variability among different inbred mouse strains. *Journal of Dental Research 81*,794-798.

Floyd RA (1997). The effect of peroxides and free radicals on body tissues. *JADA 128*;37S-40S.

Geurtsen W, Leyhausen G (1997). Biological aspects of root canal filling materials-histocompatibility,cytotoxicity, and mutagenicity. *Clinical Oral Investigation 1*,5-11.

Ghosh D, Das Sarkar S, Maiti R, Jana D, Das UB (2002). Testicular toxicity in sodium fluoride treated rats, association with oxidative stress. *Reprodutive Toxicology 16*,385-390.

Grassi TF, Camargo EA, Salvadori DM, Marques, Ribeiro DA (2007). DNA damage in multiple organs after oral exposure to chlorhexidine in Wistar rats. *International Journal of Hygiene and Environmental Health, in press.*

Guan ZZ, Xiao KQ, Zeng XY, Long YG, Cheng YH, Jiang SF, Wang YN (2000). Changed cellular membrane lipid composition and lipid peroxidation of kidney in rats with chronic fluorosis. *Archives of Toxicology 74*,602-608.

Hagiwara M, Watanabe E, Barrett JC, Tsutsui T (2006). Assessment of genotoxicity of 14 chemical agents used in dental practice, Ability to induce chromosome aberrations in Syrian hamster embryo cells. *Mutation Research 603*,111-120.

Hamaguchi F, Tsutsui T (2000). Assessment of genotoxicity of dental antiseptics, ability of phenol, guaiacol, p-phenolsulfonic acid, sodium hypochlorite, p-chlorophenol, m-cresol or formaldehyde to induce unscheduled DNA synthesis in cultured Syrian hamster embryo cells. *Japanese Journal of Pharmacology 83*,273-276.

Hansen MG (1998). Relative efficacy of solvents used in endodontics. *Journal of Endodontics 24*,38-40.

He LF, Chen JG (2006). DNA damage, apoptosis and cell cycle changes induced by fluoride in rat oral mucosal cells and hepatocytes. *World Journal of Gastroenterology 12*,1144-1148.

Heil J, Reifferscheid G, Waldmann P, Leyhausen G, Geurtsen W (1996). Genotoxicity of dental materials. *Mutation Research 368*,181-194.

Huang FM, Tai KW, Chou MY, Chang YC (2002). Cytotoxicity of resin-, zinc oxide-eugenol-, and calcium hydroxide-based root canal sealers on human periodontal ligament cells and permanent V79 cells. *International Endodontic Journal 35*,153-158b.

Huang TH, Ding SJ, Hsu TZ, Lee ZD, Kao CT (2004). Root canal sealers induce cytotoxicity and necrosis. *Journal of Materials Science Materials in Medicine 15*,767-771.

Huang TH, Lee H, Kao CT (2001). Evaluation of the genotoxicity of zinc oxide eugenol-based, calcium hydroxide-based, and epoxy resin-based root canal sealers by comet assay. *Journal of Endodontics; 27*,744-748.

Huang TH, Yang JJ, Li H, Kao_CT (2002). The biocompatibility evaluation of epoxy resin-based root canal sealers in vitro. *Biomaterials 23*,77-83a.

Jones, CA, Callaham MF, Huberman E (1988). Sodium fluoride promotes morphological transformation of Syrian hamster cells. *Carcinogenesis 9*,2279-84.

Kaplowitz GJ (1991). Evaluation of the ability of essential oils to dissolve gutta-percha. *Journal of Endodontics 17*, 448-9.

Kleinsasser NH, Schmid K, Sassen AW, Harreus UA, Staudenmaier R, Folwaczny M, Glas J, Reichl FX (2006). Cytotoxic and genotoxic effects of resin monomers in human salivary gland tissue and lymphocytes as assessed by the single cell microgel electrophoresis (Comet) assay. *Biomaterials 27*,1762-1770.

Kleinsasser NH, Wallner BC, Harreus UA, Kleinjung T, Folwaczny M, Hickel R, Kehe K, Reichl FX (2004). Genotoxicity and cytotoxicity of dental materials in human lymphocytes as assessed by the single cell microgel electrophoresis (comet) assay. *Journal of Dentistry 32*,229-234.

Kleinsasser NH, Weissacher H, Wallner BC, Kastenbauer ER, Harreus UA (2001). Cytotoxicity and genotoxicity of fluorides in human mucosa and lymphocytes. *Laryngorhinootologie 80*,187-190.

Klimm W, Janz S, Gabert A (1989). Experimental research on the genotoxicity of various root canals antiseptics in the SOS chromotest. *Dtsch Zahn Mund Kieferheilkd Zentralbl 77*,27-30.

Kubota K, Lee DH, Tsuchiya M, Young CS, Everett ET, Martinez-Mier EA, Snead ML, Nguyen L, Urano F, Bartlett JD (2005). Fluoride induces endoplasmic reticulum stress in ameloblasts responsible for dental enamel formation. *Journal of Biology and Chemistry 280*,23194-2202.

Lamb JC, Brown SM (2000). Chemical testing strategies for predicting health hazards to children. *Reprodutive Toxicology 14*,83-94.

Li Y, Liang CK, Katz BP, Brizendine EJ, Stookey GK (1995). Long-term exposure to fluoride in drinking water and sister chromatid exchange frequency in human blood lymphocytes. *Journal of Dental Research 74*,1468-1474.

Li YM, Zhang W, Noblitt TW, Dunipace AJ, Stookey GK (1989). Genotoxic evaluation of chronic fluoride exposure, sister-chromatid exchange study. *Mutation Research 227*,159-165.

Loe H, Schiott CR (1970). The effect of mouthrinses and topical application of chlorhexidine on of dental plaque and gingivitis in man. *Journal of Periodontal Research 5*,79-83.

Martin GR, Brown KS, Matheson DW, Lebowitz H, Singer L, Ophaug R (1979). Lack of cytogenetic effects in mice or mutations in Salmonella receiving sodium fluoride. *Mutation Research 66*,159-167.

Matsuda A (1980). Cytogenetic effects of fluoride on human lymphocytes in vitro. *Koku Eisei Gakkai Zasshi 30*,312-328.

Merck O, Speit G (1999). Detection of crosslinks with the comet assay in relationship to genotoxicity and cytotoxicity. *Environmental and Molecular Mutagenesis 39*,167-172.

Mitchell AD, Auletta AE, Clive D, Kirby PE, Moore MM, Myhr BC (1997). The L5178Y/rk+/- mouse lymphoma specific gene and chromosomal mutation assay. A phase III report of the US environmental protection agency gene-tox program. *Mutation Research 394*,177-303.

Miyachi T, Tsutsui T (2005). Ability of 13 chemical agents used in dental practice to induce sister-chromatid exchanges in Syrian hamster embryo cells. *Odontology 93*,24-29.

Mohamed H, Chandler ME (1977). Cytological effects of sodium fluoride on mice, presented during hearings. *The National Cancer Program. Part 2. Fluoridation of public drinking water*. Washington, 95th US Congress 21,42-60.

Morgan KT, Ni H, Brown HR, Yoon L, Qualls CW Jr, Crosby LM, Reynolds R, Gaskill B, Anderson SP, Kepler TB, Brainard T, Liv N, Easton M, Merrill C, Creech D, Sprenger D, Conner G, Johnson PR, Fox T, Sartor M, Richard E, Kuruvilla S, Casey W, Benavides G (2002). Application of cDNA microarray technology to in vitro toxicology and the selection of genes for a real-time RT-PCR-based screen for oxidative stress in Hep-G2 cells. *Toxicology Pathology 30*,435-451.

Muller BP, Eisentrager A, Jahnen-Dechent W, Hollender J (2003). Effect of sample preparation on the in vitro genotoxicity of a light curable glass ionomer cement *Biomaterials 24*,611-617.

Negrelo Newton AP, Cadena SM, Merlin Rocha ME, Skare Carnieri EG, Martinelli de Oliveira MB (2004). New data on biological effects of chlorhexidine, Fe2+ induced lipid peroxidation and mitochondrial permeability transition. *Toxicology Letters 151*,407-416.

Otsuki S, Morshed SR, Chowdhury SA, Takayama F, Satoh T, Hashimoto K, Sugiyama K, Amano O, Yasui T, Yokote Y, Akahane K, Sakagami H (2005). Possible link between glycolysis and apoptosis induced by sodium fluoride. *Journal of Dental_Research 84*,919-923.

Paranjpe A, Bordador LC, Wang MY, Hume WR, Jewett A (2005). Resin monomer 2-hydroxyethyl methacrylate (HEMA) is a potent inducer of apoptotic cell death in human and mouse cells. *Journal of Dental Research 84*,172-177.

Prasad I (1970). Mutagenic effects of the herbicide 3', 4' dichloropropionanilide and its degradation products. *Canadian Journal of Microbiology 16*,369-72.

Ribeiro DA, Scolastici C, Marques ME, Salvadori DM (2004a). Fluoride does not induce DNA breakage in Chinese hamster ovary cells in vitro. *Pesquisa Odontologica Brasileira 18*,192-196.

Ribeiro DA, Marques ME, de Assis GF, Anzai A, Poleti ML, Salvadori DM (2004b). No relationship between subchronic fluoride intake and DNA damage in Wistar rats. *Caries Research 38*,576-579.

Ribeiro DA, Bazo AP, da Silva Franchi CA, Marques ME, Salvadori DM (2004c). Chlorhexidine induces DNA damage in rat peripheral leukocytes and oral mucosal cells. *Journal of Periodontal Research 39*,358-361.

Ribeiro DA, Marques ME, Salvadori DM (2004d). Lack of genotoxicity of formocresol, paramonochlorophenol, and calcium hydroxide on mammalian cells by comet assay. *Journal of Endodontics 30*,593-536.

Ribeiro DA, Scolastici C, De Lima PL, Marques ME, Salvadori DM (2005a). Genotoxicity of antimicrobial endodontic compounds by single cell gel (comet) assay in Chinese hamster ovary (CHO) cells. *Oral Surgery Oral Medicine Oral Pathology Oral Radiology Endodontology 99*,637-640.

Ribeiro DA, Duarte MA, Matsumoto MA, Marques ME, Salvadori DM (2005b). Biocompatibility in vitro tests of mineral trioxide aggregate and regular and white Portland cements. *Journal of Endodontics 31*,605-607.

Ribeiro DA, Marques ME, Salvadori DM (2005c). Assessment of genetic damage induced by dental bleaching agents on mouse lymphoma cells by single cell gel (comet) assay. *Journal of Oral Rehabilitation 32*,766-771.

Ribeiro DA, Matsumoto MA, Duarte MA, Marques ME, Salvadori DM (2005d). In vitro biocompatibility tests of two commercial types of mineral trioxide aggregate. *Pesquisa Odontologica Brasileira 19*,183-187.

Ribeiro DA, Alves de Lima PL, Marques MEA, Salvadori DMF (2006a). Lack of DNA damage induced by fluoride on mouse lymphoma and human fibroblast cells by single cell gel (comet) assay. *Brazilian Dental Journal 2*,27-31.

Ribeiro, DA, Sugui MM, Matsumoto MA, Duarte MAH, Marques MEA, Salvadori DMF (2006b). Genotoxicity and cytotoxicity of mineral trioxide aggregate and regular and white Portland cements on Chinese hamster ovary (CHO) cells in vitro. *Oral Surgery Oral Medicine Oral Pathology Oral Radiology Endodontology 101*,258-261.

Ribeiro DA, Matsumoto MA, Duarte MA, Marques ME, Salvadori DM (2006c). Ex vivo biocompatibility tests of regular and white forms of mineral trioxide aggregate. *International Endodontic Journal 39*,26-30.

Ribeiro DA, Marques MEA, Salvadori DMF (2006d). Study of DNA damage induced by dental bleaching agents in vitro. *Pesquisa Odontologica Brasileira 20*,47-51.

Ribeiro, DA, Marques MEA, Salvadori DMF (2006e). Genotoxicity and cytotoxicity of glass inomer cements on chinese hamster ovary (CHO) cells. *Journal of Materials Science Materials in Medicine 17*,495-500.

Ribeiro DA, Marques ME, Salvadori DM (2006f). Antimicrobial endodontic compounds do not modulate alkylation-induced genotoxicity and oxidative stress in vitro. *Oral Surgery Oral Medicine Oral Pathology Oral Radiology Endodontology 102*,32-36.

Ribeiro DA, Marques ME, Salvadori DM (2006g). Biocompatibility of glass-ionomer cements using mouse lymphoma cells in vitro. *Journal of Oral Rehabilitation 33*,912-917.

Ribeiro DA, Marques ME, Salvadori DM (2006h). In vitro cytotoxic and non-genotoxic effects of gutta percha solvents on mouse lymphoma cells by single cell gel (comet) assay. *Brazilian Dental Journal 17*, 228-232.

Sakagami Y, Yamazaki H, Ogasawara N, Yokoyama H, Ose Y, Sato T (1988). The evaluation of genotoxic activities of disinfectants and their metabolites by UMU test. *Mutation Research 209*,155-160.

Sato M, Tsuchiya H, Kato M, Yamamoto K, Nakazato G, Takagi N, Namikawa I (1989). Effects of Tween 80 and sodium fluoride on extracellular glucosyltransferase production and membrane lipids of Streptococcus mutans. *International Journal of Biochemistry 21*,751-754.

Satoh R, Kishino K, Morshed SR, Takayama F, Otsuki S, Suzuki F, Hashimoto K, Kikuchi H, Nishikawa H, Yasui T, Sakagami H (2005). Changes in fluoride sensitivity during in vitro senescence of normal human oral cells. *Anticancer Research 25*,2085-2090.

Schweikl H, Schmalz G, Bey B (1994). Mutagenicity of dentin bonding agents. *Journal of Biomedical Materials Research 28*,1061-1067.

Schweikl H, Schmalz G, Rackebrandt K (1998). The mutagenic activity of unpolymerized resin monomers in Salmonella typhimurium and V79 cells. *Mutation Research 415*,119-130.

Silva GN, Braz MG, Camargo EA, Salvadori DM, Ribeiro (2006). Genotoxicity in primary human peripheral lymphocytes after exposure to regular and white mineral trioxide aggregate. *Oral Surgery Oral Medicine Oral Pathology Oral Radiology and Endodontology 102*, e50-54.

Slamenova D, Gabelova A, Ruppova K (1992). Cytotoxicity and genotoxicity testing of sodium fluoride on Chinese hamster V79 cells and human EUE cells. *Mutation Research 279*,109-115.

Spahl W, Budzikiewicz H, Geurtsen W (1998). Determination of leachable components from four commercial dental composites by gas and liquid chromatography/mass spectrometry. *Journal of Dentistry 26*,137-145.

Stea S, Visentin M, Cervellati M, Verri E, Cenni E, Savarino L, Stea S, Pizzoferrato A (1998). In vitro sister chromatid Exchange induced by glass ionomer cells. *Journal of Biomedical Materials Research 40*,545-550.

Tai KW, Huang FM, Huang MS, Chang_YC (2002). Assessment of the genotoxicity of resin and zinc-oxide eugenol-based root canal sealers using an in vitro mammalian test system. *Journal of Biomedical Materials Research 59*,73-77.

Uemura M, Hata G, Toda T, Weine FS (1997). Effectiveness of eucalyptol and d-limonene as gutta-percha solvents. *Journal of Endodontics 23*, 739-41.

US Environmental Protection Agency (USEPA) (1986). Guidelines for mutagenicity risk assessment. *Federal register 51*,34006-34012.

Velazquez-Guadarrama N, Madrigal-Bujaidar E, Molina D, Chamorro G (2005). Genotoxic evaluation of sodium fluoride and sodium perborate in mouse bone marrow cells. *Bulletin of Environmental Contamination and Toxicology 74*,566-572.

Voegel E (1973). Strong antimutagenic effects of fluoride on mutation induction by trenimon and 1-hyenyl-3,3-dimethyltriazene in Drosophila melanogaster. *Mutation Research 20*,239-252.

Wang AG, Xia T, Chu QL, Zhang M, Liu F, Chen XM, Yang KD (2004). Effects of fluoride on lipid peroxidation, DNA damage and apoptosis in human embryo hepatocytes. *Biomedical Environmental Science 17*,217-222.

Warner RR, Myers MC, Burns J, Mitra S (1993). Analytical electron microscopy of chlorhexidine-induced tooth stain in humans, direct evidence for metal-induced stain. *Journal of Periodontal Research 28*,255-265.

Wennberg A, Orstavik D (1989). Evaluation of alternatives to chloroform in endodontic practice. *Endodontic Dental Traumatology 5*, 234-7.

Wilson AD, Kent BE (1972). A new translucent cement for dentistry. The glass ionomer cement. *British Dental Journal 132*,133-135.

World Health Organization (WHO). Available from URL, http,//home.iae.nl/users/lightn.et/health/fluoride.htm. 1994.

Wtihrow TJ, Brown NT, Hitchins VM, Strickland AG (1989). Cytotoxicity and mutagenicity of ophtalmic solution preservatives and UVA radiation in L5178Y cells. *Photochemistry Photobiology 50*,385-89.

Wourns D, Campbell AD, Hicks ML, Pelleu GB (199). Alternative solvents to chloroform for gutta-percha removal. *Journal of Endodontics 16*, 224-6.

Zouain-Ferreira SL, Zouain-Ferreira TR, da Silva CR, Cervantes Dias KR, Caldeira-de-Araujo A, Bernardo-Filho M (2002). Radiation induced-like effects of four home bleaching agents used for tooth whitening, effects on bacterial cultures with different capabilities of repairing deoxyribonucleic acid (DNA) damage. *Cellular and Molecular Biology (Noisy-le-grand) 48*,521-524.

In: Progress in Oral Cancer Research
Editor: Frederik L. Nielsen, pp 157-172
ISBN 978-1-60021-865-1

Chapter VIII

SYSTEMIC RISK FACTORS FOR ORAL CANCER: ESTROGEN DEFICIENCY AND INSULIN RESISTANCE

Zsuzsanna Suba*

Department of Oral and Maxillofacial Surgery, Oral Pathology Unit, Semmelweis University, Budapest, Hungary.

ABSTRACT

Oral cancer (OC) is a tumor with a fairly large male to female sex ratio in most populations. Moreover, OC develops in older age in females as compared with males. The conspicuously larger incidence of this tumor among women than men may suggest some endocrine involvement in its development. Till now there are no available literary data, which explain definitively this gender specific incidence rate of OC.

A case-control study was performed to analyse separately the data of the male and female OC patients to clarify the role of the suspected endogenous risk factors, namely estrogen deficiency and elevated fasting glucose (>5.5mmol/L).

Significantly older mean age of OC females as compared with OC males, significantly lower ratio of young (<45 yrs) OC women as compared with OC men may allow an assumption that women are defended against OC in their reproductive period. Almost exclusively postmenopausal state of OC women and a long interval (17 yrs) between their menopause and tumor diagnosis suggest also an important role of estrogen deficiency in OC epidemiology. The mean age at tumor diagnosis of OC women with premature ovarian failure was significantly lower as compared with that of all OC women. Hysterectomy, with or without oophorectomy was significantly more frequent among OC women as compared with those of control female cases, which supports also the estrogen deficiency hypothesis. The results of the present study underline that

* Correspondence concerning this article should be addressed to: Prof. Dr. Zsuzsanna Suba, Department of Oral and Maxillofacial Surgery, Semmelweis University, H-1085 Budapest Mária str. 52, Hungary. Phone: 36-1-266-0457; Fax: 36-1-266-0456; E-mail: suba@szajseb.sote.hu.

elevated fasting glucose is also a strong risk factor for OC among estrogen deficient postmenopausal women, but not in men.

The presented results raise a new concept: not estrogen but its deficiency may provoke OC initiation, especially in postmenopausal insulin resistant women. The estrogen deficiency theory may explain the lower ratio and older age of female cases among OC patients. On the other hand, the continuously increasing prevalence of insulin resistant states (metabolic syndrome, type-2 diabetes) all over the world and the close correlation of glucose intolerance and OC risk among women may explain the increasing ratio of non-smoker non-drinker female cases among OC cases.

Introduction

Oral cancer (OC) is a serious and growing problem being the sixth most common malignancy in the world [1,2,3,4,5]. In the majority of therapeutic centers survival rates are under 50% and have not improved in the last decades. In most European countries, OC morbidity and mortality has been rising appreciably until the late 1980s, with a conspicuous excess of male cases [5]. Upwards trend in oral cancer mortality until the early 1990s were registered also in the USA, Thailand and India.

Since alcohol and tobacco are the major risk factors for OC, in developed countries advantageous reduction of alcohol and tobacco consumption may have appreciably favorable trends in OC morbidity and mortality over the last decade [6]. Persisting rises are continuously observed for most central and eastern European countries, reaching exceedingly high rates in Hungary [7]. In the last century OC incidence was markedly lower in women, but have recently a moderately upward trend in many countries. Consequently the male to female ratio has declined over the last decade. These trends were essentially interpreted in terms of patterns and changes in exposure of alcohol and tobacco among women, and call for urgent control of these factors [2].

However, in many developed countries an increasing trend in the ratio of non-smoker and non-drinker OC cases has been observed, especially among women [8,9]. The declined male to female ratio raises two different assumptions. First, there are strengthening noxious factors affecting selectively only the female patients, and second, increasing common OC risk factors may affect both genders, but female patients are more susceptible owing to their special hormonal and metabolic features.

Though OC is a multicausal disease, till now the exogenous harmful noxae (tobacco, alcohol and environmental factors) were overemphasized in its epidemiology [1,2,3,4,5,6]. However, these exogenous factors have not only local carcinogenic effects on the oral mucosa, but may also induce systemic changes. Recently, our working group revealed that some systemic factors; such as glucose intolerance, metabolic syndrome and type-2 diabetes are also strong risk factors for oral tumors [10,11,12].

The aim of the present case-control study was to examine the role of some systemic risk factors in OC epidemiology. The decreasing frequency of tobacco and alcohol intake and the increasing ratio of women among OC cases focused the attention to search for further possible risk factors, such as hormonal and metabolic disorders.

Materials and Methods

Patients

2660 inpatients (530 females and 2130 males) at the Department of Oral and Maxillofacial surgery with histologically confirmed squamous cell oral carcinoma (OC) were included into a case-control study between 1 January 1997 and 30 June 2006. The controls were complain-free adults (530 females and 2450 males) who volunteered to participate in stomato-oncological screening in the same period. The data of the oral cancer patients and their controls were collected through questionnaires and the case reports of the inpatients. All patients gave informed consent to participate in the study. Refused the participation 18 of the tumor patients and 42 of the controls.

The age of female patients was especially important in this study. For each interviewed OC women controls were chosen who matched to the patient's age (within 5 months) at the time of cancer diagnosis. The mean age of control male patients was chosen so as to be similar to OC males within 1 year.

Age of Patients

The mean ages of male and female OC patients and the rate of young (45 years and under) cases at the time of OC diagnosis were separately registered. Mean ages of male and female OC cases in the groups of the prevailing tumor locations were also established.

Tumor Locations

Frequencies of the different tumor locations among the male and female OC cases were compared.

Smoking Habits

Smoking habits and the rate of smokers among the male and female patients OC cases and their controls were separately evaluated. Mean ages of smokers and non-smokers among the male and female patients at the OC diagnosis were evaluated. The rates of smokers were established in the groups with the prevailing OC locations both of the male and female OC cases.

Alcohol Consumption

Regular alcohol consumption among OC and control male patients and among OC and control women was registered within which moderate and excessive drinking was separately evaluated. Regular <25-30 g/die alcohol intake was regarded as moderate, >30 g/die was regarded as excessive alcohol consumption. Correlations of drinking and tumor locations were also evaluated in both the male and female OC groups.

Elevated Fasting Glucose (EFG)

Ratios of EFG cases among male and female OC and control cases were established. Fasting blood glucose levels were determined repeatedly within 4 days. All determinations were made by means of Hitachi 717/912 automatic analyzers (Roche Diagnostics Boehringer

Mannheim, Germany). The level was regarded as elevated only if it was repeatedly >5.5 mmol/l. These EFG groups comprised symptom-free insulin resistant cases, newly diagnosed and known, treated or untreated type-2 diabetes cases. Correlations of EFG ratio and tumor location were also studied in the male and female groups.

Menopausal History of the OC and Control Female Patients

Ratio of the postmenopausal cases and the mean age at menopause in the OC and control groups were established. The rate of early menopause (<45 yrs) due to either unidentified ovarian failure or hysterectomy/ovarectomy and late menopause (>51 years) were also registered both in the OC and control female groups. The mean time-intervals between menopause and OC diagnosis (M-OC) were established in the early, the normal, and the late menopausal case groups. M-OC intervals were estimated in the smoker and non-smoker OC patients. Ratio of postmenopausal hormone replacement therapy and its length was registered.

Statistical Methods

Association of OC with various risk factors was measured by Odds rates and their corresponding 95% CIs. The chi-square test and Fisher exact was also used for statistical analysis. Mean ages of the different groups were compared by two-sided Student-t test. A probability level of 5% was the limit of statistical significance.

RESULTS

Male: Female Ratio

A total of 2660 newly diagnosed and histologically verified oral squamous cell carcinoma cases 2130 were males and 530 females, with a male to female ratio of 4:1.

Table I. Mean age of oral cancer (OC) cases at the time of tumor diagnosis and ratio of young OC patients

	Males	Females	p
Mean age of all OC cases (years)	55.1±10.8 (range:33-85)	63.5±10.9 (range:36-91)	p<0.001
Mean age of gingival cancer cases (years)	56.9±11.1	66.9±11.4	p<0.01
Mean age of Sublingual cancer cases (years)	54.7±10.9	56.5±10.1	p>0.05 NS
Ratio of young OC cases (<45yrs)	16.5%	4.6%	p<0.001

Age of Patients

(Table I.) The mean age of female OC patients upon admission was significantly higher as compared with the male OC patients. Young oral cancer patients aged 45 years and under were significantly more frequent among men as compared with women. Concerning the tumor site, the highest mean age was registered among the female gingival cancer cases. In the male gingival cancer group the mean age was moderately elevated as compared with all male OC cases. The lowest mean ages were observed in the sublingual cancer groups both among males and females.

Tumor Location

Regarding the male OC patients the most common tumor site was the floor of the mouth (41.6%). This was followed in decreasing order by the tongue (24.6%), lower lip (15.3%), gingiva (12.9%), palate (2.5%), bucca (2.1%) and other rare locations (1.0%). In respect to the female patients, the site prevalence was quite different. The most common OC location was the gingiva (28.3%), followed in decreasing order by the floor of the mouth (26.4%), the tongue (18.3%), lower lip (8.4%), bucca (7.1%) palate (6.1%), and other rare locations (0.6%).

Smoking

Table II. Correlations of smoking, oral cancer incidence, and mean age of patients at tumor diagnosis

	Smokers	Non-smokers
Male cases		
Male OC cases	75.1%	24.9%
Male control cases	53.0%	47.0%
	$p<0.01$	OR=3.67
Mean age of male OC cases	54.2 yrs	62.9 yrs
	$p<0.01$	
Female cases		
Female OC cases	57.2%	42.8%
Female control cases	38.3%	61.7%
	$p<0.01$	OR=2.15
Mean age of female OC cases	56.1 yrs	68.5 yrs
	$p<0.001$	

(Table II.) In the male OC group the ratio of active smokers and earlier smokers was significantly higher as compared with the male control patients. From the female oral cancer patients the ratio of smokers was also significantly higher, as compared with the smoking histories of the female control cases.

Considering the age of the patients at the OC diagnosis (Table III.), in the male OC group smokers had a significantly lower mean age as compared with the non-smoker cases. Among the female OC cases, smokers exhibited also significantly lower mean age when compared with the female non-smoker OC group.

Table III. Correlations of smoking and the prevalent OC locations in the male and female OC groups

	Smokers	Non-smokers
Male cases		
Male sublingual cancer cases	84.5%	15.5%
Male control cases	53.0%	47.0%
	$p<0.01$	OR=4.80
Male gingival cancer cases	68.2%	31.8%
Male control cases	53.0%	47.0%
	$p<0.05$	OR=1.89
Female cases		
Female sublingual cancer cases	75.9%	24.1%
Female control cases	38.3%	61.7%
	$p<0.01$	OR=5.04
Female gingival cancer cases	45.4%	54.6%
Female control cases	38.3%	61.7%
	$p>0.05$	OR=1.33 NS

Table IV. Correlations of alcohol consumption and oral cancer (OC) incidence

	All alcohol consumer OC cases	Moderate alcohol consumer OC cases	Excessive alcohol consumer OC cases
Male cases			
Male OC cases	47.7%	6.6%	41.1%
Male control cases	21.0%	3.4%	17.6%
	$p<0.01$ OR=3.26	$p<0.05$ OR=2.02	$p<0.01$ OR=3.44
Female cases			
Female OC cases	12.0%	2.8%	9.2%
Female control cases	5.5%	2.7%	2.8%
	$p<0.05$ OR=2.36	$p>0.05$ OR=1.00 NS	$p<0.01$ OR=3.72

In regard to tumor location (Table IV), the rate of smokers was the highest in the sublingual cancer subgroups both among the male and female OC cases. Accordingly, tobacco exhibited a high cancer risk to the sublingual mucosa in both genders. The rate of smokers was relatively lower in the gingival cancer groups both among males and females.

Alcohol Consumption

(Table V). In the male OC group near the half of the cases were regular alcohol consumers, within which a small part of them were moderate drinkers, whereas the majority were excessive drinkers. A significantly lower regular alcohol consumption rate was registered in the male control group, however the great majority of them were excessive drinkers. In men alcohol consumption proved a high risk factor for OC, though the risk was lowered among moderate drinkers.

Table V. Correlations of regular alcohol consumption and oral cancer (OC) location

	Sublingual cancer ratio	Gingival cancer ratio
Male cases		
Male alcohol consumer OC cases	58.1%	46.7%
Male alcohol consumer control cases	21.0%	21.0%
	$p<0.01$ OR=5.22	$p<0.01$ OR=3.30
Female cases		
Female alcohol consumer OC cases	20.4%	11.3%
Female alcohol consumer control cases	5.5%	5.5%
	$p<0.001$ OR=4.46	$p>0.05$ OR=0.93 NS

In the female OC group, the rate of regular alcohol consumption was significantly lower as compared with the male OC group. Among the female drinker OC patients the excessive drinkers predominated. Regarding the female control cases, the regular alcohol consumption rate was significantly lower as compared with the female OC cases. Regular excessive alcohol consumption proved also to be a high risk for OC among women; however, regular moderate alcohol consumption was not an OC risk for them.

Considering tumor location (Table VI.), alcohol consumption proved to be a higher risk for sublingual cancer when compared with all OC cases in both genders. Among males with gingival cancer the rate of regular drinkers was similar as compared with all male OC cases. Among female gingival cancer cases, drinking proved to be slightly lower risk factor, as compared with all OC women.

Non-Smoker, Non-Drinker (NSND) OC Cases

Of all male OC patients 20.8%, and of the male controls 44.1% were NSND cases (OR:0.34). Of all female OC patients 47.9%, and of the female controls 60.5% were NSND cases. The highest rates of NSND cases were found in the gingival cancer groups both among OC males and females. Near one third (29.4%) of the male group with gingival cancer, and more than half (54.5) of the female gingival cancer group were registered as NSND cases (OR:0.80 and OR:0.53, respectively).

Table VI. Ratio of non-smoker, non-drinker (NSND) cases among male and female patients

	NSND cases	Smoker and/or drinker cases
Male cases		
Male **OC** patients	20.1%	79.9%
Male **control** patients	44.1%	55.9%
	$p<0.01$ OR=0.33	
Male **sublingual** cancer patients	14.3%	85.7%
Male **control** patients	44.1%	55.9%
	$p<0.01$ OR=0.21	
Male **gingival** cancer patients	29.3%	70.7%
Male **control** patients	44.1%	55.9%
	$p<0.05$ OR=0.52	
Female cases		
Female **OC** patients	43.1%	56.9%
Female **control** patients	60.0%	40.0%
	$p<0.05$ OR=0.48	
Female **sublingual** cancer patients	24.1%	75.9%
Female **control** patients	60.0%	40.0%
	$p<0.05$ OR=0.21	
Female **gingival** cancer patients	54.7%	45.3%
Female **control** patients	60.0%	40.0%
	$p>0.05$ OR=0.80 NS	

Elevated Fasting Glucose (EFG)

(Table VII). In the male OC group EFG rate was quite similar to that of control men. However, among female OC cases EFG proved to be a risk factor as EFG rate was significantly lower among female controls.

As regards tumor location, EFG rates of sublingual and gingival cancer groups were examined separately in both genders because of the primacy of these locations among the male and female OC patients.

The EFG rate in the group of *male sublingual cancer* cases was similar both to the male controls and all the male OC cases. EFG proved to be no risk factor for sublingual cancer in men. In contrast, regarding the *female sublingual cancer* cases, the EFG rate was significantly higher as compared with the female controls. EFG was a demonstrable risk factor for sublingual cancer in women.

Table VII. Elevated fasting glucose (EFG) and oral cancer risk

	All oral cancer cases	Sublingual cancer cases	Gingival cancer cases
Male cases			
EFG ratio of male OC patients	51.9%	51.6%	56.8%
EFG ratio of male control patients	52.5%	52.5%	52.5%
	OR=0.97 NS	OR=0.96 NS	OR=1.19 NS
Female cases			
EFG ratio of female OC patients	55.4%	53.7%	56.9%
EFG ratio of female control patients	43.5%	43.5%	43.5%
	OR=1.61 p<0.05	OR=1.51 p<0.05	OR=1.69 p<0.05

The EFG rate was found slightly higher in the *male gingival cancer* group as compared with the rate found in controls and with all the male OC patients. EFG proved to be no risk factor for gingival cancer in males. In the *female gingival cancer* group the EFG rate was significantly elevated as compared with the controls and moderately elevated in comparison with all female OC cases. EFG proved to be an even higher risk for gingival cancer in women when compared with all female OC cases.

Table VIII. History of menopause of OC females and controls

	OC females	Control females	
Postmenopausal cases	98%	74%	p<0.001
Mean age at menopause	43.5 yrs	50.9 yrs	p<0.01
Early menopause (<45 yrs) cases	31.4%	16.0%	p<0.05 OR=2.36
Late menopause (>50 yrs) cases	14.3%	23.1%	p<0.05 OR=0.78
Hysterectomy cases	35.1%	18.4%	p<0.05 OR=1.69

History of Menopause in the Group of Female Patients

(Table VIII.) Female OC patients were near all postmenopausal, whereas among control women in the same age group a quarter of them were premenopausal. Mean age at menopause was significantly lower among the female OC patients as compared with the female controls. The rate of early menopause (<45 yrs) due to unidentified ovarian failure or hysterectomy and/or ovarectomy was significantly higher among OC women, as compared with the control patients. Hysterectomy and/or ovarectomy occurred significantly more frequently in the history of female OC cases as compared to the controls. The mean time interval between menopause and OC diagnosis (M-OC) among the female OC patients was 16.9 years (range: 3-35 years). The mean M-OC interval in the female OC group with early menopause was significantly lower (13.4 yrs) and in the female OC group with late menopause significantly longer (23.5 yrs) as compared with all OC women ($p<0.05$, and $p<0.05$, respectively). Separated evaluation of M-OC intervals related to smoker and non-smoker OC females resulted in significant differences: 11.9 years for smokers and 19.2 years for non-smokers ($p<0.01$). Postmenopausal hormone replacement therapy was relatively rare both in the OC group (8.4 %) and in the control group (10.5%), and showed no significant difference ($p>0.05$). The hormone therapy was relatively short; the mean length was 1.6 yrs in the OC group, and 1.9 yrs in the control group.

Discussion

Estrogen deficiency and insulin resistance are well-known, concordant disorders with a mutual interrelationship [13]. Today the role of insulin resistance in the initiation and progression of cancer is undoubtedly justified [14,15,16,17,18], however, the role of estrogen deficiency in the development of malignancies is completely obscure. Separated analysis of the well known exogenous and the suspected endogenous OC risk factors in male and female patients yielded striking differences. Apart from the well-known risk of tobacco and alcohol, elevated fasting glucose and postmenopausal sex hormone deficiency in women proved to b e strong factors affecting OC incidence.

Nowadays, a prevailing concept is the positive correlation between female sexual steroid hormones and risk for cancers [19,20,21]. However, unexplained, beneficial anticancer effects of hormone replacement therapy (HRT) of postmenopausal women were reported against esophageal, gastric, colorectal, cervical and liver cancers [22,23,24].

A protective role of HRT use for smoking associated cancers, such as OC, was justified among smoker postmenopausal women [25]. The authors supposed that HRT postpones the smoking associated cancers by a transitory maintenance of epithelial thickness and integrity in the upper aero-digestive tract.

In the present study, the significantly older mean age of female OC patients as compared with male OC patients, further, the significantly lower ratio of young (<45 yrs) female OC cases as compared with male OC cases may allow the assumption that women are defended against OC in their reproductive period. Almost exclusively postmenopausal state of the female OC patients and the long mean interval (17 yrs) between their menopause and tumor diagnosis also suggest an important role of estrogen deprivation in OC epidemiology. The significantly younger mean age at menopause and the considerably higher rate of hysterectomy and/or ovarectomy among the female OC patients in comparison with the control women also support the estrogen deficiency hypothesis.

Similarly to our observations, a statistically significant increase of bladder cancer was associated with the postmenopausal state and the early menopause in female cases [26]. An increased risk for renal cell carcinoma was also reported among women who had been submitted to a hysterectomy with or without oophorectomy [27]. Unfortunately, menopausal history of the cases was not reported in this study. Similar gynecological surgeries were significantly more frequent in our group of female OC cases when compared with the control females. These observations also support the correlations between estrogen deficiency and cancer.

The results of the present study raise a new concept concerning OC initiation. Not estrogen but its deficiency may provoke malignant transformation. This new theory may explain many controversial associations of female sexual steroids and malignancies [28]. At the same time supplies an explanation for the lower ratio and older age of women among OC patients

The postmenopausal state is an excellent physiological model to study the hormonal and metabolic effects of estrogen deprivation in women [29]. On the other hand, estrogen deficiency in males occurs in extremely rare cases. Nevertheless, it is a well-known fact that estrogen deficiency has a close association with insulin resistance both in males and females [30].

Insulin resistance is a disturbance of the peripheral glucose uptake and has currently of great importance as it is spreading as an epidemic in the developed countries [31]. The western lifestyle (obesity, fat-rich diet, and lack of physical exercise) favors this metabolic disorder and is likely to lead to future increases in the incidence of serious diseases, such as cardiovascular complications and malignancies.

In the partially compensated first phase of insulin resistance, a reactive hyperinsulinemia strives to maintain the normal serum glucose level. Insulin plays a crucial role in the carbohydrate and lipid metabolism, and at the same time it is a growth factor, which can provoke an increased production and enhanced mitogenic activity of other insulin-like growth factors (IGFs) [32]. Recent data support that both hyperinsulinemia and IGFs have proven associations with cancer promotion [33,34].

In the uncompensated phase of insulin resistance, the secretor activity of the β-cells becomes exhausted, and with a detectable elevation in blood glucose level type 2 diabetes develops. Hyperglycemia itself leads to tissue derangement by several pathways. Excessive deliberation of free radicals, increased production of cytokines, protein glycation and tissular hypoxia caused by microangiopathy adversely affect the gene regulation and may provoke neoplastic proliferation [35,36,37]. Otherwise, the excessive glucose supply is rather advantageous for the unrestrained DNA-synthesis of the tumor cells through the pentose phosphate pathway. There are a number of data indicative of associations among hyperglycemia, tumor incidence and tumor progression [14,15,16,17].

All phases of insulin resistance (hyperinsulinemia, hyperglycemia, metabolic syndrome and type-2 diabetes) are proven risk factors for pancreas, liver, colon, urinary bladder, prostate and oral cavity cancers [11,12,38,39,40,41,42] and even for malignancies of highly estrogen dependent tissues [43,44,45].

Elevated fasting glucose is an easily accessible mirror to reflect the different stages of the glucose metabolism disorder. The results of the present study underline that EFG is a strong risk factor for OC in estrogen deficient postmenopausal women, especially in gingival cancer cases. In contrast, among male OC patients EFG is not a marked risk factor. These results supply some explanation of the increasing ratio of female cases among OC patients, as they are fairly susceptible for the glucose intolerance compared with the male cases.

Results of clinical and experimental investigations suggest that pre- or postmenopausal decrease of female sexual steroid hormone levels enhance the prevalence of insulin resistant states [13,46,47]. Polycystic ovarium syndrome (PCOS) in young, premenopausal women is a pathologic example of the correlations between estrogen deficiency and insulin resistance

[13]. Its cardinal symptoms are anovulation, infertility, hirsutism and obesity, and predict the risk of type-2 diabetes. In PCOS cases hyperinsulinemia overregulates ovarian androgen production at the expense of reduction of estrogen synthesis [48]. In young PCOS cases the combination of estrogen deficiency and insulin resistance is also in close association with cancer risk for the highly hormone-sensitive breast, endometrium and ovary [13,49].

Premenopausal or postmenopausal decrease of the estrogen level, relative excess of androgens, hyperinsulinemia and elevated IGF-I bioavailability exert a cross fire at cellular level and may induce serious gene alterations, even malignant transformation.

Oral mucosa and especially the gingiva are thoroughly affected by hormonal influences [50]. Type-2 diabetes is associated with increased prevalence of gingivitis and periodontitis in both genders. In postmenopausal women reduced estrogen level results in atrophic, desquamative gingivitis.

In the present study the conspicuous difference of the prevailing OC locations between male and female patients supplied a further key to reveal the gender specific risks.

Among the female OC patients the gingiva was the most prominent tumor location (28.3%), however in the male OC group gingival cancer incidence was significantly lower (13.0%). In the female gingival cancer group, EFG proved to be a stronger risk factor as compared with all OC women. Exogenous carcinogenic noxae (alcohol and tobacco) were not demonstrated in near one third of the male and in more than half of the female gingival cancer group! These results suggest that a combined estrogen deficiency and insulin resistance play etiologic role in gingival cancer epidemiology in postmenopausal women.

Alcohol consumption is a well-known, strong risk factor for OC [51]. However, it has contradictory metabolic effects. Mild to moderate alcohol consumption is associated with improved insulin sensitivity, while the two extremes: complete abstinence and excessive drinking are risks for insulin resistance in both genders [52,53]. In postmenopausal women, regular moderate alcohol consumption mediates the increase of estrogen synthesis in the peripheral adipose tissue [54].

In the present study, excessive alcohol consumption proved to be a high risk for OC both in the male and female cases. Among male patients moderate alcohol intake was a lower OC risk as compared with heavy drinkers. However, in postmenopausal women moderate drinking was not an OC risk factor, which may be attributed to both increased insulin sensitivity and elevated estrogen level.

Smoking is a double cancer risk for the oral mucosa by means of its local toxic derivatives and systemic metabolic effects [51]. However, Mediterranean dietary habits, such as high fruit, vegetable, fish consumption and red wine mean a decreased risk for oral cancer even in heavy smokers [55]. This protective dietary effect in smokers was also observed against breast, female genital tract, urinary tract and other epithelial neoplasms due to a systemic antioxidant effect of this advantageous diet.

Primacy of sublingual cancers among male OC patients may be explained by the higher rate of smoking and alcohol consumption as compared with the OC women. These well-known carcinogenic noxae are dissolved and concentrated in the saliva of the floor of mouth, which results in strong, local carcinogenic effect [1].

In the present study smoking was a high risk for oral cancer both among men and women in concordance with the results of earlier studies [1,2,3,4,5,6]. On the other hand, smoking seemed to be an anticipating factor for OC initiation in the group of both male and female OC patients as the mean age of smokers was significantly lower as compared with the non-smoker cases.

Conclusion

The theory of estrogen deficiency as OC risk factor may explain the conspicuously lower incidence and the significantly older age of OC women as compared with men. On the other hand, the continuously increasing prevalence of insulin resistant states (metabolic syndrome, type-2 diabetes) all over the world and the close correlation of glucose intolerance and OC risk among women may explain the increasing ratio of non-smoker non-drinker female cases among OC cases.

This novel hypothesis of estrogen deficiency and elevated fasting glucose as risks for OC may provide new insights into the etiology of oral malignancies and leads to new strategies for cancer prevention.

References

[1] Neville BW, Day TA. Tumors and precancerous lesions of the oral cavity. *CA Cancer J Clin* 2002; 52:195-215

[2] La Vecchia C, Lucchini F, Negri E, Levi F. Trends in oral cancer mortality in Europe. *Oral Oncol* 2004; 40:433-439

[3] Krolls SO, Hoffman S. Squamous cell carcinoma of the oral soft tissues: a statistical analysis of 14,253 cases by age, sex and race of patients. *JADA* 1976; 92: 571-574

[4] Rich AM, Radden BG. Squamous cell carcinoma of the oral mucosa: a review of 244 cases in Australia. *J Oral Pathol* 1984;13:459-471

[5] Levi F, Lucchini F, Negri E, Zatonsky W, Boyle P, La Vecchia C. Trends in cancer mortality in the European Union and accession countries, 1980-2000. *Annals of Oncology* 2004; 15:1425-1431

[6] Johnson NW. Etiology and risk factors for oral cancers and their correlations with smoking and alcohol consumption. *Hung Oncology (in Hungarian)* 2001; 45:115-122

[7] Döbrőssy L. Cancer mortality in central-eastern Europe: Facts behind the figures. *Lancet Oncol* 2002; 3:374-381

[8] Llewellyn CD, Johnson NW, Warnakulasuriya KA. Risk factors for oral cancer in newly diagnosed patients aged 45 years and younger: a case-control study in Southern England. J *Oral Pathol Med* 2004; 3:525-532

[9] Iype EM, Pandey M, Mathew A, Thomas G, Sebastian P, Nair MK. Oral cancer among patients under the age of 35 years. *J Postgrad Med* 2001; 47:171-176

[10] Suba Zs, Ujpál M. Correlations of insulin resistance and cancer (in Hungarian). *Hungarian Oncology* 2006; 50:127-135

[11] Suba Zs, Barabás J, Szabó Gy, Takács D, Ujpál M. Increased prevalence of diabetes and obesity in patients with salivary gland tumors. *Diabetes Care* 2005; 28:228

[12] Ujpál M, Matos O. Bíbok Gy, Somogyi A, Szabó Gy, Suba Zs. Diabetes and oral tumors in Hungary: Epidemiological correlations. *Diabetes Care* 2004; 27:770-774

[13] Bloomgarden ZT. Second World Congress on the Insulin Resistance Syndrome: Mediators, pediatric insulin resistance, the polycystic ovary syndrome, and malignancy. *Diabetes Care* 2005; 28:1821-1830

[14] Jee SH, Ohrr H, Sull JW, Yun JE, Ji M, Samet JM. Fasting serum glucose level and cancer risk in Korean men and women. *JAMA* 2005; 293:194-200

[15] Cowey S, Hardy RW. The metabolic syndrome: A high-risk state for oral cancer? *Am J Pathol* 2006; 169:1505-1522

[16] Kuriki K, Hirose K, Tajima K. Diabetes and cancer risk for all and specific sites among Japanese men and women. *Eur J Cancer Prev* 2007; 16:83-89

[17] Nagel JM, Goke B. Colorectal carcinoma screening in patients with type-2 diabetes mellitus. (in german) *Z Gastroenterol* 2006; 44:1153-1165

[18] Ujpál M, Barabás J, Kovalszky I, Szabó Gy, Németh Zs, Gábris K, Suba Zs. A preliminary comparative study of the prognostic implications of type 2 diabetes mellitus for patients with primary gingival carcinoma treated with surgery and radiation therapy. *J Oral Maxillofac Surg* 2007; 65:452-456

[19] Huber JC, Schneeberger C, Tempfer CB. Genetic modelling of the estrogen metabolism as risk factor of hormone-dependent disorders. *Maturitas* 2002; 42:1-12

[20] Liehr JG. Is estradiol a genotoxic mutagenic carcinogen? *Endocrine Reviews* 2000; 21: 40-54

[21] Diamanti-Kandarakis E. Hormone replacement therapy and risk of malignancy. *Curr Opinion Obstet Gynecol* 2004; 16:73-78

[22] Gallus S, Bosetti C, Franceschi S, Levi F, Simonato L, Negri E, La Vecchia C. Oesophageal cancer in women: tobacco, alcohol, nutritional and hormonal factors. *Br J Cancer* 2001; 85:341-345

[23] La Vecchia C, D'Avanzo B, Franceschi S, Negri E, Parazzini F, Decarli A. Menstrual and reproductive factors and gastric-cancer risk in women. *Int J Cancer* 1994; 59:761-764

[24] Parazzini F, La Vecchia C, Negri E, Franceschi S, Bolis G. Case-control study of estrogen replacement therapy and risk of cervical cancer. *British Med J* 1997; 315:85-88

[25] Olsson H, Bladström AM, Ingvar C. Are smoking-associated cancers prevented or postponed in women using hormone replacement therapy? *Obstetrics and Gynecology* 2003; 102:565-570

[26] McGrath M, Michaud DS, De Vivo I. Hormonal and reproductive factors and the risk of bladder cancer in women. *Am J Epidemiol* 2006; 163:236-244

[27] Gago-Domingez M, Castelao JE, Yuan JM, Ross RK, Yu MC. Increased risk of renal cell carcinoma subsequent to hysterectomy. Cancer *Epidemiol Biomark & Prev* 1999; 8:999-1003

[28] Ettinger B, Friedman GD, Bush T, Quesenberry CP Jr. Reduced mortality associated with long-term postmenopausal estrogen therapy. *Obstet Gynecol* 1996; 87:6-12

[29] Reckelhoff JF. Sex steroids, cardiovascular disease, and hypertension. *Hypertension* 2005; 45:170-180

[30] Faustini-Fustini M, Rochira V, Carani C. Oestrogen deficiency in men: where are we today? *Eur. J. Endocrinol* 1999; 140:111-129

[31] Ford ES, Giles WH, Mokdad AH. Increasing prevalence of the metabolic syndrome among U.S. adults. *Diabetes Care* 2004; 27:2444-2449

[32] Gupta K, Krishnaswamy G, Karnad A, Peiris AN. Insulin: A novel factor in carcinogenesis. *Am J Med Sci* 2002; 323:140-145

[33] Yu H, Rohan T. Role of the insulin-like growth factor family in cancer development and progression. *J Natl Cancer Inst* 2000; 92:1472-1489

[34] Smith GD, Gunnell D, Holly J. Cancer and insulin-like growth factor-I. *BMJ* 2000; 321:847-848

[35] Hussain SP, Hofseth LJ, Harris CC. Radical causes of cancer. *Nat Rev Cancer* 2003; 3:276-285

[36] Vlassara H. Recent progress in advanced glycation, end products and diabetic complications. *Diabetes* 1997; 46: S19-S25

[37] Cho E, Spiegelman D, Hunter DJ et al. Premenopausal dietary carbohydrate, glycemic index, glycemic load and fiber in relation to risk of breast cancer. *Cancer Epidemiol Biomark & Prev* 2003; 12:1153-1158

[38] McKeown-Eyssen G. Epidemiology of colorectal cancer revisited: are serum triglycerides and plasma glucose associated with risk? *Cancer Epidemiol Biomark & Prev* 1994; 3: 687-695

[39] Everhart J, Wright D. Diabetes mellitus as a risk factor for pancreatic cancer: a meta-analysis. *JAMA* 1995; 273:1605-1609

[40] Balkau B, Kahn H, Courbon D, Eschwege E, Ducimetiere P: Hyperinsulinemia predicts fatal liver cancer but is inversely associated with fatal cancer at some other sites: The Paris Prospective Study. *Diabetes Care* 2001; 24:843-849

[41] Yeung NG, Husain I, Waterfall N. Diabetes mellitus and bladder cancer – An epidemiological relationship? *Pathol Oncol Res* 2003; 9:30-31

[42] Barnard RJ, Aronson WJ, Tymchuk CN, Ngo TH. Prostate cancer: another aspect of the insulin-resistance syndrome. *Obesity Reviews* 2002; 3:303-308

[43] Muti P, Quattrin T, Grant BJB, Krogh V, Micheli A, Schünemann HJ, Ram M, Freudenheim JL, Sieri S, Trevisan M, Berrino F. Fasting glucose is a risk factor for breast cancer. *Cancer Epidemiol Biomark & Prev* 2002; 11:1361-1368

[44] Key TJ, Applyby PN, Reeves GK. Body mass index, serum sex hormones and breast cancer risk in postmenopausal women. *J Natl Cancer Inst* 2003; 95:1218-1226

[45] Soliman PT, Oh JC, Schmeler KM, Sun CC, Slomovitz BM, Gershenson DM, Burke TW, Lu KH. Risk factors for young premenopausal women with endometrial cancer. *Obstet Gynecol* 2005; 105:575-580

[46] Solomon CG, Hu FB, Dunaif A, Rich-Edwards J, Willett W, Hunter DJ, Colditz GA, Speizer FE, Manson JE. Long or highly irregular menstrual cycles as a marker for risk of type-2 diabetes mellitus. *JAMA* 2001; 286:2421-2426

[47] Godsland IF. Oestrogens and insulin secretion. *Diabetologia* 2005; 48:2213-2220

[48] Nestler JE. Obesity, insulin, sex steroids and ovulation. International Journal of Obesity & Related Metabolic Disorders: *J Internat Assoc for the Study of Obesity* 2000; 24 Suppl 2: 571-573

[49] Gadducci A, Gargini A, Palla E, Fanucchi A, Genazzani AR. Polycystic ovary syndrome and gynccological cancers: is there a link? *Gynecol Endocrinol* 2005; 20:200-208

[50] Mealey BL, Moritz AJ. Hormonal influences: effects of diabetes mellitus and endogenous female sex steroid hormones on the periodontium. *Periodont 2000* 2003; 32:59-81

[51] Poschl G, Seitz HK. Alcohol and Cancer. *Alcohol & Alcoholism* 2004; 39:155-165

[52] Sierksma A, Patel H, Ouchi N, Kihara Sh, Funahashi T, Heine RJ, Grobbe DE, Cluft C, Hendriks HF. Effect of moderate alcohol consumption on adiponectin, tumor necrosis factor alpha and insulin sensitivity. *Diabetes Care* 2004; 24:184-189

[53] Beulens JW, Stolk RP, van der Schouw YT, Grobbee DE, Hendriks HF, Bots ML. Alcohol consumption and risk of type 2 diabetes among older women. *Diabetes Care* 2005; 28:2933-2938

[54] Onland-Moret NC, Peeters PHM, van der Schouw YT, Grobbee DE, van Gils CH. Alcohol and endogenous sex steroid levels in postmenopausal women: A cross-sectional study. *J Clin Endocrinol Metab* 2005; 90:1414-1419

[55] Tavani A, Gallus S, La Vecchia C, Talamini R, Barbone F, Herrero R, Franceschi S. Diet and risk of oral and pharyngeal cancer. An Italian case-control study. *Eur J Cancer Prev* 2001; 10:191-195

In: Progress in Oral Cancer Research
Editor: Frederik L. Nielsen, pp 173-186
ISBN 978-1-60021-865-1

Chapter IX

THE PROGNOSTIC AND PREDICTIVE VALUE OF ECM PROTEINS IN ORAL CANCER. CLINICOPATHOLOGICAL AND IMMUNOHISTOCHEMICAL ASPECTS

***Z.S' Nemeth*[*1], *Zs. Suba*[1], *M. Mathe*[2], *I. Kovalszky*[2], *S. Bogdan*[1] and *G.Y. Vegso*[3]**

[1]Department of Oral and Maxillofacial Surgery and Dentistry, Semmelweis University Budapest, Hungary
[2]Department of Pathology and Experimental Cancer Research, Semmelweis University Budapest, Hungary
[3]Department of Transplantation and Surgery, Semmelweis University Budapest, Hungary

ABSTRACT

During the past 30 years, great emphasis has been placed on the determination of prognostic and predictive factors in cases of oral squamous cell tumors. Numerous systems have been devised, and numerous investigations have been performed, not only on the clinical parameters relating to the patient and the tumor, but also on histological, immunohistochemical and biological markers.

In our present study, 60 patients with tumors of the floor of the mouth or of the tongue ($T_2N_{0\text{-}1\text{-}2}M_0$) were randomized into three treatment groups. The first two groups participated in low dose inductive chemotherapy, surgery and then radiotherapy, while the third, control group underwent only surgery and radiotherapy. In all three groups, studies were made of the stage, grade, gender, the localization, the extents of expression of the pretreatment laminin and syndecan-1 and the disease-free survival rate, and the correlations between these.

* Correspondence concerning this article should be addressed to: Dr. NEMETH Zsolt, MD, PhD, Dept. of Oral and Maxillofacial Surgery, Semmelweis University, Budapest, Faculty of Dentistry, H-1085 Budapest, Mária u. 52. Tel/Fax: 00-36-1-2660-456; e-mail: nemeth@fok.usn.hu

The response to neoadjuvant chemotherapy was assessed by means of a method that we ourselves developed, involving measurement of the degree of histological regression observed in response to chemotherapy.

Immunhistochemical methods were applied to investigate the changes in degree of expression of laminin and syndecan-1 in response to the medication, and their correlations with the survival.

As concerns the overall tumor-free survival rate a significant difference was not found between the two chemotherapeutic groups. However, there was a significant difference between the survival indices of those who participated in cytostatic treatment (70%) and the control group. (40%).

In the clinical and immunhistochemical examinations the initial laminin and syndecan-1 levels obtained from biopsy samples could be used as *prognostic factors.*

Our model measuring the extent of histological regression clearly demonstrated that the survival indices of the patients who responded to the neoadjuvant cytostatic treatment with adequate tissue regression were better than those of the patients who responded to the treatment to only a decreased extent or not at all.

The changes in the expressions of laminin and syndecan-1 in response to cystostatic treatment proved to be important *predictive factors*. The increase or stagnation of these clearly forecast a good prognosis, whereas their decrease was a definite indication of poor prognosis.

Keywords: prognostic and predictive factors, basement membrane, oral cancer, laminin, syndecan-1

INTRODUCTION

Of all the different tumor types, tumors of the oral cavity have recently displayed the most dynamic increase in incidence in Hungary. Between 1948 and 1999, the rate of death from all types of tumors in Hungary increased „only" 2.8-fold, whereas the rate of death from tumors of the lip, the oral cavity and the pharynx increased nearly 6-fold. After 1970, there was a rise of 4.5-fold and after 1980, a rise of 2.5-fold, while even in the 1990s the rate increased by around 70%.

During the past 30 years, great emphasis has been placed on determination of the prognostic factors in cases of malignant tumors of the head and neck. Many systems have been considered, but it now appears that only the histological type, the localization, the stage and the grade are of significance from this respect.

Despite surgery, chemotherapy and radiotherapy, some patients with tumors of the head and neck die from a locoregional relapse. As concerns the elements of this complex therapy, the possibilities for repetition of the radiotherpy and surgery are limited or zero.

During the past 20 years, there has been no breakthrough as regards the survival indices in spite of the facts that the radicality of the operations has increased and the possibilities for reconstruction have been broadened substantially. Since nearly 70% of the patients who present for care are already in stage III or IV, many authors consider that the solution lies in the early recognition of the disease and in prevention. In a narrower sense, however this is not so much a professional as a professional-political question, and it is by no means a bedside problem.

Accordingly, it appears obvious that an improvement in the survival is to be expected in part from an extension of the available chemotherapeutic tools, and from the elaboration of more effective chemotherapeutic schemes including the optimization of neoadjuvant treatment, which is of promise.

Head and neck squamous cell carcinoma (HNSCC) is the sixth most prevalent cancer in developed countries and its management would be greatly improved by the identification of molecular markers for prediction of disease course and outcome as recurrent disease is common and major cause of mortality.

Thus we have to focuse our efforts on identifying novel or previously characterized molecules that show altered expression in cells, derived from HNSCC and that might have potential future use as prognostic indicators or for pharmacologic intervention of HNSCC.

PATIENTS AND METHODS

The examinations were performed on patients, with biopsy-confirmed squamous cell cancer (SCC) in clinical stage $T_2N_{0-1-2}M_0$. Localisation, gender, age, TNM and clinical stage were noted [1]. 60 patients were enrolled into the prospective, randomized study, in 3 groups each containing 20 subjects.The patients, 46 men and 14 women, had an avarage age of 55.1 years (range: 43-69 years).

The tumors affected the tongue and the sublingual region; they did not extend over the midline, the patients had not received any previous treatment. The circulatory, respiratory and renal functions were satisfactory, and no pathological change was observed in the bone marrow function.

Patients were checked monthly postoperatively, for an average time of 35 months overall: 33, 36 and 36 months in the groups of PF, ME and S patients, respectively. On these occasions, the oral cavity and the cervical regions were examined. Most of the patients regularly attended these check-ups, but a few of them had to be motivated via telephone, by post, or by a personal visit.

After randomization (performed by an independent person) three treatment groups were created.

In the PF-group the patients received neoadjuvant cytostatic treatment, involving 60 mg/m^2 Cisplatin (P), followed by 600 mg/m^2 5-Fluorouracil (F) on day 1, and then with 600 mg/m^2 5-Fluorouracil, intravenously, on days 2, 3, 4 and 5. Between days 8 and 10, the tumor was excised, supraomohyoidal neck dissection was performed, and the patient then received a total dose of 60 Gy irradiation in a dose of 2 Gy/day.

In the ME-group, the patients were given 30 mg/m^2 Methotrexate (M) on days 1, 3 and 5, and 30 mg/m^2 Epirubicine (E) on days 2 and 4. Between days 8 and 10, the tumor was excised, supraomohyoidal neck dissection was performed, and the patient then received a total dose of 60 Gy irradiation in a dose of 2 Gy/day.

In the the thrid group (group S) chemotherpy was not administered. The tumor was first excised, supraomohyoidal cervical dissection was performed, and the patients then received a total dose of 60 Gy irradiation in a dose of 2 Gy/day.

A biopsy excision was made before each of these treatment modes, for a histological diagnosis. Immunohistochemical examinations were performed for detection of the laminin and syndecan-1 expressions before and after chemotherapy. Correlations between the prognosis and the extent of the changes in their expression were investigated, and the survival indices in groups PF and ME were compared with the corresponding parameters for group S, who did not paticipate in cytostatic treatment.

In only 34 of the 40 cases (in groups PF and ME) immunhistochemical examinations could be performed: in 4 cases complete remission occured, and 2 cases immunohistochemical reaction did not worked.

Only one cycle of treatment was applied in both groups which participated in chemotherapy; because of the brief treatment period and the low doses we paid attention to the extent of the histological regression rather than to the degree of clinical remission.

Histomorphological Analysis

40 patients participated in the prospective, randomized investigation; as far as tumor localisation, the applied treatment and the histological classification of the tumors were concerned, these patients comprised a fairly homogenous population. Histological evaluation of the effect of low-dose neoadjuvant chemotherapy was performed on surgically removed tumors. A study was further made of the resulting data with the subsequent fate and survival prospects of these tumorous patients.

The operation was always performed 3-5 days after the completion of chemotherapy, wich is of great importance in judging the histological reactions. The surgery involved supraomohyoidal neck-dissection, primary tumor exstirpation.

The surgical samples were processed together in a uniform manner; thus, it was not possible to include further cases in the histological study retrospectively. Measurements were made of the three diameters of the tissue specimens, and of the dimensions of the macroscopically recognizable tumor residues. The exstirpated tumor was completely embedded in blocks about 0.3 mm thick, numbered in sequence. Complete tumor regression was established only if every serial section from all blocks proved to bee tumor-free.

Evaluations were made on 4- to 5 μm-thick sections stained with haematoxylin/eosin. This basic principles in the histological processing applied with those in the modified method of *Sulfaro* [2].

The tumor regression (R) was evaluated in our modified method [2], quantitatively on a scale ranging between 1 and 4. In the case of histologically complete regression, the tumor received a value R1 for the sake of statistical evaluability. A value R2 was given if only microscopically perceptible, small tumor cell groups were found. The size of the residue was examined in comparison with the estimated size of the original tumor. In our experience, the residual tumor is bordered by marginal scarring corresponding to the extent of the untreated tumor, since the adjacent, tumorously infiltrated oral cavity structures (striated musculature, salivary glands) are not capable of regeneration after destruction of the tumor.

If it was found that the two diamaters of the residual tumor in the serial section s were less than 50% of the estimated diameter of the original tumor, the regression was classified as R3. If the tumor regression did not attain 50%, it was classified as R4. In the interest of a relatively simple statistical evaluation, good responder (R1 and R2) and moderate-responder (R3 and R4) groups were formed.

Immunohistochemistry

Laminin-Staining

5-μm thick step sections were mounted on glass slides covered with Vectabond™ bonding agent (Vector Laboratories Inc.) and stained with a standard three-step avidin-biotin-complex method (Vectastain ABC kit). Deparaffinized and rehydrated tissue sections were immersed in 1.5% H_2O_2 for 10 min. in dark place, in order to block endogenous peroxidase activity. After washing in tris-buffered saline (TBS, pH 7.6) the sections were digested with 2 mg/ml pepsin in 0.2 M HCL for 30 min., at 37 ^{0}C, for optimal antigen retrieval. Further washing was followed by saturation of the sections with nonimmune serum diluted in TBS supplemented with 1% bovine serum albumin (BSA).

Incubation with mouse monoclonal antibodies to human laminin diluted at 1:2000 and 1:50, respectively, in TBS – 1% BSA, was performed overnight at 4-5 ^{0}C. The sections were washed in TBS, incubated with the biotinylated secondary antibody, diluted in TBS – 1% BSA, washed again in TBS and treated with the ABC complex, diluted in TBS – 1% BSA. Antibody binding was visualized with 60 mg/100 ml 3.3'-diaminobenzidine tetrahydrochloride (DAB) and 0.003% H_2O_2. Sections were counterstained with Harris' haematoxylin, dehydrated, cleared and mounted [3].

Syndecan-1 Staining

The sections were stained using a polyclonal affinity-purified rabbit antibody and the avidin-biotin immunperoxidase (ABC) technique. After fixing with acetone for 5 min. at 4 ^{0}C, the slides were incubated with 2% normal goat serum in 0.01 M Tris-buffered saline, pH 8.0 (TBS), for 30 min. at room temperature, followed by rabbit antibody (5μg ml^{-1}) in 1% (w/v) BSA-TBS overnight at 4 ^{0}C. Normal rabbit IgG, incubated in the same way, was used as a negative control.

After washing, the slides were incubated with Vectastain (Vector Laboratories) biotinylated horseradish peroxidase H mixture for 30 min. at room temperature. For colour reaction, the slides were incubated with 0.02% hydrogen peroxide, and 0.1% (w/v) diaminobenzidine tetrahydrochloride (DAB) in 0.1 M Tris buffer, pH 7.2, for 5 min., counterstained with heamatoxylin and mounted [4].

The intensity of staining for syndecan-1 was classified as: +/-, negative; +, weak staining of tumor cells; ++, intermediate intensity of staining; or +++, strong staining similary of that of epithelial cells of the normal mucosa. The staining pattern of laminin was examined in the basement membrane at the tumor-stroma border and graded as follows: +/-, almost negative;

+, less than 50% of positive staining; ++, more than or equal to 50% of positive staining; +++, continous linear staining (compatible with normal epithelia).

The integrity or damage of the basement membrane is an important indicator of the invasivness of epithelial cancers in the oral cavity. The intact or impaired nature of the basement membranc can be revealed by the continuity or fragmentation of the linear deposition of laminin. In the course of the inductive chemotherapy, we examined possible changes in the expression of laminin and syndecan-1. With a view to simpler evaluability, as concerns both laminin and syndecan-1, we divided the patients into two groups, denoted +/- and +, and ++ and +++.

A decrease, stagnation or an increase, of the expression of laminin or syndecan-1 as a result of the chemotherapy is indicated by the symbol ↓, → or ↑ respectively. Classifications were performed by the author without knowledge of the survival informations or other clinical data.

Statistical Methods

Statistical evaluation was performed with Origin 7.0. Univariate analysis was performed using the log rank test and multivariate analysis was performed using the Cox proportional hazards model, with booth forward and backward stepvise procedures.

In all cases, statistical significance was claimed for $p < 0.05$.

Results

Since none of the patients died from any cancer-independent reason, we considered it sufficient to discribe the fate of the patients in terms of the cancer-free survival, the CSS: cancer-specific survival (Table 1.). In none of the cases was it necessary to interrupt treatment because of side-effects for any other reason; similarly it did not prove necessary to exclude any of the patients from the study. There were no unexpected deaths, and distant metastases were not observed.

We have found that the CSS was 28/40 (70%) in both group PF and group ME, whereas it was 8/20 (40%) in group S. For the three groups combined, the CSS was 36/60 (60%), which is in accordance with the unfortunately poor prognosis for tumors of the oral cavity *(p=0.1737)*

When the correlation between the CSS and the localization of the tumor was considered for the patients overall (n=60), it was found that in the sublingual tumor cases the CSS was 73.3% (22/30), and in the lingual tumor cases it was 46.6% (14/30). Using the Cox analysis, this relation was not significant *(p=0.6956)*.

Examination of the correlation between the CSS and the stage for the three patient groups combined (n=60) revealed that in stage II the CSS was 71.4% (10/14), while in stages III and IV together it was 56.5% (26/46). Using the Cox analysis, this relation was close to significant *(p=0.0566)*.

Table 1. The correlation between CSS and the examined prognostic factors

	CSS (at 36 months)		*p-value*
Type of protocol			**0.1737**
PF+ME+S	36/60	60%	
PF+ME	28/40	70%	
S	8/20	40%	
Location (**PF+ME+S**)			**0.6956**
Floor of mouth	22/30	73.3%	
Tongue	14/30	46.6	
Stage (**PF+ME+S**)			**0.0566**
II	10/14	71.4%	
III+IV	26/46	56.5%	
Grade (**PF+ME+S**)			**0.0001**
I+II	30/36	83.3%	
III+IV	6/24	25%	
Lamstart (**PF+ME**)			**0.0492**
+/- and +	22/32	68.7%	
++ and +++	2/2	100%	
Synstart (**PF+ME**)			**0.0314**
+/- and +	18/22	81.8%	
++ and +++	6/12	50%	
Lamchange (**PF+ME**)			**0.0394**
↑ and →	22/26	84.6%	
↓	2/8	25%	
Synchange (**P+ME**)			**0.0475**
↑ and →	22/26	84.6%	
↓	2/8	25%	
Histological (**PF+ME**) regression			**0.0383**
R_1 and R_2	20/22	90.9%	
R_3 and R_4	8/18	44.4%	

As concerns the degree of histological regression in groups PF and ME (n=40), it proved that the CSS among the good responder patients (R1 and R2) in group PF was 87.5% (14/16), while all of the patients who exhibited virtually no regressions in response to medication (R3 and R4) died (0/4, 0%). In group ME, the CSS for the responders was 100% (6/6), while for the moderate-responders it was 57.1% (8/14). For the two chemotherapeutic groups combined, the CSS for the responders was 90.9% (20/22), whereas for the moderate-responders it was 44.4% (8/18). The correlation between CSS and the degree of histological regression in the two chemotherapy-group was significant *(p=0.0383)*.

Correlation between CSS and the grade for the three groups combined (n=60) demonstrated that in grade I the CSS was 87.5% (14/16), in grade II it was 80% (16/20), in grade III it was 16.6% (2/12), and in grade IV it was 33.3% (4/12). From another aspect, for the patients with a good prognosis (grades I and II) the survival rate was 83.3% (30/36) while for those with a less favourable prognosis (grades III and IV) it was only 25% (6/24). Using the Cox analysis, this relation was strongly significant *(p=0.0001)*.

The correlations were investigated between the survival indices and the extents of expression of laminin and syndecan-1.

When laminin levels were determined in the biopsy samples taken prior to treatment in the two chemotherapeutic groups (n=34) combined, it was revealed that in the +/- and + cases together the CSS was 68.7% (22/32), while in the ++ and +++ cases it was 100% (2/2); from a statistical aspect, it is clear that little can be concluded from this two individual cases *(p=0.0492)*. As regards the syndecan-1 levels, the corresponding data were 81.8% (18/22) and 50% (6/12), respectively *(p=0.0314)*.

In our study, we explored whether there are associations between the changes of laminin and syndecan expression during chemotherapy and survival. The aim here was to establish whether the changes in expression of these extracellular proteins in response to treament can be regarded as predictive factors.

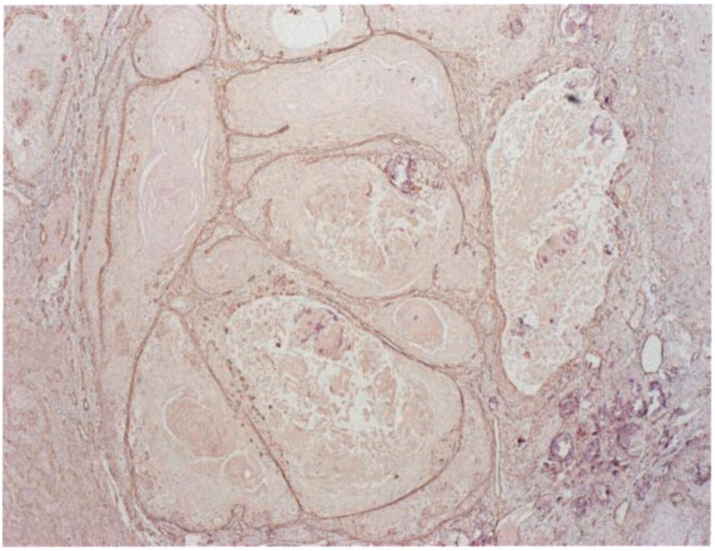

Figure 1. Immunohistochemical appearence of laminin prior to chemotherapy.

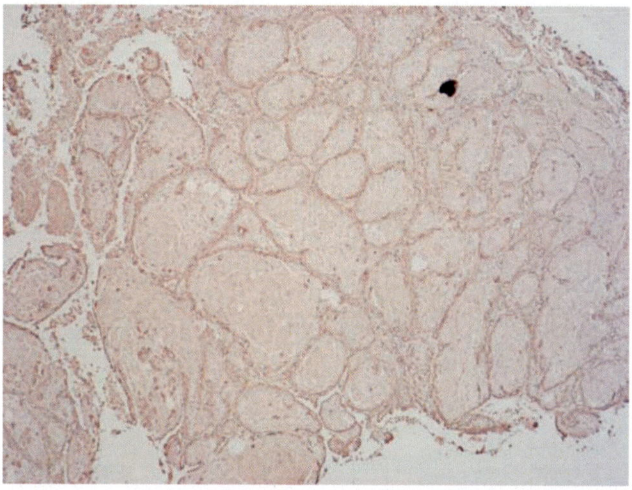

Figure 2. Increased laminin expression in the same patient after chemotherapy.

For groups PF and ME together (n=34), the CSS correlated closely with the change in laminin expression in response to chemotherapy. For these cases where the extent of laminin experession increased or stagnated, the overall CSS was 84.6% (22/26); for those where the expression decreased, it was 25% (2/8) *(p=0.0394)* (Figures 3.-4.). The data for the change in syndecan-1 expression paralleled those for laminin, with overall CSS data of 84.6% (22/26) and 25% (2/8), respectively *(p=0.0475* (Figures 1, 2).

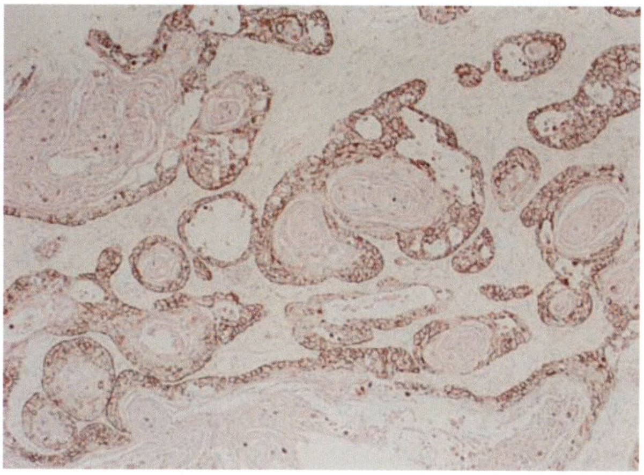

Figure 3. Immunohistochemical expression of syndecan-1 prior to chemotherapy in oral squamous cell tumor.

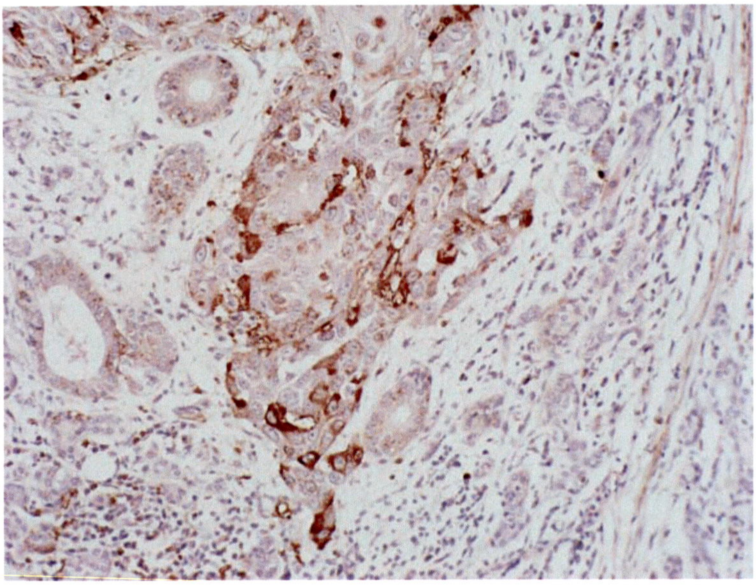

Figure 4. The same case after chemotherapy. The increased syndecan-1 expression is visible.

Discussion

The constant development of tumor therapy and the ever-extending application of chemotherapeutical possibilities have led to a need for the effect of such treatment to be evaluated not only quantitatively but also qualitatively [5,6] .The resulting data could assist the clinician in the planning of further treatment, the assessment of the prognosis and the standardized evaluation of the results.

Few publications have appeared so far on the histological evaluation of the regression of tumors of the head and neck treated by chemotherapy [7,8,9,10].

A standardized pathological method was devised by *Sulfaro* and his team for evaluation of the responses of tumors of the oral cavity to intra-arterial treatment [11]. This procedure was adapted to check on the efficacy of the systemic treatment.

Systemic neoadjuvant therapy plays an important role in the improvement of the survival prospects of patients with tumors of the head and neck. In spite of this, the result vary within a rather wide scale, ranging from histologically confirmed total tumor regression to a minimal response, stable or progressive disease. It is clear that, even in cases that are clinically similar and are treated in accordance with identical principles, the result are influenced by the immunological reactivities of the individual patients and by the individual characteristics of their tumors [5]. Cell surface and extracellular matrix molecules mediating cell adhesion play a role in cell migration, their interaction providing traction and direction for movement [12]. The progression of malignancy includes detachment from the adhesive interactions in the epithelium, invasion through the underlaying basement membrane, and migration of neoplastic cells through the stroma.

Therefore, alteration of epithelial cell adhesion to adjacent cells and to the basament membrane may be advantageous for the early stages of tumor growth [13,14].

Laminins are a family of glycoproteins that consists of one heavy α chain and two light β and γ chains. The laminin molecule is a major component of the basement membrane wich performs multiple biologic roles, including cell attachement [15], spread and migration as well as beeing involved in cellular proliferation and differentation [16]. In normal mucosa, basement membrane laminin was found distributed in linear pattern in the epithelial-stromal junction, around the blood vessels, the nerve fibers and the skeletal muscle bundles. In the cancerous tissues a variety in the linear staining around the cancer cell nests was seen. Laminin is frequently localized in the cytoplasm of invading cancer cells, wich suggests that laminin may be involved in tumor invasion. Extreme attenuation or complete loss of the linear staining of laminin means an unfavourable course of the malignant disease [17]. The basement membrane (BM) appears to be an important component of cellular structure, playing a key role in epithelial carcinogenesis particulary during invasion and metastasis [18].

In normal tissues it provides physical support and cell attachement, and also acts as a selective barrier separating the epithelium from underlaying connective tissue. The basement membrane is composed of several ECM proteins including laminin, collagen IV, fibronectin, heparane sulphate, proteoglycans, nidogen and entactin [19]. Because alterations in expression of these proteins can occur during carcinogenesis, they have been used as markers to study the involvement of basement membrane in cancer promotion [20].

Differentiated lesions showed a more conspicuous BM than less differentiated lesions. Previous observations in tumors of oropharyngeal regions have also shown that the expression of BM proteins is related to differentation status of the tumors. It has also been postulated that well-differentiated cells may secrete BM glycoproteins more rapidly than poorly differentiated ones [21]. Besides the fundamental biological importance of studying the pattern of distribution of basement membrane in malignant conditions, the information also has value in diagnostic and prognostic pathology. Patterns of basement membrane protein staining and prognosis or survival rate have been correlated with different types of tumours, including head and neck, oesophagus, cervix, colorectum and breast [21].

The study of *Sakr et al.* reported that BM was usually present in invasive squamous cell carcinomas with well-defined tumor-host borders, whereas invasive carcinomas with irregular small cords or single cells distributed through the stroma invariably lacked BM at the tumor-stromal interface [22].

Harada et al. found that in highly invasive primary tumors, the expression of laminin in the basement membrane along the tumor-stromal borderline was significantly decreased [23].

In a study of *Tosios et al.* it was reported about a significant linear trend for discontinous laminin distribution with the increasing grade of dysplasia ($p<0.05$) [3].

Kumagai et al. found that the distribution pattern of the basement membrane (BM) around tumour cells was determined in 72 oral squamous cell carcinomas. Statistical analysis showed that the degree of BM loss was correlated with the degree of differentation of tumor cells, but not with tumor size, and most significantly, with the mode of cancer invasion and the incidence of lymph node metastasis [24].

Syndecans form a group of cell-surface proteoglycans, wich can interact with various effector molecules, such as extracellular matrix molecules and growth factors. Syndecan-1 expression is induced during keratinocyte differentation and reduced in squamous cell carcinomas [25]. The syndecan family has four members, of wich syndecan-1 is the most studied and best characterized.

Syndecan-1 is found by immunohistochemistry in keratinizing cells of the horn pearls in well-differentiated carcinomas. Syndecan-1 expression is SCC is reduced compared with that in normal epithelium, and in addition its expression correlates with histological differentation grade of the tumors, lacking often in poorly differentiated tumors [26,27].

Inki et al. reported that the intermediate or strong staining for syndecan-1 was associated with small primary tumor size (p=0.0005). However, no association between syndecan-1 expression and the presence of cervical nodal metastases was found. Tumors that expressed syndecan-1 were more often well differentiated than those that did not express it (p=0.006).

Syndecan-1 expression did not correlate significantly with the age at diagnosis, WHO performance status or gender. In a univariate analysis syndecan-1 staining intensity correlated well with overall survival and patients with a syndecan-1-positive tumor had a more favourable prognosis [4].

Pulkkinen et al. found that there is a significant correlation between syndecan-1 expression and overall survival (p=0.048). The positive syndecan-1 immunostaining correlated with lack of metastasis (p=0.001), grade of keratinisation (p=0.001) and with histological grade (p=0.004) [27].

Studies, involving 29 and 89 invasive SCC head and neck carcinomas have suggested that reduced syndecan-1 expression is associated with poor survival in HNSCC but syndecan-1 expression has not been shown to have independent prognostic value in any type of human cancer, including cancer of the head and neck [27,28].

Anttonen et al. investigated syndecan-1 expression in a homogenously treated patients with HNSCC with a minimum follow up of 2 years and they found syndecan-1 expression to have prognostic value that was independent of clinical stage and histologic grade [29].

CONCLUSION

In the present study there was a close correlation between the CSS and grade and degree of histological regression of tumor.

One purpose of our study was to analyze laminin and syndecan-1 expression immunohistochemically prior and after chemotherapy in lingual and sublingual SCC as well as the relationship between laminin/syndecan-1 expression and the clinical outcome in patients with SCC of the tongue and sublingual region. We compared their prognostic value with that of conventional prognostic factors, such as grade, clinical stage, location, the degree of histological regression etc..

There have been a number of publications that have reported a more favourable prognosis in the event of an elevated syndecan-1 and/or laminin expression [30,31]. In our own material, we first investigated the correlations between the prognosis and the initial levels of syndecan-1 and laminin. We concluded that booth are useful prognostic factors to determine the course of disease.

We have supposed that the degree of their expression could be increased with neoadjuvant chemotherapy.

In this study it was clarified whether there are associations between the changes of laminin and syndecan expression during chemotherapy and survival. To our knowledge, there are no data available on the prognostic influence of the changes in laminin (Figures 1 and 2) and syndecan-1 (Figures 3 and 4) expression (after induction chemotherapy) in oral cancer patients. It was found that increases in the levels of these proteins unambiguously indicated a good prognosis, whereas decreases in their production were associated with a poor prognosis.

REFERENCES

[1] Hermanek P, Hutter RVP, Sobin LH et al. (Eds): *TNM Atlas Illustrated Guide to the TNM/pTNM Classification of Malignant Tumours*. UICC, 4th Edition 1997, Springer

[2] Suba Z, Szabó G, Barabás J, Németh ZS: Histological evaluation of chemotherapeutically induced tumour regression. *Reg Cancer Treat.* 1992; 4:313-319.

[3] Tosios KI, Kapranos N, Papanicolaou SI: Loss of basement membrane components laminin and type IV collagen parallels the progression of oral epithelial neoplasia. *Histopathology* 1998;33:261-268.

[4] Inki P, Joensuu H, Grenman R et al.: Association between syndecan-1 expression and clinical outcome in squamous cell carcinoma of the head and neck. *Br J Cancer* 1994;70:319-323.

[5] Friedmann Nervi C, Casale C, Starace G et al.: Significance of growth rates cell kinetics and histology in the irradiation and chemotherapy of squamous cell carcinoma of the mouth. *Cancer* 1973;31:10-16.

[6] Jacobsson PA, Eneroth CM, Killander D et al.: Histologic classification and grading of malignancy in carcinoma of the larynx (a pilot study). *Acta Radiol Ther Phys Biol.* 1973;12:1-8.

[7] Micheau C, Richard JM, Marandas P, Bosq J, Cailland JM: La regression tumorale apres chimiotherapie locale dans les carcinomes des voies aero-digestives superieues: le point de vue pathologiste. *Ann Otolaryngol.* 1983;100:577-580.

[8] Richard J, Domenge C: La chimiotherapie intra-arterielle d'induction dans les tumeurs des voies aero-digestives superieures. In: Jaquillat C, Weil M, Khayat M (eds) *Neo-adjuvant chemotherapy*. John Libbey Eurotext, London, 1986,447-453.

[9] Shapsay SM, Hong WK, Incze JS, Yamaguchi K, Bhutani R, Waughan ChW, Strong MS: Histopatologic findings after cis-platinum beleomycin therapy in advanced previously untreated head and neck carcinoma. *Am J Surg*. 1987;136:534-538.

[10] Shimosato Y, Oboshi S, Baba K: Histological evaluation of effects of radiotherapy and chemotherapy for carcinomas. *Jpn J Clin Oncol*. 1971;1:19-35.

[11] Sulfaro S, Frustaci S, Volpe R et al.: A pathologic assessment of tumour residue and stromal changes after intra-arterial chemotherapy for head and neck carcinomas. *Cancer* 1989;64:994-1001.

[12] Ruoslathi E, Giancotti FG: Integrins and tumor cell dissemination. *Cancer Cells* 1989;1:119-126.

[13] Albelda SM: Role of integrins and other cell adhesion molecules in tumor progression and metastasis. *Lab Invest.* 1993;68:4-17.

[14] Gianelli G, Milillo L, Marinosci F et al..: Altered expression of integrins and basement membrane proteins in malignant and pre-malignant lesions of oral mucosa. *J Biol Regul Homeost Agents* 2001;15:375-80.

[15] Pirila E, Sharabi A, Salo T et al: Matrix metalloproteinases process the laminin-5 gamma2-chain and regulate epithelial cell migration. *Biochem Biophys Res Commun.* 2003;18:303:1012-1017.

[16] Patel V, Aldridge K, Ensley JF et al.: Laminin-γ_2 overexpression in Head and Neck squamous cell carcinoma. *Int J Cancer* 2002;99:583-588.

[17] Moriya Y, Niki T, Yamada T et al: Increased expression of laminin-5 and its prognostic significance in lung adenocarcinomas of small size. *Cancer* 2001;91:1129-1141.

[18] Liotta LA: Tumor invasion and metastases: role of basement membrane. *Am J Pathol.* 1984;117:339-348.

[19] Abrahamson DR: Recent studies on the structure and pathology of basement membranes. *J Pathol.* 1986;149:257-278.

[20] Birumbaut P, Caron Y, Adnet JJ et al.: Usefulness of basement membrane markers in tumoral pathology. *J Pathol.* 1985;145:283-296.

[21] Kannan S, Balaram P, Chandran G.J. et al: Alterations in expression of basement membrane proteins during tumour progression in oral mucosa. *Histopathology* 1994;24:531-537.

[22] Sakr WA, Zarbo RJ, Jacobs JR et al.: Distribution of basement membrane in squamous cell carcinoma of the head and neck. *Hum Pathol.* 1987;18:1043-1050.

[23] Harada T, Shinohara M, Nakamura S et al.: An immunohistochemical study of extracellular matrix in oral squamous cell carcinoma and its association with invasive and metastatic potential. *Virchows Arch.* 1994;424:257-266.

[24] Kumagai S, Kojima S, Imai K et al.: Immunohistologic distribution of basement membrane in oral squamous cell carcinoma. *Head Neck* 1994;16:51-57.

[25] Soukka T, Pohjola J, Inki P et al.: Reduction of syndecan-1 expression is associated with displastic oral epithelium. *J Oral Pathol Med.* 2000;29:308-313.

[26] Inki P, Kujari H, Jalkanen M: Syndecan in carcinomas produced from transformed epithelial cells in nude mice. *Lab Invest.* 1992;66:314-323.

[27] Pulkkinen JO, Penttinen M, Jalkanen M et al.:Syndecan-1: A new prognostic factor in Laryngeal Cancer. *Acta Otolaryngol. (Stockh)* 1997;117:312-315.

[28] Inki P, Gomez M, Quintanilla M et al: Expression of syndecan in transformed mouse keratinocytes. *Lab Invest.* 1992;67:225-33.

[29] Anttonen A, Heikkila P, Kajanti M et al.: High syndecan-1 expression is associated with favourable outcome in squamous cell lung carcinoma treated with radical surgery. *Lung Cancer* 2001;32:297-305.

[30] Carter RL: Pathology of squamous carcinomas of the head and neck. *Curr Opin Oncol.* 1991;3:507-511.

[31] Anttonen A, Kajanti M, Heikkilä P et al: Syndecan-1 expression has prognostic significance in head and neck carcinoma. *Br J Cancer* 1999;79:558-564.

In: Progress in Oral Cancer Research
Editor: Frederik L. Nielsen, pp 187-197
ISBN 978-1-60021-865-1

Chapter X

Opinions in Oral Carcinogenesis Prevention

Zeng-Tong Zhou*, Wei-Wen Jiang and Yu-Feng Wang
Department of Oral Medicine, The Ninth People's Hospital, School of Medicine, Shanghai Jiao Tong University, China.

Abstract

Oral epithelial carcinogenesis is multifocal carcinogenesis and multistep carcinogenesis. This concept decides the biologic rationale for chemoprevention in oral cancer. We demonstrated the strategies for clinical treatments of oral premalignancies. We reviewed the current status of chemoprevention and addressed a new approach of integrating traditional Chinese medicine (TCM) and western medicine in the chemoprevention of oral carcinogenesis.

Keywords: Chemoprevention, traditional Chinese medicine, oral, cancer, premalignancy

Abbreviation:

TCM	traditional Chinese medicine;
13cRA	retinoid 13-cis-retinoic acid;
SM-470	*Salvia miltiorrhiza*;
Cam-300	*Camellia sinensis*;
Sal B	Salvianolic acid B;
DMBA	7,12-dimethylbenz[a]anthracene;
GP	*Gynostema pentaphyllum mak*

* Correspondence concerning this article should be addressed to: Zeng-Tong Zhou, Department of Oral Medicine, Institute of Stomatology, The Ninth People's Hospital, Shanghai Jiao Tong University; 639 Zhizaoju Road, Huangpu District, Shanghai China. 200011; email:zhouzengtong@hotmail.com.

INTRODUCTION

Oral epithelial carcinogenesis is field carcinogenesis and multistep carcinogenesis. In field carcinogenesis, diffuse epithelial damage in tissues, results from generalized carcinogen exposure throughout the field and clonal proliferation of mutated cells. Genetic changes exist throughout the field and increase the likelihood that one or more premalignant and malignant lesions may develop within that field [1,2]. Multistep carcinogenesis describes a stepwise accumulation of alterations, both genotypic and phenotypic [3,4]. Although various molecular predictors of oral cancer progression have been identified, histological diagnosis of dysplasia remains the best marker and is used routinely in clinical practice to guide the management of patients with oral cancer. The dysplasia of lesion was catalogued into 3 degrees: mild, moderate and severe by the WHO criteria [5]. Three principal modalities are currently used to control this disease: 1) smoking cessation programs as primary prevention; 2) local therapy including local medication and surgical removal; and 3) systemic chemopreventive therapy (Figure 1). The management recommendation for patients with mild epithelial dysplasia is offered a chemopreventive medication. The moderate epithelial dysplasia patients are provided with a discussion of diagnosis and treatment plan, which usually involving an intensive follow-up every 3 months and a combined chemopreventive medication and physical therapy. The patients with severe dysplasia are recommended surgical removal of the oral lesion. All of patients with premalignancies are recommended smoking cessation.

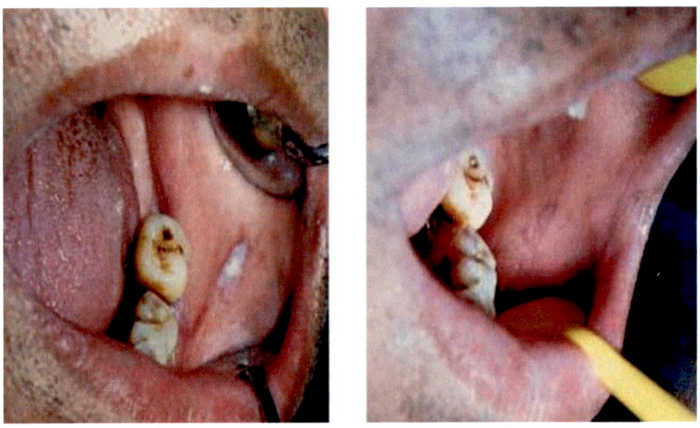

A B

Figure 1. Systemic chemopreventive therapy on oral premalignant lesion. Patient with premalignant lesion (leukoplakia) on the left buccal micusa is treated by Eb formula, which including *Erigeron Breviscapus vant Hand-Mazz*. A, before treated with Eb formula; B, after treated with Eb formula 3months.

COVENTIONAL CANCER CHEMOPREVENTION

The concepts of multistep epithelial cancer development and field carcinogenesis decide the primary biologic rationale for chemoprevention in oral cancer. Sporn in 1976, as first defined, cancer chemoprevention, uses natural, synthetic, or biologic chemical agents to reverse, suppress, or prevent carcinogenic progression [6]. For decades, the researchers and oncologists have been fighting to find effective agents with relatively little or no toxicity for preventing cancer in relatively healthy people. In pursuing this goal, trials big and small of a myriad of agents with relatively less or more toxicity were carried out. However, it reached at least a temporary plateau with the double edged results. In 1998, the results of the Breast Cancer Prevention Trial were published [7] Tamoxifen reduced the risk of breast cancer by almost 50% among the 13,388 randomized women (moderately high risk) but also increased these women's risk of endometrial cancer. In 2003, Thompson et al showed the results of the Prostate Cancer Prevention Trial [8]. Finasteride produced a 25% overall reduction in prostate cancer prevalence among the 18,882 randomized men but also surprisingly seemed to increase these men's risk of high-grade prostate cancer.

The climactic results were obtained in work carried out by Hong's group with retinoids in oral leukoplakia, or intraepithelial neoplasia, and other cancers of the upper aerodigestive tract. This project provided the proof of principle of human cancer chemoprevention when it showed that a high dose of the retinoid 13-cis-retinoic acid (13cRA) could prevent second primary tumors associated with head and neck cancer [9-11]. This high dose was intolerably toxic, however, and a subsequent trial of a low, tolerable dose of 13cRA was not effective second primary tumor prevention [12].

With a better understanding of relevant molecular changes in each carcinogenic step of oral cancer, the availability of specific molecular targeting agents are increased, which including COX inhibitors, EGFR tyrosine kinase inhibitors, farnesyl transferase inhibitors, and others [13]. COX-2 catalyzes prostanoid synthesis from arachidonic acid. COX-2 is undetectable (or at low levels) in most normal tissues but is rapidly induced in response to inflammatory or mitogenic stimuli, including cytokines, growth factors, and tumor promoters [14,15]. In oral cancer, there is a stepwise increase in COX-2 expression through the normal, hyperplastic, dysplastic, and invasive carcinoma stages, suggesting its carcinogenic role in oral cancer [16-18]. Studies in preclinical models have clearly showed that COX-2 inhibitors repressed tumor growth, including oral cancer [19-24]. Based on these promising results, many clinical trials of chemoprevention using various COX-2 inhibitors have been conducted in various organs. However, notable cardiovascular toxicity was reported, which resulted in reevaluation of the clinical use of COX-2 inhibitors [25]. In April 2005, the Food and Drug Administration announced restricted use of nonsteroidal anti-inflammatory drugs, including celecoxib (COX-2 inhibitor), by providing revised labels to include more specific information about the potential cardiovascular and gastrointestinal risks [26].

EGFR, a surface receptor with intrinsic tyrosine kinase activity, is one of several known pivotal intermediates in many epithelial malignancies [27]. Dysplastic lesions overexpress EGFR, and invasive cancer displays a more jumped-up pattern of overexpression [28,29]. All this implicates the EGFR signaling pathway in the early stages of oral carcinogenesis and progression. In oral cancer, EGFR inhibition also showed growth inhibition and inhibition of metastasis in *in vitro* and *in vivo* experiments [30-35]. Likewise, EGFR inhibitor toxicity was reported. The main toxic effects of EGFR tyrosine kinase inhibitors, such as OSI-774 and ZD1839, include headache, diarrhea, and skin rash [36-38]. Rare association with interstitial lung disease was also observed using ZD1839 [39,40].

TCM and Chemoprevention in Oral Carcinogenesis

Selection of chemopreventive agents requires consideration of several criteria. Biological efficacy impeding the carcinogenic process, selectivity for transformed tissue, minimal toxicity, and the ability to obtain good patient compliance are essential. Traditional Chinese medicine (TCM) has been available for centuries and is widely used in China for a variety of indications, including anti-cancer. Experimental evidences explored several possible mechanisms of anti-cancer. Ikezoe et al. demonstrated PC-SPES decreasing proliferation and inducing differentiation and apoptosis in acute myeloid leukemia and prostate cancer [41,42]. In a study reported by Hong-Fen et al., tumor metastasis in rat was inhibited by ACNO, which is a Chinese herb formula, through regulating NK cell activity [43]. The biological function of TCM in enhancing the immune system, inhibiting angiogenesis and reversing multi-drug resistance also have been assessed [44,45].

Several studies support the application of TCM in combination with routine chemical agents. Huang et al. showed the apoptosis rates and the Bcl-2 phosphorilation levels were much higher in asiaticoside plus vincristine groups than that in vincristine or asiaticoside groups in the KBv200, MCF-7 and MCF-7/ADM lines [46]. Plouzek et al. reported the extract of *Rosemarinus officinalis labiatae* increased the intracellular accumulation of the chemotherapeutic agents, doxorubicin and vinblastine in the drug resistant-MCF-7 line [47].

In our group, we chose four compounds representing two functional classes of botanicals, the purified plant flavins scutellarin and baicalin, and two extracts purified from *Salvia miltiorrhiza* (SM-470) and *Camellia sinensis* (Cam-300), examined their anti-proliferation affects in the human breast cancer cell lines MCF-7 and T-47D. All four compounds inhibited MCF-7 and T-47D cell proliferation, baicalin being the most potent inhibitor. Moreover, the combination of the compounds from different classes showed enhanced potential therapeutic benefits; the combination of SM-470 with scutellarin, Cam-300 or baicalin, augmented the inhibition of cell proliferation. In the contrast, inhibition of T-47D cell proliferation using the same combination was dependent on baicalin only [48].

Angiogenesis, the growth of new capillaries from preexisting blood vessels, is essential for cancer to grow beyond minimal size and metastasize [49,50]. Anti-angiogenesis remains a prime therapeutic target. Increasing experimental evidences suggest that angiogenic switch occurs in premalignant lesions, and angiogenesis persists during progression to expansive solid tumors and invasive carcinomas [51-53]. Blocking angiogenic switch before the initial formation of solid tumor may be a promising cancer prevention modality. Therefore, we used Salvianolic acid B (Sal B), a pure compound extracted from *Salvia miltiorrhiza* to investigate the chemopreventive effect of Sal B on 7, 12-dimethylbenz[a]anthracene (DMBA)-induced oral carcinogenesis in hamsters with respect to angiogenesis. Seventy male Syrian golden hamsters were randomly divided into five groups, with two of 20 and three of 10. DMBA solution (0.5% in acetone) was applied topically to the left cheek pouch of male Syrian golden hamsters in Groups A and B, while animals in Group C were painted with acetone, three times a week for 6 weeks. For the next 18 weeks, animals in Groups B and D received Sal B daily (10 mg/kg body wt/day) by gavage, animals in Groups A and C received same volume of saline. Animals in Group E received no treatment and served as blank control. At the end of the experiment, animals were killed and tissue samples were collected for histopathological and immunohistochemical examinations. The results showed that Sal B significantly decreased the squamous cell carcinoma incidence from 64.7 (11/17) to 16.7% (3/18) (P = 0.004); angiogenesis was inhibited in dysplasia and SCC ($P < 0.01$), with a simultaneous decrease in the immunostaining of hypoxia-inducible factor 1_α and vascular endothelium growth factor protein ($P < 0.05$). The results suggested that Sal B had inhibitory effect against the malignant transformation of oral precancerous lesion and such inhibition may be related to the inhibition of angiogenesis [54] (Table I). In the similar animal model, we studied the association of oral carcinogenesis and Genistein, an isoflavone present in soy at high concentrations. DMBA solution (0.5% in mineral oil) was applied and two days after the last treatment of DMBA, genistein suspended in distilled water (10 mg/kg body Wt/day) or same volume of distilled water was administered into the animals by gavage daily for 12 weeks. The genistein treatment decreased the incidence of visible oral tumor to 40.7 (11/27), in comparison with 53.6% (15/28) of that in the positive control. However, the difference was not statistically significant (P = 0.34). And no significant difference in the average number of tumors/tumor-bearing hamster, the average volume of tumor or latency was observed between the control and the genistein-treated group. Vascular density in oral cancer of the genistein-treated group and that of the control group was similar and there was no significant difference. Interestingly, three animals in the genistein-treated group produced poorly differentiated fibrosarcomas in the DMBA-painted cheek pouches. Genistein appeared to promote oral submucosa stroma tumorigenesis in concert with DMBA. Caution should be warranted for people with predisposition to oral cancer [55].

Table I. Microvessel density data of different groups

Group	Treatment	MVD Normal	Inflammation	Hyperplasia	Dysplasia	OSCC
A	DMBA+saline			372±21.21	402±18.06	504±17.24
B	DMBA+Sal B			304±29.40	311±27.77	392±24.81
C	Acetone+saline	279±19.94	288±27.27			
D	Sal B only	269±21.63				
E	Blank control	273±17.2				

MVD (vessels/mm) quantitated at 200x magnification. Mean ± SE.
(cited from Zhou ZT et al / Carcinogenesis. 2006;27(4):826-832.)

Telomerase is a specialized ribonucleoprotein polymerase composed of RNA and protein components and is thought to compensate for the loss of telomere during cell division. Telomerase activity has been detected in immortalized and cancer cell lines, germ line cells, and most human malignancies, including head and neck squamous cell carcinomas. Recent findings suggest that the activation of telomerase is a crucial step in the continuous proliferation of cancer cells, which allows them to attain immortality and therefore may be considered as a marker for tumor progression [56-58]. We investigated the influence of another Chinese herb, *Gynostema pentaphyllum mak* (GP) (Figure 2), on telomerase activity during oral carcinogenesis. The above DMBA-induced animal model was used again. We found the positivity of pathology and telomerase was significantly different in the GP administration groups and the control groups ($p<0.05$; $p<0.01$). The phase during which GP most inhibits telomerase activity is in the duration of moderate dysplsia ($p<0.05$) [59].

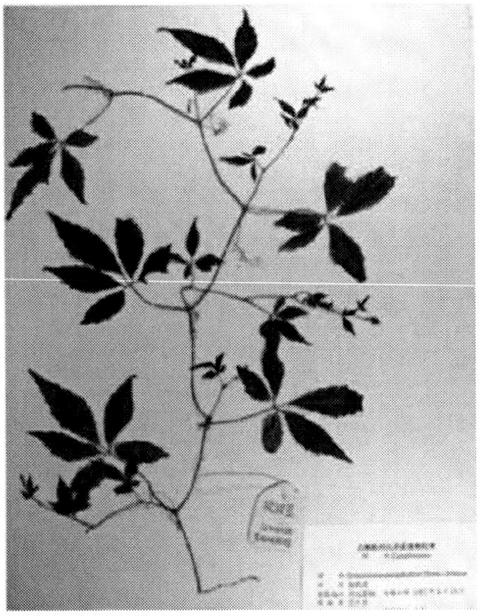

Figure 2. Photograph of Chinese herb *Gynostema pentaphyllum mak.* GP formula, which *Gynostema pentaphyllum mak* being main component, is well used in TCM.

Over 400 Chinese herbs were showed to have anticancer function [60-62]. To obtain the potential chemopreventive drugs from Chinese herbs, we screened 7 candidates, which were *Radix et Rhizoma Thalictri, Radix Sophorae Tonkinesis, Pseudobubus Cremastrae appendiculate, Rhizoma Acori Tatarinowii, Radix Angelicae Dahuricae, Rhizoma Curcumae* and *Fructus Tricosanthis*. DMBA-animal model was used. Four hundred and ten golden hamsters were randomly divided into control groups and Chinese herb groups. The results showed that the prevalence of dysplasia was significantly reduced in the *Radix Sophorae Tonkinesis* treated group and in the *Radix Angelicae Dahuricae* treated group. Further work is needed to explore their biological function and the mechanism.

ISSUES AND STRATEGIES

One concerning is the risks and side-effects as a long-term chemopreventive agent. These risks include increasing the incidence of different organ's carcinogenesis and intolerably toxic of high dosage. The emergence of a new class of chemopreventive agents, known as TCM with a more favorable side-effects profile has introduced the potential for long-term use. However, TCM has fundamental difference from any other medical systems. It has its own holistic concept, ethnic and social backgrounds. The opposition and inter-dependence, inter-promoting and inter-consuming as well as inter-transforming are applied to explain the human physiology, pathology, disease diagnosis and treatment. The composition of the formula and the dosage of the individual ingredients of Chinese herb depend on the signs and symptoms of the patient and the experience of the practician. On the contrast, western modern medicine is based on "the evidence". It is an "evidence-based medicine". The drug developing requires *in vitro* and *in vivo* experimental evidence through genomic, proteomic and pharmacological means by targeting disease's pathways, followed by clinic trails. This main difference makes TCM reaches its plateau, which is also the major reason preventing TCM from being accepted worldwide.

Integrating TCM and western medicine is the strategy to achieve a new era of chemoprevention. First of all, it should be understood the holistic concept of TCM; With the development of modem science and medicine, TCM modernization is the way to go. Using the state-of-art technology, basic experiments in different systems should be conducted to explore the underlying mechanism of TCM. The rigorously controlled clinical trials are required to better define the objective effects of TCM, eventually, to resolve the myth of TCM "black box"; Lastly, standardizing the clinical TCM therapy.

With such an integrated approach and strategies, they may ultimately lead to major improvements in the prevention of oral cancer.

References

[1] Slaughter, DP; Southwick, HW; Smejkal, W. Field cancerization in oral stratified squamous epithelium; clinical implications of multicentric origin. *Cancer* 1953;6:963-968.

[2] Braakhuis, BJ; Tabor, MP; Kummer, JA; et al. A genetic explanation of Slaughter's concept of field cancerization: evidence and clinical implications. *Cancer Res* 2003;63:1727-1730.

[3] Califano, J; van der Riet, P; Westra, W; et al. Genetic progression model for head and neck cancer: implications for field cancerization. *Cancer Res* 1996;56:2488-2492.

[4] Jiang, WW; Fujii, H; Shirai, T; Mega, H; Takagi, M. Accumulative increase of loss of heterozygosity from leukoplakia to foci of early cancerization in leukoplakia of the oral cavity cancer. *Cancer* 2001;92:2349-2356.

[5] Pinborg, JJ; Reichart, PA. Histological typing of cancer and precancer of the oral mucosa. Second Edition. *WHO*:1997:21-31.

[6] Sporn, MB. Approaches to prevention of epithelial cancer during the preneoplastic period. *Cancer Res* 1976;36:2699-2702.

[7] Fisher, B; Costantino, JP; Wickerham, DL; et al. Tamoxifen for prevention of breast cancer: report of the National Surgical Adjuvant Breast and Bowel Project P-1 Study. *J Natl Cancer Inst* 1998;90:1371-88.

[8] Thompson, IM; Goodman, PJ; Tangen, CM; et al. The influence of finasteride on the development of prostate cancer. *N Engl J Med* 2003;349:215-24.

[9] Hong, WK; Endicott, J; Itri, LM; et al. 13-cis Retinoic acid in the treatment of oral leukoplakia. *N Engl J Med* 1986;315:1501-5.

[10] Hong, WK; Lippman, SM; Itri, LM; Karp, DD; Lee, JS; Byers, RM; Schantz, SP; Kramer, AM; Lotan, R; Peters, LJ; et al. Prevention of second primary tumors with isotretinoin in squamouscell carcinoma of the head and neck. *N Engl J Med* 1990;323:795-801.

[11] Lippman, SM; Batsakis, JG; Toth, BB; Weber, RS; Lee, JJ; Martin, JW; Hays, GL; Goepfert, H; Hong, WK.. Comparison of low-dose isotretinoin with beta carotene to prevent oral carcinogenesis. *N Engl J Med* 1993;328:15-20.

[12] Papadimitrakopoulou, VA; Hong, WK; Lee, JS; Martin, JW; Lee, JJ; Batsakis, JG; Lippman, SM. Low-dose isotretinoin versus beta-carotene to prevent oral carcinogenesis: long-term follow-up. *J Natl Cancer Inst.* 1997;89(3):257-8.

[13] Papadimitrakopoulou, VA; Shin, DM; Hong, WK. Chemoprevention of head and neck cancer. In: Harrison LB, Sessions RB, Hong WK, editors. HNC, A multidisciplinary approach. Philadelphia (PA): *Lippincott Williams & Wilkins*; 2004;p.985-1000.

[14] Turini, ME; Dubois, RN. Cyclooxygenase-2: a therapeutic target. *Annu Rev Med* 2002;53:35-57.

[15] Dannenberg, AJ; Subbaramaiah, K. Targeting cyclooxygenase-2 in human neoplasia: rationale and promise. *Cancer Cell* 2003;4:431-6.

[16] Chan, G; Boyle, JO; Yang, EK; et al. Cyclooxygenase-2 expression is up-regulated in squamous cell carcinoma of the head and neck. Cancer Res 1999;9:991-994.

[17] Renkonen, J; Wolff, H; Paavonen, T. Expression of cyclooxygenase-2 in human tongue carcinoma and its precursor lesions. *Virchows Arch* 2002;440:594-597.

[18] Choe, MS; Rogatko, A; Tighiouart, M; et al. Role of cyclooxygenase-2 (Cox-2) expression in tumor progression and survival in the squamous cell carcinoma of the head and neck (HNSCC). *Proc Am Soc Clin Oncol* 2005;23:502s

[19] Subbaramaiah, K; Dannenberg, AJ. Cyclooxygenase 2: a molecular target for cancer prevention and treatment. *Trends Pharmacol Sci* 2003;24:96-102.

[20] Peng, JP; Liu, LT; Chang, HC; Hung, WC. Enhancement of chemotherapeutic drug-induced apoptosis by a cyclooxygenase-2 inhibitor in hypopharyngeal carcinoma cells. *Cancer Lett* 2003;201:157-63.

[21] Hashitani, S; Urade, M; Nishimura, N; et al. Apoptosis induction and enhancement of cytotoxicity of anticancer drugs by celecoxib, a selective cyclooxygenase-2 inhibitor, in human head and neck carcinoma cell lines. *Int J Oncol* 2003;23:665-72.

[22] Minte, HA; Eveson, JW; Huntley, S; Elder, DJ; Hague, A. The cyclooxygenase 2-selective inhibitor NS398 inhibits proliferation of oral carcinoma cell lines by mechanisms dependent and independent of reduced prostaglandin E2 synthesis. *Clin Cancer Res* 2003;9:1885-97.

[23] Zweifel, BS; Davis, TW; Ornberg, RL; Masferrer, JL. Direct evidence for a role of cyclooxygenase 2-derived prostaglandin E2 in human head and neck xenograft tumors. *Cancer Res* 2002;62:6706-11.

[24] Sumitani, K; Kamijo, R; Toyoshima, T; et al. Specific inhibition of cyclooxygenase-2 results in inhibition of proliferation of oral cancer cell lines via suppression of prostaglandin E2 production. J Oral Pathol Med 2001;30:41-7.

[25] Bannwarth, B. Do selective cyclo-oxxygenase-2 inhibitors have a future? *Drug Safety* 2005;28:183-9.

[26] The Food and Drug Administration announces series of changes to the class of marketed nonsteroidal anti-inflammatory drugs. *Food and Drug Administration News,* April 7, 2005. Available at http://www.fda.gov/bbs/topics/news/2005.

[27] Raymond, E; Faivre, S; Armand, JP. Epidermal growth factor receptor tyrosine kinase as a target for anticancer therapy. *Drugs* 2000;60:15-23.

[28] Shin, DM; Ro, JY; Hong, WK; Hittleman, WN. Dysregulation of epidermal growth factor receptor expression in premalignant lesions during head and neck tumorigenesis. *Cancer Res* 1994;54:3153-9.

[29] Grandis, JR; Tweardy, DJ; Melhem, MF. Asynchronous modulation of transforming growth factor and epidermal growth factor receptor protein expression in progression of premalignant lesions to head and neck squamous cell carcinoma. *Clin Cancer Res* 1998;4:13-20.

[30] Matheny, KE; Barbieri, CE; Sniezek, JC; Arteaga, CL; Pietenpol, JA. Inhibition of epidermal growth factor receptor signaling decreases p63 expression in head and neck squamous carcinoma cells. *Laryngoscope* 2003;113:936-9.

[31] Di Gennaro, E; Barbarino, M; Bruzzese, F; et al. Critical role of both p27KIP1 and p21CIP1/WAF1 in the antiproliferative effect of ZD1839 (''Iressa''), an epidermal growth factor receptor tyrosine kinase inhibitor, in head and neck squamous carcinoma cells. *J Cell Physiol* 2003;195:139-50.

[32] Shintani, S; Li, C; Mihara, M; et al. Gefitinib (''Iressa'', ZD1839), an epidermal growth factor receptor tyrosine kinase inhibitor, up-regulates p27KIP1 and induces G1 arrest in oral squamous cell carcinoma cell lines. *Oral Oncol* 2004;40:43-51.

[33] Shintani, S; Li, C; Mihara, M; Nakashiro, K; Hamakawa, H. Gefitinib (''Iressa''), an epidermal growth factor receptor tyrosine kinase inhibitor, mediates the inhibition of lymph node metastasis in oral cancer cells. *Cancer Lett* 2003;201:149-55.

[34] Faust, RA; Tawfic, S; Davis, AT; Ahmed, K. Apoptosis and growth inhibition of head and neck tumor cell line induced by epidermal growth factor receptor tyrosine kinase inhibitor. *Oral Oncol* 1999;35:290-5.

[35] Modjtahedi, H; Affleck, K; Stubberfield, C; Dean, C. EGFR blockade by tyrosine kinase inhibitor or monoclonal antibody inhibits growth, directs terminal differentiation and induces apoptosis in the human squamous cell carcinoma HN5. *Int J Oncol* 1998;13:335-42.

[36] Soulieres, D; Senzer, NN; Vokes, EE; Hidalgo, M; Agarwala, SS; Siu, LL. Multicenter phase II study of erlotinib, an oral epidermal growth factor receptor tyrosine kinase inhibitor, in patients with recurrent or metastatic squamous cell cancer of the head and neck. *J Clin Oncol* 2004;22:77-85.

[37] Barlesi, FA; Tchouhadjian, CA; Doddoli, C; et al. Gefitinib [(ZD1839), Iressa (R)] in non-small-cell lung cancer: a review of clinical trials from daily practice perspective. *Fund Clin Pharm* 2005;19:385-93.

[38] Hidalgo, M; Siu, LL; Nemunaitis, J; et al. Phase I and pharmacologic study of OSI-774, an epidermal growth factor receptor tyrosine kinase inhibitor, in patents with advanced solid malignancies. *J Clin Oncol* 2001;19:3267-79.

[39] Inoue, A; Saijo, Y; Maemondo, M; et al. Severe acute interstitial pneumonia and gcfitinib. *Lancct* 2003;361:137-9.

[40] Forsythe, B; Faulkner, K. Overview of the tolerability of gefitinib (IRESSA2) monotherapy. *Drug Safety* 2004;27:1081-92.

[41] Ikezoe, T; Chen, S; Saito, T; Asou, H; Kyo, T; Tanosaki, S; Heber, D; Taguchi, H; Koeffler, HP. 2003a. PC-SPES decreases proliferation and induces differentiation and apoptosis of human acute myeloid leukemia cells. *Int J Oncol.* 2003;23(4):1203-1211.

[42] Ikezoe, T; Chen, S; Yang, Y; Heber, D; Taguchi, H; Koffler, HP. 2003b. PC-SPES: molecular mechanism to induce apoptosis and down regulate expression of PSA in LNCaP human prostate cancer cells. *Int J Oncol.* 2003;23(51):l46l-l470.

[43] Hong-Fen, L; Waisman, T; Maimon, Y; Shakhar, K; Rosenne, E; Ben-Eliyahu, S. The effects of a Chinese herb formula, anticancer number one (ACNO), on NK cell activity and tumor metastasis in rats. *Int Immunopharmacol.* 2001;1(11):1947-1956.

[44] Hsieh, TC; Lu, X; Guo, J; Xiong, W; Kunicki, J; Darzynkiewicz, Z; Wu, JM. Effects of herbal preparation Equiguard on hormone-responsive and hormone-refractory prostate carcinoma cells : mechanistic studies. *Int J 0ncol.* 2002;20(4):681-689.

[45] Wartenberg, M; Budde, P; de Marees, M; Grunheck, F; Tsang, SY; Huang, Y; Chen, ZY; Hescheler, J; Sauer, H. Jnhibition of tumor induced angiogenesis and matrix-metalloproteinase expression in confrontation cultures of embryoid bodies and tumor spheroids by plant ingredients used in additional chinese medicine. *Lab Invest.* 2003;83(11):87-98.

[46] Huang, YH; Zhang, SH; Zhen, RX; Xu, XD; Zhen, YS. Asiatieoside inducing apoptosis of tumor cells and enhancing anti-tumor activity of vincristine. *Ai Zheng.* 2004;23(12):1599-l604.

[47] Plouzek, CA; Ciolino, HP; Clarke, R; Yeh, GC. Inhibition of P-glycoprotein activity and reversal of multi-drug resistance in vitro by rosemary extract. *Eur Cancer* 1999;35(10):154l-1545.

[48] Franek, KJ; Zhou, ZT; Zhang, WD; Chen, WY. In vitro studies of baicalin alone or in combination with *Salvia miltiorrhiza* extract as a potential anti-cancer agent. *Int J Oncol.* 2005;26:217-224.

[49] Fox SB. Tumor angiogenesis and prognosis. Histopathology. 1997;30:294-301.

[50] Folkman J. Introduction angiogenesis and cancer. *Semin. Cancer Biol.*, 1992;3:47-48.

[51] Folkman, J; Watson, K; Ingber, D; *et al.* Induction of angiogenesis during the transition from hyperplasia to neoplasia. *Nature.* 1989;339:58-61.

[52] Pazouki, S; Chrisholm, DM; Adi, MM;. *et al.* The association between tumour progression and vascularity in the oral mucosa. *J. Pathol.*1997;183:39-43.

[53] Jin, Y; Tipoe, GL; White, FH; *et al.* A quantitative investigation of immunocytochemically stained blood vessels in normal, benign, premalignant and malignant human oral cheek epithelium. *Virchows Aich.* 1995;427:145-151.

[54] Zhou, ZT; Yang, Y; Ge, JP. The preventive effect of salvianolic acid B on malignant transformation of DMBA-induced oral premalignant lesion in hamsters. *Carcinogenesis*. 2006;27(4):826-832.

[55] Yang, Y; Zhou, ZT; Ge, JP. Effect of genistein on DMBA-induced oral carcinogenesis in hamster. *Carcinogenesis*. 2006;27(3):578-583.

[56] Kim, NW; Piatyszek, MA; Prowse, KP; Harley, CB; West, MD; Ho, PL; Coviello, GM; Wright, WE; Weinrich, SL; Shay, JW. Specific association of human telomerase activity with immortal cells and cancer. *Science* 1994;266:2011-15.

[57] Mutirangura, A; Supiyaphun, P; Trirekapan, S; Sriuranpong, V; Sakuntabhai, A; Yenrudi, S; Voravud, N. Telomerase activity in oral leukoplakia and head and neck squamous cell carcinoma. *Cancer Res* 1996;56:3530-3.

[58] Califano, J; Ahrendt, SA; Meininger, G; Westra, WH; Koch, WM; Sidransky, D. Detection of telomerase activity in oral rinses from head and neck squamous cell carcinoma patients. *Cancer Res* 1996;56:5720-2.

[59] Zhou, ZT; Lou, JN. Experimental study of Gynostema pentaphyllum mak on telomerase activity during oral leukoplakia carcinogenesis. *Chin J Dent Res*. 2000;6(1):47-53.

[60] Li, PW. Practical clinical anti-cancer drug. Shengyang: *Liaoning Science & Technology Publisher*. 2001:1-365.

[61] Zhao, CQ; Xu, YL; Wang, YZ. Anti-cancer herb drugs and effective compounds. Beijing: *China Chinese Medicine Drug Publisher*.1999:1-219.

[62] Ji, YB. Pharmacology and application of anti-cancer Chinese medicine. Haerping: *Heilongjiang Science & Technology Publisher*. 1999:1-1334.

INDEX

A

D

E

F

G

H

I

J

K

L

M

Q

R

S

T

U

V

W

X

Y

Z